Professional and Therapeutic Communication

Second edition

Melanie Birks, Jenny Davis and Ysanne B. Chapman

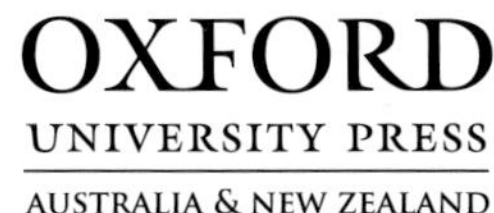

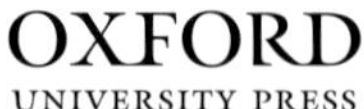

Oxford University Press is a department of the University of Oxford.
It furthers the University's objective of excellence in research, scholarship, and education by publishing worldwide. Oxford is a registered trademark of Oxford University Press in the UK and in certain other countries.

Published in Australia by
Oxford University Press
8/737 Bourke Street, Docklands, Victoria 3008, Australia

First edition published 2015
Second edition published 2020

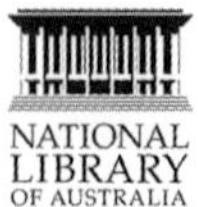

A catalogue record for this book is available from the National Library of Australia

ISBN 9780190323462

Typeset by Newgen KnowledgeWorks Pvt. Ltd., Chennai, India
Edited by Anne Mulvaney
Proofread by Carolyn Leslie, AE
Indexed by Mei Yen Chua
Printed in China by Leo Paper Products Ltd.

CONTENTS

LIST OF FIGURES

LIST OF TABLES

PREFACE

We are excited to bring you this second edition of *Professional and Therapeutic Communication*. The success of the first edition reinforced the need for a text that provides a comprehensive understanding of communication for students, novice and experienced practitioners working in complex and diverse multidisciplinary healthcare environments.

As with the first edition, this text focuses on all aspects of interpersonal interaction that are essential to safe, high-quality healthcare. The therapeutic nature of engagement with patients, clients and consumers of healthcare cannot be detached from the professional elements of communication. This second edition provides a practical approach to concepts fundamental to both the professional and therapeutic elements of the caring relationship in all its forms. In response to feedback from the first edition, we have added additional content focusing on the important use of self in communication, extending into concepts of reflection and supervision. The importance of self-care for healthcare professionals as an adjunct to effective communication is also examined.

Updated content throughout the text aims to promote skill development for healthcare students and professionals from all health disciplines. The contemporary and pragmatic approach ensures broad applicability and relevance. Once again this text is written for Australian and New Zealand contexts, yet it has relevance for students and practitioners of healthcare more broadly. Contributors to the text represent a wide range of professional groups, further increasing the reach of the text and reinforcing the interprofessional nature of healthcare delivery in the contemporary context.

The book features comprehensive consideration of all aspects of communication relevant to the healthcare professional. Part 1 commences with an introduction to concepts of professional and therapeutic communication. Principles and practices in communication are then explored, followed by an exploration of communication and self. Part 1 concludes with a chapter on the important practices of reflection and clinical supervision.

Part 2 applies concepts of professional and therapeutic communication to interprofessional, culturally diverse, organisational and community contexts. Part 3 focuses on ethical and supportive communication, commencing with the important and often overlooked concepts of safety and quality in communication, before examining confidentiality, advocacy and the management of conflict. Part 4 addresses communication and health literacy, with special attention given to academic writing and communicating electronically.

The pedagogical features employed in this text ensure that the reader is able to grasp and reflect on key concepts. Learning objectives are included in each chapter to guide the reader through the sections that follow. Key terms embedded in the discussion ensure that the reader remains orientated throughout each chapter. The use of features such as focus boxes and authentic case activities, and opportunities to reflect on the application of content through 'Skills in practice' and 'Reflect and apply' activities, encourage the reader to relate concepts to practice. Summary points and critical thinking questions at the conclusion of each chapter serve to pull together the content and promote consolidated understanding. Each chapter in this new edition also includes a group activity to assist consolidation of knowledge in the classroom context. Referral to relevant weblinks further enhances the experience for the reader. The text also includes a Glossary to promote understanding of less familiar concepts.

Once again in this edition, the contemporary content, supplemented by pedagogical features, ensures the relevance and application of key concepts of both professional and therapeutic communication for use by multidisciplinary healthcare practitioners in all clinical contexts. We trust that you will enjoy reading through this text and find it of ongoing value and relevance in your professional career.

Melanie Birks,
Jenny Davis and
Ysanne B. Chapman

ABOUT THE AUTHORS

Professor Melanie Birks is an experienced academic with an extensive track record in research and publication, having authored numerous peer-reviewed journal articles as well as textbooks and book chapters. She has more than 25 years' experience in academia. Professor Birks currently occupies the position of Professor and Head of Nursing and Midwifery at James Cook University. She is passionate about learning and teaching, and believes that quality education can be a life-changing experience. Her research interests are in the areas of accessibility, innovation, relevance and quality in healthcare professional education.

Dr Jenny Davis is a nurse, midwife and health information manager with extensive experience in the Australian health and higher education sectors as clinician, manager, educator and researcher. Jenny is currently a senior lecturer at La Trobe University in Melbourne. Jenny has a big-picture perspective and is passionate about system and clinical practice improvement through contemporary education, strategic knowledge management and translational research. Jenny's research interests include health workforce education, practice and sustainability; information/knowledge management; and research ethics.

Ysanne B. Chapman is a retired Professor of Nursing and has been in the profession for over 50 years. While she is retired, enjoying the wonders and freedom of beachside living in Victoria, she is still active in professional work, as she continues to write for publication, researches with colleagues, teaches and facilitates higher-degree students. Ysanne believes that effective communication is central to compassionate and efficient healthcare.

Dr Narelle Biedermann is a senior lecturer at James Cook University, Townsville, and is the course coordinator of the Master of Nursing (JCU Online) program. She received her PhD in nursing in 2001 from James Cook University. She also holds a Postgraduate Certificate in Nursing Science (majoring in clinical teaching) awarded by James Cook University in 2010, a Master of Defence Studies awarded by University of New South Wales in 2008, and a Bachelor of Nursing Sciences (Honours) awarded by James Cook University in 1993. Her broad research interests include military nursing, nursing history, online learning pedagogies and gender in healthcare.

Dr Beryl Buckby is a clinical psychologist, lecturer and supervisor in the Clinical Psychology Program at James Cook University. In the early 2000s, she worked on the Queensland beyondblue National Postnatal Depression Program at James Cook University. Dr Buckby was also a working group member in establishment of interprofessional clinics at James Cook University and is currently researching interprofessional education methodologies. She also teaches, supervises and researches primarily in mental health, well-being and resilience with a focus on trauma, stress-related disorders, suicide prevention, stigma and dementia. Dr Buckby was instrumental in establishing the multidisciplinary Australasian Mental Health in Higher Education Conference (AMHHEC) in 2017/18 and the AMHHEC 2019 Conversations on Building Resilient Communities hosted at James Cook University that reflected on collaborative strengths of individuals and organisations of Townsville regional communities after devastating floods in February 2019.

Dr Maria Carbines is a registered nurse in operating rooms throughout the Auckland District Health Board in New Zealand. She has links to nursing education at several Auckland-based nursing schools, having taught for many years across a wide variety of health-related subjects and contributed to support of postgraduate students who are using grounded theory as a research approach. In particular, Maria has a passion for teaching and exploring topics related to the sociology of health and the diverse ways in which people view and manage their health.

Associate Professor Sophia Couzos is a public health physician and general practitioner with the College of Medicine and Dentistry, James Cook University. She has nearly 30 years' experience working within Aboriginal community-controlled health services in remote Australia, the Canberra-based National Aboriginal Community Controlled Health Organisation (NACCHO), and the Queensland Aboriginal and Islander Health Council. She has led multi-centre award-winning research, specialising in community-based participatory research, and is editor and author of *Aboriginal Primary Health Care: An Evidence-based Approach* (Oxford University Press), and the *National Guide to a Preventive Health Assessment for Aboriginal and Torres Strait Islander Peoples* (NACCHO and Royal Australian College of General Practitioners). She is a GP educator and coordinator of an undergraduate medical curriculum teaching health systems science and patient-centred care.

Professor Karen Francis is currently Professor of Nursing and Head, School of Nursing University of Tasmania. She is an experienced nurse academic and researcher, with qualifications in nursing, primary healthcare and education. Her research program targets rural health, chronic and complex illness and nursing and midwifery workforce. She has significant publications and research reflecting her expertise in rural nursing and midwifery. She is a Fellow of the Australian College of Nursing and Joanna Briggs Institute.

Michelle Francis has worked in health and human services for over 10 years as a clinician, supervisor, researcher and manager and holds a Masters in Addiction. She has worked in a variety of domains including mental health, drug treatment, homelessness, emergency and youth services, and has a passion for developing programs and initiatives that reach the most vulnerable in the community.

Professor Susan Gordon worked as a clinical physiotherapist for more than 20 years, mostly in rural and remote South Australia. She moved to James Cook University in 2006 to contribute to the development of a new physiotherapy program and led the program from 2009 to 2015, as well as being the Deputy Dean of the College of Healthcare Sciences from 2014 to 2015. She is currently a Strategic Professor at Flinders University as the Chair of Restorative Care in Ageing, a position co-funded by Aged Care Housing Group.

Sue Lim QSM is the eCALD® national programme director, Waitemata DHB's Institute for Innovation and Improvement. Sue is the founder of the eCALD® national cultural competency programme and services. She has been developing culturally and linguistically diverse (CALD) education resources since 2006, collaborating with stakeholders and experts in the cultural education field. She and her team have recently won a major award at the Diversity Awards NZ 2018 event for the development of a digital education programme delivering cultural competency courses to the New Zealand health workforce.

Professor Jane Mills is the Pro Vice Chancellor, College of Health at Massey University, New Zealand. Considered one of Australia's foremost primary healthcare academics with extensive experience leading and managing teams in both government and tertiary sectors, her research portfolio focuses on rural and public health, health workforces and health system strengthening. With a career vision to improve the health and well-being of individuals, families and communities, Professor Mills believes education and research are powerful vehicles for change that makes a positive difference.

Associate Professor Clint Moloney is a doctoral qualified registered nurse with a Masters of Health Research. He has experience with the conduct of systematic reviews as the previous Associate Director of the Australian Centre for Rural and Remote Practice, Queensland Health. His post-doctoral research has targeted research utilisation practices within acute care and aged care organisations. He is often sought after to assist clinicians in the application of evidence to practice, and is the primary author of the 'Spillway Model', a controlled, integrated risk management approach to research utilisation. Clint now targets research that considers the increasing economic burden of chronic disease on emergency departments and acute hospital settings.

Dr Annette Mortensen is a registered nurse who has worked for the past 19 years to improve the health of newcomers to New Zealand from ethnically diverse backgrounds. From 2000 to 2007, she worked as the Refugee Health Coordinator for the Auckland Regional Public Health Service. In 2007, Annette received the Supreme Harmony Award for her contributions to Muslim relations in New Zealand by the Federation of Islamic Associations of New Zealand (FIANZ). In 2008, Annette received a doctorate from Massey University on the topic of integrating refugees into the NZ health system. From 2007, Annette worked as the Asian, refugee and migrant health program manager for the Northern Regional Alliance on behalf of the Auckland Region District Health Boards and as the project manager research and development for eCALD services. Currently, she is the nurse consultant for Auckland Regional Public Health Service.

Associate Professor Nicholas Ralph is employed at the University of Southern Queensland's Centre for Health Research. He has over 50 peer-reviewed publications, has co-authored numerous textbook chapters, and has attracted over $2 million in research funding to date. He served as the Editor in Chief for the *Journal of Perioperative Nursing* and as editor for *Collegian*, worked as the Senior Research Fellow at St Vincent's Hospital, Toowoomba, and is a member of the National Health and Medical Research Council's Centre for Research Excellence in Prostate Cancer Survivorship. He is currently the Senior Manager for Cancer Control and Survivorship at the Cancer Council Queensland.

Associate Professor Suzanne Robertson-Malt is the program lead for Health at the University of Wollongong in Dubai. Suzanne has a proven ability to lead people of diverse backgrounds and motivate interprofessional teams to achieve strategic goals and objectives relative to the provision of excellent patient care.

Amy Salmon is a social worker who holds a Masters of Social Work (Forensic Studies) and a Graduate Certificate in Counselling Skills. Amy has worked in a variety of roles in the alcohol and other drug, forensic, mental health and education sectors for over 12 years. She has a passion for quality supervision, training, clinician development and supporting those who are most disconnected and disadvantaged in the community.

Julie Shepherd is a registered nurse and lecturer at James Cook University. She is the Subject Coordinator for Communication in Nursing and Midwifery and the First Year Nursing and Midwifery Student Advisor. She holds a Graduate Certificate in Education majoring in Academic Practice awarded by James Cook University in 2019. She has worked clinically over the past 34 years specialising in perioperative, pain management and palliative care nursing fields. She has special interests in communication skills and empathy in healthcare and is a reviewer for the PCC4U (Palliative Care Curriculum for Undergraduates).

Dr John Solas is Senior Lecturer in Social Work at the University of Bradford. While Coordinator of Social Work and Welfare Studies at Charles Darwin University, John was a representative on the Northern Land Council, and his research and advocacy were instrumental in improving the delivery of primary healthcare services to Indigenous communities in central and northern regions of Australia. John has published widely on social justice and is a reviewer for *Australian Social Work* and the *British Journal of Social Work*.

Professor Lee Stewart is currently Dean of the College of Healthcare Sciences at James Cook University. Professor Stewart completed a Master of Dispute Resolution degree in 2002. Her PhD, completed in 2008, concerned clinical governance and health industry leadership in a developing country. Professor Stewart has presented 'lessons about leadership', including managing conflict and negotiation skills, both nationally and internationally to a wide range of audiences.

Dr Jessica H. Stone is an author, marketing consultant and long-distance sailor. She holds a PhD in Communication from the University of Washington, where she enjoyed a lengthy career teaching marketing, strategic planning and business communications. She served as the Director of Columbia College in Washington State and as the Executive Director of Academic Product Development at NSTS in Malta. As a sought-after public speaker, she has presented to businesses and schools throughout Europe, the United States and Australia. Her programs focus on marketing, sailing and the writing life.

Associate Professor Louise Young is employed in rural medical education in the College of Medicine and Dentistry at James Cook University. This role encompasses Postgraduate Education Co-ordinator for a suite of health professional education courses and clinical education preceptor support for James Cook University's GP training program. She also provides supervisor training for health professionals in Pacific island nations and is a program external assessor for the University of Malaya. Research and publication interests include innovations in teaching and learning, development of clinical teacher skills, mentoring, at-risk students and rural recruitment and retention. Louise has been awarded a Fellowship by Health Workforce Australia and was a member of a team that won a Carrick Award for university programs that enhance learning.

ACKNOWLEDGMENTS

We wish to acknowledge the work of the authors of each of the chapters in this text and thank them for their collaborative contribution. We also wish to acknowledge staff at Oxford University Press. In particular, the efforts of the Publisher, Sarah Fay, who encouraged and supported us throughout the development of this second edition with the assistance of Alex Chambers. We also gratefully acknowledge the work of the copyeditor, Anne Mulvaney, and the proofreader, Carolyn Leslie. Finally, we thank our families for their continued support of our work.

Every effort has been made to trace the original source of copyright material contained in this book. The publisher will be pleased to hear from copyright holders to rectify any errors or omissions.

OXFORD UNIVERSITY PRESS

PART 1

COMMUNICATING PROFESSIONALLY AND THERAPEUTICALLY

OXFORD UNIVERSITY PRESS

CHAPTER 1

AN INTRODUCTION TO PROFESSIONAL AND THERAPEUTIC COMMUNICATION

MELANIE BIRKS, YSANNE B. CHAPMAN AND JENNY DAVIS

CHAPTER FOCUS

After reading this chapter and completing the activities, you will be able to:

- define the terms 'professional' and 'therapeutic' communication
- critically examine the need for the study of professional and therapeutic communication by students of the health professions
- examine factors that promote professional and therapeutic communication in differing contexts and at various life stages.

KEY TERMS

Client
Communication literacy
Consumer
Fourth Industrial Revolution
Othering
Patient
Professional communication
Therapeutic communication

Introduction

Communication is an activity we engage in almost every day. As it is such a significant part of everyday life, you might be asking, 'Why do I need to learn about it?'. While you will no doubt already be a communicator, are you an effective communicator? Will your existing communication skills serve you well in your role as a healthcare professional? In this chapter, we provide an overview of the essential elements presented in each part of this text. This first chapter also explores factors that impact on effective communication with individuals at different life stages. You can use this chapter to orientate (and where necessary, reorientate) yourself to the concepts presented throughout the text in the context of the relevant stage of your learning. As learning is a lifelong journey, we also encourage you to revisit this foundation chapter and its core communication concepts whenever you encounter a communication challenge.

What is professional and therapeutic communication?

Professional communication The exchange of information in the context of inter- and intra-professional relationships with the aim of achieving positive outcomes for the recipients of healthcare services.

Therapeutic communication The exchange of information between healthcare providers and patients, clients or consumers of healthcare services, with the aim of developing a relationship that benefits the well-being of the individual.

Henderson (2019) describes communication as a vital aspect of our personal, professional and social lives. But what exactly do we mean by 'professional' and 'therapeutic' communication? For healthcare professionals, are they the same thing? While professional and therapeutic communication are built on similar theoretical principles and rely on many of the same skills, each term is distinguished by the particular aim of the communication process.

We describe **professional communication** in healthcare as the exchange of information in the context of inter- and intra-professional relationships with the aim of achieving positive outcomes for the recipients of healthcare services.

Therapeutic communication, while having elements of professional communication, is the exchange of information between healthcare providers and patients, clients or consumers of healthcare services, with the aim of developing a relationship that benefits the well-being of the individual.

Reflect and apply

Think about the types of interactions you engage in on a day-to-day basis. Beyond the healthcare setting, what instances of professional communication might you engage in? Can you think of any examples of therapeutic communication that occur in your everyday life?

Why do we need to study professional and therapeutic communication?

Based on the definitions provided in the preceding section, it may be easy to assume that the distinction between professional and therapeutic communication is absolute. From a reductionist perspective, professional communication may be considered transactional and practical. Conversely, therapeutic communication may be viewed as inherent and an extension of natural human qualities such as empathy and compassion. While there may be some truth in these assertions, in practice it is not that simple. There is an unfathomable number of factors (individual, environmental, psychosocial, etc.) that influence every single exchange that occurs between ourselves and others. While it is not possible to fully control these factors, having an understanding of their possible influence enables us to manage their potential impact on a given situation.

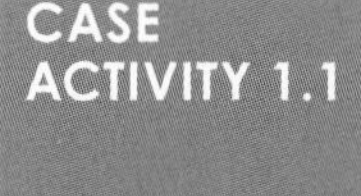

The need to study communication

Christopher is a 38-year-old student who recently enrolled in a medical imaging degree. He has spent the past 20 years working in the hospitality industry and is looking for a change. Christopher has commenced his first year of study and is frustrated to find that he needs to complete a communication subject. He expresses this frustration during the tutorial activities and states that someone of his age and with his life experience should be exempt from studying concepts and principles of communication that he believes are 'common sense'.

1. Do you agree with Christopher's assertion that communication is 'common sense'? Why, or why not?
2. How would you respond to Christopher if you were a fellow student?
3. How might his life and professional experience be used to best effect in studying this subject?

Christopher's belief that his existing communication skills are adequate for his future role as a health professional is not uncommon. Students often feel overwhelmed by the intensity of study and may therefore rank subjects such as communication as being a lower priority than those requiring mastery of more concrete skills (Birks, Cant, Al-Motlaq & Jones 2011). Any reflective practising health professional can confirm, however, that technical skills are of limited value in the absence of effective communication.

Othering
The identification of people as being different from oneself and responding accordingly.

Communication is the mechanism by which we connect with others. A failure to make such a connection can result in '**othering**', where we identify people as being different from ourselves and interact with them accordingly. The process of othering is often based on bias and stereotypical beliefs. In the healthcare context, the application of such beliefs can negatively impact on relationships with both patients and other health professionals (Roberts & Schiavenato 2017).

Othering is often an unconscious process and one that can get in the way of how we engage with others. Failing to engage in a positive, meaningful way can prevent us from understanding the perspective of those with whom we interact.

How do we ensure communication is professional and therapeutic?

This book is structured around four main areas: communicating professionally and therapeutically; professional and therapeutic communication in context; ethical and supportive communication; and communication literacy. Each of these areas reinforces the need to consider the study of communication as a continuous process that is critical to quality outcomes in healthcare practice. We assert that effective communication is contingent on an understanding of these areas.

Communicating professionally and therapeutically

How do we know how to communicate? Where do we develop the skills needed to effectively convey a message to others? Like so many life skills, our approach to communication is the product of our biology, our history, our life experiences and our education. These influences usually provide us with fundamental skills that enable us to function in our everyday personal and professional lives. For some professional groups, however, the complexity of the interactions in which they engage make skills in professional and therapeutic communication critical to effective performance in their role.

Skills in practice

Communicating therapeutically

Christopher attends his first clinical experience placement where he is observing the work of a sonographer in a health service. The sonographer shows Christopher around the facility and explains that they have a very busy day ahead. The first patient the sonographer sees is a middle-aged woman who has been referred by her doctor following detection of a lump in her breast. Christopher is surprised that the sonographer spends quite some time with the woman reassuring her and gently explaining the procedure. The woman, who was visibly anxious on arrival, becomes more at ease as the sonographer takes the time to speak with her ahead of the procedure. After the patient leaves, Christopher asks whether these procedures 'always take so long' given that there are a number of patients to see that day.

What's happening here?

The sonographer in this case understands the importance of assessing each individual's needs, and modifies their communication style accordingly. This health professional has the communication skills necessary to reduce the woman's anxiety and ensure the procedure is undertaken without causing her any unnecessary additional stress. In these circumstances, the outcomes are positive for both the patient and the health professional.

Healthcare professionals work with individuals of various life stages and with diverse experiential histories. Communication skills that may carry us through familiar day-to-day interactions are rarely adequate to deal with the complexity of experiences confronted by healthcare professionals in professional practice. People who seek out health services are often at their most vulnerable. At best they will find themselves in uncertain and often uncomfortable situations. An understanding of the principles of professional and therapeutic communication, as we will discover in the following chapters, provides a foundation on which skills can be further developed through practice in the clinical environment.

Of all the techniques available in the communication toolkit, perhaps none is more important than the use of self. Individual characteristics, both of the patient and healthcare professional, can act as barriers to effective communication in the clinical environment (Amoah et al. 2019). If we add uncertainty, pain and distress, among other variables to this fear, it is no surprise that miscommunication and consequential misinterpretation can occur. By using the self as an effective, therapeutic tool in the communication process, we can constantly develop as empathetic professional and therapeutic practitioners. Reflection is also an important tool in developing as a professional practitioner and, by extension, clinical supervisor. As with the study of communication generally, students may find concepts such as the use of self and reflection as abstract ideals that have no relevance in the real world. Usually with time and experience, however, even the most sceptical practitioner will come to realise that these practices are some of the most powerful tools available to support them in their practice. These concepts are explored in detail in Chapters 3 and 4.

Reflect and apply

The role of the self and the use of reflection are widely discussed in the literature. However, these practices can take many forms. What do you think of when you read these terms? Make a few notes to record your thoughts and revisit these when you have read through Chapters 3 and 4.

Professional and therapeutic communication in context

Consideration of the skills needed for professional and therapeutic communication cannot be undertaken without reference to the context in which communication occurs. Health professionals work in various diverse contexts—clinical environments, schools, workplaces and even people's private homes. The skills we use to communicate, and how we employ them, will vary considerably depending on the context. Even the language we use to describe the people we work with will vary, depending on the nature of the relationship we have with them, which in turn is shaped by context. Throughout this text we will use terms to describe recipients of healthcare as appropriate to the relationship between them and the health professional. Most commonly we think of the term **patient** in the context of healthcare. This term is appropriate for people receiving healthcare in a clinical environment, often to address a deviation from their usual state of wellness. The term **client** is more commonly used when referring to a person who is engaging with a health service for the purpose of maintaining or promoting health. The term **consumer** is used in some settings, particularly where an individual has a high level of engagement in decision making in respect of their own care.

Patient
A person receiving healthcare, usually in a clinical environment.

Client
A person engaging with a health service, usually for the purpose of maintaining or promoting health.

Consumer
A person engaging with healthcare, usually with a high level of involvement and decision making in their own care.

Reflect and apply

Review these definitions of patient, client and consumer. What connotations are associated with these terms? How might this terminology influence interactions between health professionals and recipients of healthcare?

Clearly healthcare professionals do not just engage with the recipients of care. Whatever the contexts in which they work, healthcare professionals will invariably interact with other health professionals on a regular basis. The nature of the relationships that exist within an interdisciplinary team will ultimately affect the quality of communication (Lee & Doran 2017). Building positive relationships within the team is therefore essential if desired outcomes are to be achieved. This may be easier said than done, given the different philosophical perspectives of nurses, doctors and allied health professionals (Foronda, MacWilliams & McArthur 2016). As discussed in Chapter 5, an understanding of these perspectives is best achieved through mutual respect and a spirit of cooperation based on a commitment to shared professional goals.

An important consideration in respect of context is culture. In Chapter 6 we explore culture and communication in depth. In that chapter, culture is defined as 'a cluster of societal elements held in common by a particular group of people'. While we commonly consider the term 'culture' as being applicable to groups who share a racial or religious connection, this perspective is quite narrow. Societies are becoming increasingly diverse, and contemporary definitions of culture extend beyond more traditional understandings of diversity as synonymous with multiculturalism. Any group that commonly shares values, beliefs, language, symbolism, clothing, etc. can be considered as being representative of a culture. As an example, different disciplinary groups in the health professions can be considered as having their own culture, often sharing a uniform, specific terminology and customary practices. These elements contribute to the broader context and therefore impact on the effectiveness of communication in the healthcare organisation, or in the broader community in which healthcare services are delivered. For this reason, it is important to explore factors that influence effective communication within the organisation (Chapter 7) and the community (Chapters 8).

Ethical and supportive communication

As discussed earlier in this chapter, health professionals often work with people when they are most vulnerable. In such circumstances, there is a need to be conscious of the ethical elements of all communication exchanges. Furthermore, the interactions between healthcare professionals and the quality of their communication have direct implications for patient safety (Lee & Doran 2017). In Chapter 9 we look closely at these concepts. We discuss accountability for safety and quality when communicating in the clinical setting and examine ways to minimise risk that can arise in such a complex environment.

In the healthcare context, communication is often exchanged on the understanding that it will be held in confidence. In Chapter 10 we examine confidentiality and privacy in the context of healthcare communication. Given the significance of accurate information in ensuring appropriate plans of care are devised and implemented, those with whom we work must feel comfortable in disclosing information that may be deeply sensitive or personal.

The vulnerability inherent in the patient role means that we are often required to act as advocates on their behalf. This situation does not suggest a paternalistic approach to decision making for a patient. Rather, such advocacy aims to ensure that individuals, families, groups and communities retain their agency in respect of decision making about their care. We examine advocacy as an element of the health professional role in Chapter 11. Being able to work with others in such a capacity is a privilege, and it is essential that health professionals understand the responsibilities associated with such privilege.

When determining an appropriate approach to providing healthcare, conflict may result where two or more people disagree on the best way forward. Disputes, disagreements and simple differences of opinion may occur between healthcare professionals and even between healthcare professionals and patients or relatives. Conflict is inevitable in any environment where individuals are principled and passionate about an issue. While conflict need not be a bad thing, if poorly managed it can impact negatively on relationships, communication processes and, ultimately, patient outcomes. Chapter 12 discusses strategies for the management of conflict with particular reference to the healthcare setting. The very essence of ethical and supportive communication is respect; a factor that is discussed throughout Part 3 of the book.

Communication literacy

Communication literacy
The ability to understand and apply principles of communication in order to effectively convey meaning.

Communication literacy is the ability to understand and apply principles of communication in order to effectively convey meaning. Communication literacy in healthcare relies on healthcare professionals' ability to read, write and speak with clarity and accuracy. Depending on the role of the individuals involved in a communication exchange, there may be a need to adapt communication through the use of particular language, tools or symbols.

In the healthcare setting, decisions are made by patients and other health professionals on the basis of information available to them. Understanding and applying principles of effective communication is therefore the best way of promoting positive outcomes in all exchanges in the clinical setting. For consumers of healthcare services, the amount of information provided in a single interaction with a health professional may be overwhelming. In addition to this, while it may be convenient to assume a base level of understanding of information provided to those who engage with the healthcare service, the consequences of overestimating health literacy can be significant, even life-threatening. Health literacy is an essential element in healthcare, whether individuals seek to promote, maintain or restore their health. Any form of communication, in the absence of health literacy, cannot achieve the desired outcomes. In Chapter 13 we explore health literacy, its assessment and management.

While it is important to take account of the health literacy skills of those who engage with healthcare services, health professionals must also have a level of communication literacy that will enable them to adapt and function effectively in the workplace. Academic writing and communication skills are not simply the remit of academics—they apply to all health professionals, regardless of their role. A key feature of any professional group is their ability to contribute to the disciplinary evidence base. This contribution can only be achieved through skills in scholarly communication. In Chapter 14, skills in academic writing and communication are examined. Whether to make a case for a new procedure, to advocate for a patient, to interpret or present evidence, academic and scholarly communication skills are essential aspects of the health professional's role.

BOX 1.1

THE ROLE OF HEALTHCARE PROFESSIONALS IN GENERATING EVIDENCE

Health professionals often regard themselves as simply consumers of evidence (e.g. research, policy documents, discussion papers) that are produced by others. Clinicians are, however, often the best placed to identify and investigate issues of contemporary relevance to the healthcare environment. Conversely, often those with the skills to investigate problems of significance are not embedded in the clinical context and thus rely on clinicians to identify areas for potential investigation. Possessing basic skills in academic writing and communication positions clinicians to be part of a broader team where the resultant skills mix enhances the potential for success.

Finally, information technology literacy is no longer optional in the healthcare setting. As we enter the **Fourth Industrial Revolution**, skills in working with electronic forms of communication are essential. In the final chapter of this text, Chapter 15, we look at the numerous ways in which we communicate with each other in the technological age, and the specific application of electronic forms of communication in the healthcare environment. All aspects of care are mediated in the modern world through electronic communication and embracing technology in the workplace is essential.

Fourth Industrial Revolution
A period of societal disruption brought about by the advent and increasing use of digital technologies.

Reflect and apply

Consider the preceding discussion about communication literacy. Would you consider yourself to be 'literate' in respect of communication? Communication literacy has several dimensions. Which of these are you strongest in? Which do you feel need improvement?

Who are we communicating with?

Earlier in this chapter we discussed the impact of context and other factors that influence the communication process. These will be elaborated on as we work through this text. It is important to remember, however, that regardless of context the nature of our work will see us interacting with people of all ages and from diverse backgrounds. Often we are working with individuals who have an altered health status. Illness, pain and fear can cause a person to communicate in ways that are out of character or inconsistent with their background and developmental stage. Tailoring our approach to communication when working with these individuals requires comprehension of the myriad influential factors that may be in play at a given point in time.

An important consideration when communicating with others is the development stage of that person. An in-depth examination of the physical, cognitive, emotional and social changes that occur across the lifespan, and that can affect the communication process, is beyond the scope of this text. There are, however, some key considerations for communicating with individuals at various stages of life that should be kept in mind when developing and applying the principles and skills discussed in the chapters that follow. The following sections present examples of these considerations as they relate to broad categories of development.

Communicating with children

Individuals at different ends of the developmental continuum are often those who are most vulnerable. Children are often unable to understand the complexity of situations that bring them in contact with healthcare professionals. When caring for a child, we usually communicate with the parent or guardian responsible for their care. Remember that in such circumstances it is still possible, indeed optimal, to include the child in the discussion as much as possible. Whatever the circumstances, keep in mind that children are experts in picking up non-verbal cues, so whether or not they are spoken to directly, they can read our body language (O'Toole 2016). It is therefore important to moderate verbal and non-verbal language using the techniques discussed throughout this text.

As children grow, so do their abilities to understand more complex language and ideas. An important development from Great Ormond Street Children's Hospital in London is the Me first communication model that allows healthcare professionals to learn about how to communicate with children and young people (Naunton, Martin & Reid 2017). The model, which has been developed with children, is the first of its kind. The authors suggest that the impetus for its development was frequent complaints from children about feeling left out of healthcare conversations. The step-by-step model takes us through what young people want from conversations with healthcare professionals. The site also gives feedback from children and tips from a range of healthcare professionals on various aspects of conversation.

Reflect and Apply

Access the Me first website at www.mefirst.org.uk and view the Me first communication model. The model has five main questions that stimulate activities and conversation. Work through the package, engage with some of the resources and make notes about what you have found to be important in this communication process.

Communicating with adolescents

Adolescence is a complex developmental stage associated with numerous physiological, social and emotional changes. At this age confidentiality is paramount as adolescents grapple with sensitive issues such as bodily changes, sexual behaviours and gender identity (English & Ford 2018). Communicating with adolescents has been examined with particular emphasis on confidentiality (Edwards et al. 2018; Gilbert et al. 2018). Gilbert et al. (2018) purport that the adolescent needs to know that all information will be treated confidentially and this needs to be stated up front in all consultations so that the adolescent feels comfortable in disclosing sensitive information. Although there are laws that protect the rights of confidentiality for adolescents and disclosure of healthcare issues, laws do not necessarily result in open and frank discussions; an environment of trust needs to be achieved. These issues are explored in Case activity 1.2.

CASE ACTIVITY 1.2

Adolescence and confidentiality

Winter and Rose met three months ago at a therapy meeting held at their local Headspace rooms. They have been cohabiting since. Winter is 18 and Rose is 17 and they both have fractured relationships with their immediate family. They both feel they have each other and really do not need other family members in their life—they seem reasonably happy with their lot in life and are attending Headspace therapy sessions to help with their addictive behaviours. At the last Headspace session, Rose announced that she and Winter are expecting their first child in six months. They appear quite delighted with the prospect of becoming parents.

As the worker facilitating the group session, you remind all group members of the confidentiality of information shared in the group. However, at the next therapy meeting Rose arrives very distressed as her parents found out that she was pregnant. They have chastised her for allowing the pregnancy to happen and not telling them her news. One of the other group members, who was excited for Winter and Rose, admits to sharing the information with her own parents and thinks they might have mentioned the pregnancy to Rose's parents.

1. What will you say and/or do in the therapy session?
2. How will you regroup and re-establish the issue of confidentiality with Winter and Rose?

Communicating with young adults

Trust and autonomy are crucial factors in facilitating good communication with young adults (Kim & White 2017). Kim and White (2017) reported that some topics were taboo for young people to discuss with healthcare professionals who were relative strangers. These include sex, childhood abuse and mood issues. Talking about private matters such as emotions and psychological struggles also prove to be troublesome, with some young people suggesting they feared being misinterpreted, demeaned or judged (Binder et al. 2011). These difficult conversations could more easily be initiated following an informal conversation to ease any tensions or awkwardness (Kim & White 2017).

As with adolescents, young adults also value a sense of trust and emotional safety; they need to feel respected, and they need humanistic engagement. Young adults want to develop their own autonomy and gain a sense of ownership of their healthcare (van Staa 2011). This search for autonomy is often shrouded in tension as the young person moves from being in a dynamic situation with their parent(s) to being self-sufficient. This area of tension is also felt by the healthcare professional, with van Staa (2011) suggesting the situation can be described as 'tricky'. For the young adult, being included in decisions about their own health is paramount (Kim & White 2017).

Communicating with adults

As adults, most healthcare professionals are experienced in communicating with other adults in workplace and social situations. When communicating with adults in a professional and therapeutic role, basic principles of communication apply. It is important to be aware, however, that people entering the healthcare setting often have limited experience of that environment and their ability to receive and respond to messages may be altered.

As has been reinforced throughout this chapter, context is a critical factor that will impact on the effectiveness of communication. Whether communicating therapeutically with adults who are the recipients of healthcare, or engaging professionally with colleagues, a 'one-size-fits-all' approach cannot be applied. Respectfully communicating with others as individuals requires empathy and self-awareness, as discussed in Chapter 3.

Communicating with older people

Communicating with the older person can be challenging due to the complications of age-related deficiencies (Noordman et al. 2019), including comorbidity, memory loss, hearing and visual problems and loss of social network. This group of individuals often relate that they forgot to ask the healthcare professional an important question, or they just did not understand what was being said to them, and rather than be a burden to others, they refrained from seeking clarification. As we will read in Chapter 2, active listening is important for effective communication, especially with this vulnerable age group.

Not only does communication with the older person need to be individualised, communication between healthcare professionals also needs to reflect what the older person wants. Communication should not be allowed to disintegrate into a one-way, linear type of communication (Hansson et al. 2018). Rather, for communication to remain open, the healthcare team should be committed to keeping communication channels interactive and respectful, involving the patient and in some instances their immediate family and/or carer.

Regardless of the nature of the exchange or the uniqueness of the people we are communicating with, there is a temptation to lapse into viewing the person in a stereotypical way. This can be particularly the case with older people, so we need to avoid making assumptions about the capability of a person to engage in decisions about their care and ensure that we employ ethical and supportive approaches to communication, as discussed in Part 3 of this text.

Conclusion

This introductory chapter provided an overview of the concepts discussed throughout the text and considerations for communicating professionally and therapeutically with people of all ages and stages of life. Each chapter in this text encourages you to develop your skills in communication, taking into account the context in which you work. The quality of your professional practice is contingent on your own communication literacy and specific skills in your communication toolkit. Investing in developing these skills will ensure that you practise to the best of your ability for the benefit of those with whom you work and, more importantly, those for whom you provide care.

SUMMARY POINTS

- Skills in professional and therapeutic communication are essential to the establishment of positive relationships that benefit the recipients of care.
- Skills used in day-to-day communication are generally not sufficient for professional and therapeutic purposes.
- Professional and therapeutic communication is contingent on the therapeutic use of self, an understanding of the context in which it occurs, an ethical and supportive approach, and strong communication literacy.
- Regardless of the purpose or form of communication, the health status, background, age and life stage of the individual needs to be taken into account.

CRITICAL THINKING QUESTIONS

Think about your own health profession.

1. How important are high-quality communication skills for this role?
2. Are there any specific communication skills that are important for this professional discipline?
3. Do your existing skills align with these requirements? Which areas in particular do you need to develop?

Group activity

Studying communication

In your study groups or via your subject discussion site, discuss how you feel about studying communication. Undertake a reverse brainstorming activity where you compile a list of the consequences of poorly developed communication skills in your professional discipline. Does this change your perspective on the importance of developing your knowledge, skills and attitudes in respect to professional and therapeutic communication?

WEBLINKS

Communication in healthcare

Institute for Healthcare Communication:
https://healthcarecomm.org/about-us/impact-of-communication-in-healthcare

University of Melbourne, Healthcare Communication:
https://medicine.unimelb.edu.au/research-groups/medical-education-research/healthcare-communication

University of Otago, ARCH: Applied Research on Communication in Health Group:
www.otago.ac.nz/wellington/research/arch/index.html

REFERENCES

Amoah, V.M.K., Anokye, R., Boakye, D.S., Acheampong, E., Budu-Ainooson, A., Okyere, E., ... Afriyie, J.O. (2019). A qualitative assessment of perceived barriers to effective therapeutic communication among nurses and patients. *BMC Nursing*, 18(1). doi:10.1186/s12912-019-0328-0.

Binder, P.E., Moltu, C., Hummelsund, D., Sagen, S.H. & Holgersen, H. (2011). Meeting an adult ally on the way out into the world: Adolescent patients' experiences of useful psychotherapeutic ways of working at an age when independence really matters. *Psychotherapy Research*, 21, 554–6. doi:10.1080/10503307.2011.587471.

Birks, M., Cant, R., Al-Motlaq, M. & Jones, J. (2011). 'I don't want to become a scientist': Undergraduate nursing students' perceived value of course content. *Australian Journal of Advanced Nursing*, 28(4), 20–7.

Edwards, L.L., Hunt, A., Cope-Barnes, D. Hensel, D.J. & Ott, M.A. (2018). Parent–child sexual communication among middle school youth. *Journal of Pediatrics*, 199, 260–2.

English, A. & Ford, C.A. (2018). Editorial: Adolescent health, confidentiality in healthcare, and communication with parents. *Journal of Pediatrics*, 199, 11–13.

Foronda, C., MacWilliams, B. & McArthur, E. (2016). Interprofessional communication in healthcare: An integrative review. *Nurse Education in Practice*, 19, 36–40.

Gilbert, A.L., McCord, A.L., Ouyang, F., Etter, D.J., Williams, R.L. & Hall, J.A. (2018). Characteristics associated with confidential consultation for adolescents in primary health care. *Journal of Pediatrics*, 199, 79–84.

Hansson, A., Svensson, A., Ahlstrom, B.H., Larsson, L.G. Forsman, B. & Alsen, P. (2018). Flawed communications: Health professionals' experience of collaboration in the care of frail elderly patients. *Scandinavian Journal of Public Health*, 46, 680–9. doi:10.1177/1403494817716001.

Henderson, A. (2019). *Communication for Health Care Practice*. Melbourne: Oxford University Press.

Kim, B. & White, K. (2017). How can health professionals enhance interprofessional communication with adolescents and young adults to improve health care outcomes?: Systematic literature review. *International Journal of Adolescence and Youth*, 23(2), 198–218.

Lee, C. T.-S. & Doran, D.M. (2017). The role of interpersonal relations in healthcare team communication and patient safety: A proposed model of interpersonal process in teamwork. *Canadian Journal of Nursing Research*, 49(2), 75–93. doi:10.1177/0844562117699349

Me first—Children and young people centered communication. (2008). Retrieved from www.mefirst.org.uk.

Naunton, R., Martin, K. & Reid, J. (2017). Me first: Promoting children and young people centered communication in health and social care using innovative educational resources. *Archives of Disease in Childhood*, 102(S3), A4.

Noordman, J., Driesenaar, J.A., Bruinessen, I.R., Portielje, J.E.A. & van Dulmen, S. (2019). Evaluation and implementation of listening time: A web-based preparatory communication tool for elderly patients with cancer and their health care providers. *JMIR Cancer*, 5(1), e11556. doi:10.2196/11556.

O'Toole, G. (2016). *Communication. Core Interpersonal Skills for Health Professionals*. Chatswood: Elsevier.

Roberts, M.L.A. & Schiavenato, M. (2017). Othering in the nursing context: A concept analysis. *Nursing Open*, 4(3), 174–81.

Van Staa, A. (2011). Unravelling triadic communication in hospital consultations with adolescents with chronic conditions: The added value of mixed method research. *Patient Education & Counselling*, 82, 455–64. doi:10.1016/j.pec.2010.12.001.

CHAPTER 2

PRINCIPLES AND PRACTICES IN COMMUNICATION

SUZANNE ROBERTSON-MALT AND YSANNE B. CHAPMAN

CHAPTER FOCUS

After reading this chapter and completing the activities, you will be able to:

- define key concepts related to communication
- identify the different models of and skills in communication
- explain why communication in healthcare settings needs to be person-centred
- analyse the key skills of effective and ineffective therapeutic and professional communication
- describe how non-verbal communication is used to support verbal communication
- apply the notion of compassionate intention to therapeutic communication.

KEY TERMS

Active listening
Communication skills
Communication triggers
Compassionate intention
Models of communication
Mutual understanding of self
Person-centred communication
Non-verbal communication
Therapeutic relationships
Verbal communication

Introduction

This chapter presents an overview of contemporary communication theories and skills to address the question: What is communication? Key concepts essential to understanding and practising effective interpersonal communication in the healthcare setting will be discussed.

Why might professional health-accrediting agencies position communication as a core skill for all healthcare professionals? This attention can at first seem excessive, particularly when communication is something that we are continuously doing. After all, **communication skills** are essential to our existence, having developed from the time we are born. Yet poor communication is one of the most common complaints made by staff and patients in healthcare settings (Pelletier, Green-Demers, Collerette & Heberer 2019). For example, speaking does not necessarily mean that communication has taken place. And just because we understand a language does not mean that we understand how to communicate effectively—and assuming otherwise can be problematic.

Communication skills
The ability to convey and share information with another effectively and efficiently using verbal, non-verbal and written skills.

Much of our communication with others occurs at an unconscious level, without careful thought. Even when we are very deliberate and careful with our communication, how it is received is completely beyond our control. Think about these limitations in an emotionally charged and stressful environment, such as a healthcare setting, and the importance of developing skills in effective communication becomes apparent. The professional caring or **therapeutic relationship** is the key to the healing process. The formation, sustenance and disengagement of the therapeutic relationship are based on the essential building blocks of communication and interpersonal skills. These important components will be examined and described in relation to the most common theories of communication.

Therapeutic relationships
Collaborative relationship between the healthcare professional and client that empowers and fulfils the client's needs.

Three models of communication

Communication theorists break communication into different components and **models**: some linear, others circular. There are three models that influence communication research and theorists: the linear model, the interactive model and the transactional model.

Models of communication
A collection of agreed terms and ideas that form a framework on which communication practice can be based.

1 Linear model of communication

As its name implies, the linear method of communication begins at point A and ends at point B. Linear communication is used extensively in mass media: television, telecommunication, radio, newspapers and some aspects of business, such as marketing. It is used to transmit ideas, information, attitudes and emotion from one person to another primarily through symbols (Boyd & Dare 2014).

Linear communication is successful when the sender and the receiver use a common language, and mutual understanding leads to correct interpretation.

There are five elements in the linear model of communication:

1. The sender.
2. The message itself.
3. The transmitter or medium of transmission.
4. The receiver.
5. The listener.

Communication occurs when a person speaks, and the listener hears what is spoken (see Figure 2.1). A breakdown in communication occurs when an error arises with one of the five elements. A common interference is termed 'noise', which can be anything that impedes the transmission or decoding of the message; for example, conflicting interests, pressure of work, too many other messages. In healthcare, noise could be the disease process, the consciousness of the person or their hearing abilities.

The linear model of communication is suitable for mass communication and can be useful in healthcare when a message needs to be delivered and understood. Airhihenbuwa and Obregon (2000) suggest that the linear model was a successful method of communication during the HIV/AIDS pandemic. It is used in health promotion and health education when a message has to be transmitted from the speaker to the receiver. The speaker has to make an impact and thus uses the main tool on offer—the voice.

FIGURE 2.1 The linear model of communication

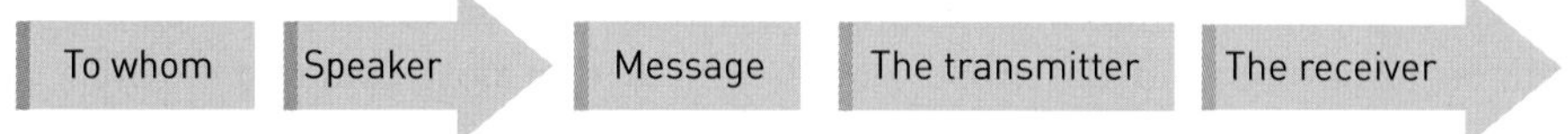

2 Interactive model of communication

If communication is only one way, as with the linear model, then how can the sender know if their message was received? The interactive model evolved from the linear model to solve this problem. Simply hearing, reading or seeing something does not mean that it has been understood or communicated as intended. Only when the receiver responds to the message sent and interacts with the sender to clarify different elements of the message, can communication be said to occur. According to Schramm (1954), communication is a two-way process, a process of interaction (see Figure 2.2) that is socially based.

The main distinction between the linear and interactive models is the positioning of 'feedback', which allows for bi-directional communication. The sender delivers the message and the receiver is no longer passive but responds with feedback about the message or the way in which it is delivered. This model of communication is important in healthcare, as it allows the healthcare professional to know if the message has been understood; it can also increase the healthcare professional's deeper understanding of the person's needs. As with linear communication, 'noise' can also interfere with messages sent and received in interactive communication. Murray et al. (2005) conducted a systematic review on the place of interactive health communication in the treatment of chronic illness. They found that using the interactive model adopted by online packages was highly successful in building consumers' knowledge and confidence and helped to develop changes in behaviour that achieved better health.

FIGURE 2.2 The interactive model of communication

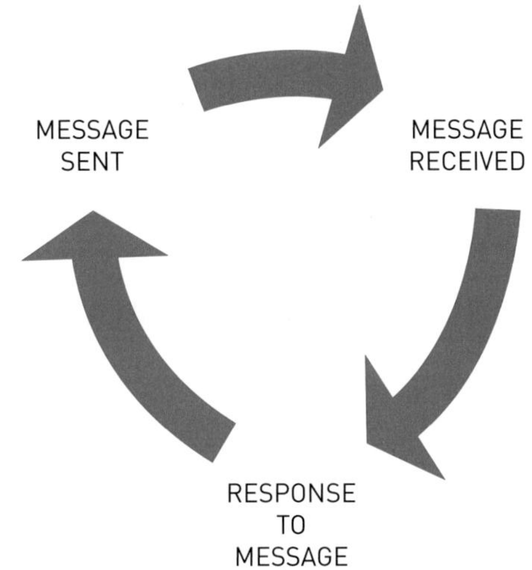

Skills for practice

'Noise' as an impediment to communication

John, aged 21, has been newly diagnosed with type I diabetes. Hilary is the registered nurse assigned to teaching him about injecting insulin before his meals. The following dialogue is an example of how 'noise' can get in the way of understanding and completing a task.

John: 'I hate needles nurse; I'll never be able to inject myself.'

Hilary: 'Don't worry John, we will do this together a few times until you get the hang of it.'

John: 'What if I make a mistake nurse; will I die?'

Hilary: 'No John, I'll check your dose and how you manage the injection each time you do it. Just try to stay calm.'

John: 'I am calm' (he yells nervously).

Hilary: 'OK John, it is nearly time for your lunch, so I want you to draw up 10 units of Actrapid insulin and give it to yourself. Remember we talked about how to give yourself an injection yesterday?'

John: (shaking) 'Do I get the insulin from the fridge now? Do I have to warm it up? There's so much to remember, I am never going to remember everything, I am so nervous about getting it wrong.' (He drops the syringe and the insulin bottle, smashing it to pieces).

What's happening here?

Hilary is being kind and encouraging, but she is ignoring John's fears. John is consumed by his fears and cannot focus on what he has to do. The 'noise' of his fears is getting in the way of completing the action. A better outcome would have been for Hilary to explore his fears rather than asking him to complete the task.

3 Transactional model of communication

Influenced by the philosophical and psychological theories of the 1970s, the third interaction of the communication model is the transactional model of communication (see Figure 2.3). Like Eric Berne's (1910–70) psychological theory of transactional analysis, the transactional model of communication states that communication occurs within a web of personal history and culture. Communication is no longer simplified as a two-way process, but as a multi-level, multifaceted process. Both the sender and receiver are actively engaged simultaneously in sending and receiving communication signals from multiple conscious and subconscious levels (Berne 2010). Contemporary models of communication capture the complexity of the circular process. Lavender (2010, p. 256–7) contends that in the transactional model 'emphasis is placed on the contexts of communication within a relationship and, in contrast to the linear model, holds that feedback and validation are interdependent and dynamic elements.'

These three communication models heralded decades of inquiry into understanding the dynamics of communication. In a systematic review of the literature, Chung, Barnett, Kim and Lackaff (2013) identified 89 different communication theories being actively used in research. However, as the review by Chung et al. was not directly related to healthcare communication, the three models so far discussed will form the basis of further elaboration and discussion about communication.

FIGURE 2.3 The transactional model of communication

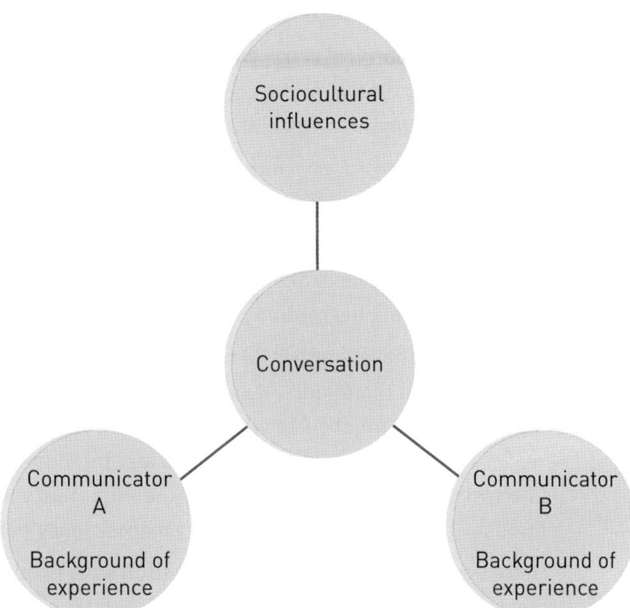

The communication process as relational

What then can the healthcare professional do to ensure that their communication efforts are as effective as possible? First, it is essential to establish an understanding or knowledge base about communication. Careful reflection on the three models of communication will help to establish this knowledge base. Each model presents communication as having a number of different components, but each component on its own does not comprise communication. For example, if a night duty nurse records a report for the morning staff to listen to after the nurse has left the healthcare setting, we cannot consider that communication has taken place until the morning staff listen to the recording. Even then, we have no evidence that the morning staff understood the recording. The quality and effectiveness of communication is limited because the morning staff lack the opportunity to ask questions and clarify their interpretation of what they heard. Efficient communication does not necessarily equate with effective communication. Communication is a process that arises from an unfolding relationship between each component; the relational nature of the communication process is vitally important.

Common sources of communication errors are our assumptions: what we say and think inside our head. Understanding communication as relational, forces us to move beyond our assumptions. Too often, the thoughts inside our head are incorrect, yet we tend to believe them more often than we question their accuracy. Through asking questions and listening to the responses given, our initial assumption is often modified.

CASE ACTIVITY 2.1

Communication as relational

Mary, a physiotherapist in a busy surgical ward, is writing reports on the 10 patients that she has seen during the day. She is at the central desk sorting through notes and writing her reports. The telephone rings and she picks it up.

Mary: 'Hello, surgical ward, physiotherapist speaking.'

Caller: 'Is that you Mary? It's Bob here (her husband). There's been a small accident and Julian (their eight-year-old son) has fallen off his bike. He is okay; there's just a large hole in his chin and he wants his mummy.'

Mary: 'Oh Bob, I just have another 30 minutes to work before I am off duty, I am in the middle of writing the reports. Is Julian okay? Is he hurt much? Are you bringing him to Accident and Emergency? When did he have his last tetanus shot? Is he bleeding very much? (Suddenly the emergency bell sounds) Oh Bob I have to go, there's an emergency here.'

Caller: 'There's an emergency here too Mary (Bob says firmly), but your patients always seem to come before us! (he slams down the phone).'

Clearly, Mary had the completion of her work duties at the foremost of her mind. However, the phone call and its message placed an added layer of concern on her, and she was thinking of getting off duty quickly so she could be with Julian. However, the emergency bell added yet another dimension of competing discourse, and in trying to explain her situation to Bob she inadvertently moved the conversation away from Bob and Julian to focus on her own work. Bob's thoughts about the conversation were incorrect. Of course, Mary was concerned about Julian' however, she had competing demands on her time and work took priority.

1. How could this interaction be managed differently?
2. What would have to happen for this interaction to have ended in a positive manner?
3. Can you think of a time when you had competing demands on your time?
   a. How did you organise your priorities?
   b. Did these demands interfere with your processes of communication?
   c. How did you deal with them?
   d. Has this experience helped you in future, similar experiences?

Understanding communication as being context-dependent helps us to appreciate the dynamic, continuously changing nature of our communication. However, it is important to be cautious here, as it is easy to fall prey to the belief that the process of communication is the avenue through which we continuously remain open to the possibilities and potentials arising within each human engagement. Sadly, this is rarely the case. Instead, communication can become the means by which we reinforce our beliefs about the world around us. For example, all patients who often ring the bell and continuously ask for different things can be seen as 'problematic patients'. Appreciating the context-bound, time-dependent nature of our communication forces us to reflect on our personal beliefs and values. Communication is not just about what we say, it can be how we say it and what our body says. We have to ask ourselves: is what we are saying (words) congruent with what our body is saying?

Verbal and non-verbal communication

Interpersonal communication has been broadly divided into two categories: **verbal communication** and **non-verbal communication**; non-verbal communication is then subdivided into vocal or non-vocal forms of communication (Chung et al. 2013). The vocal form of verbal communication refers to spoken language. It is important to acknowledge the power of words. Language in both its written and spoken forms communicates a complex mix of sociocultural institutions (Parikh 2000). Language, even without a speaker, communicates. For example, language use is often a form of social action in the case of gossip or protest (Strack & Förster 2015). The non-vocal form of verbal communication involves all written and symbolic communication, such as finger spelling and Braille. However, we can appreciate that there is a lot more to interpersonal communication than just spoken and written words.

Verbal communication All communication that is spoken (including words and other sounds).

Non-verbal communication Communication without spoken words.

Reflect and apply

Think for a moment about the clothes you wear. Each clothing option sends a message to those around you. Did you choose what you are wearing today as a means to be comfortable, to impress someone, or are you wearing a uniform?

Your choice in clothes can signal a host of information about your personal likes and dislikes, such as your favourite colour; your gender; ethnicity; generation; where you work or go to school; your favourite band, movie or sport, etc. For example, before you open your mouth to speak, the simple act of wearing a uniform can communicate:

- that you are employed
- where you are employed (if the uniform has a logo, etc.)
- the position you hold within an organisation, such as nurse, cleaner, doctor, physiotherapist
- that you possess a level of personal responsibility that enables you to hold down a regular job.

Likewise, your choice of words and tone of voice are also sending information to others. Research has revealed that as much as 90 per cent of human communication is non-verbal (Hall, Horgan & Murphy 2019; Manadal 2014). The vocal form of non-verbal communication is present in the tone, speed and pitch of spoken words. Let's consider the voice as the main instrument of communication. There are several aspects of voice that need to be considered as we learn about communicating effectively. In the linear model of communication, we usually use it to influence others, so we want them to give us their full attention. How do we use the voice to make others listen?

BOX 2.1

DIMENSIONS OF VOICE

In a TED talk presentation (2014), Julian Treasure suggests there are six dimensions to the voice; they are the 'tool box of voice'—register, timbre, prosody, pace, pitch and volume.

The six tools described in the focus box can enable us to develop a voice that can be effective in changing others' behaviour (Schaefer et al. 2016). Register denotes from where in your body you are speaking: a high falsetto versus a deep chest voice, for example. We tend to like voices that are deep and emanate from the chest rather than the nose or the throat. Timbre denotes how rich and warm the voice might be and people are attracted to voices that are possess these qualities rather than voices that are screechy and flat (Treasure 2014). Timbre has a lot to do with controlling the breath as we speak—it is the domain of voice trainers who manage politicians and others who rely on speech for their employment. Prosody is the meta-language to impart meaning—it is the 'sing-song' effect of the voice (Treasure 2014). People with a monotone voice are difficult to listen to as they sound monotonous and uninteresting. Prosody can also be used repetitively, when every sentence ends as if it were a question, rather than a statement. The pace of speaking affects the importance of what is said. If we become very excited about something, we tend to speed up our speech, but if we want to influence others, then we need to slow down our pace—then everyone will hang on every word. In harmony with pace is pitch. Practise saying the same thing at different pitches and you will find the 'sweet spot' for what you are saying—the pitch that is suited to the message. Lastly, volume is a powerful influencer on what is being said, with softer volumes often being more effective than words that are delivered loudly. These tools are at hand for almost everyone and, like most tools, they need to be used to keep them malleable and significant.

Reflect and apply

Imagine you are running a healthy eating workshop for a group of adolescents. The meaning you want to impart is 'eat sensibly from the five main groups of food'. First, make up a sentence that reflects this message and, second, using the tools listed in Box 2.1, practise saying this message in many different ways. Identify the qualities of the six different tools that makes your message meaningful.

As stated previously, non-verbal messages should be congruent with verbal messages. This means that what you are saying with words should match what you are saying with your body. What would you think if you were having a conversation with your friend and she was constantly playing with her mobile phone? Would you think she was interested in what you have to say? Or how would you feel if you were giving a presentation at a conference and people were looking at their watches or fidgeting?

Non-verbal language should be as clear as verbal language, as each deliver messages to the receiver. And as stated before, the meaning interpreted by the patient or client must be what the healthcare worker intended (Chan 2013). In Chan's study, the participants thought that their non-verbal communication was far superior in delivering a sense of support, encouragement and compassion to a patient. The participants further stated they needed to observe their patients' non-verbal communication to ensure they correctly addressed their patients' needs. Thus 'non-verbal communication is tailor-made rather than a formulistic practice' (Chan 2013, p. 1944). Positive non-verbal cues included facial expressions, in particular, smiling (Chan 2013), and patients often focused on the nurse's expression, especially when dealing with unpleasant odours like wound dressings. The power of touch is also debated in the literature with Benbenishty and Hannink (2015) conveying a case study of a patient (JH) who was hospitalised following being crushed between two buses.

> Before my parents arrived to ICU, I was very alone. I was too nervous to sleep, and I couldn't verbally communicate. One of the nurses entered my room, began speaking in English, shampooing my hair. Not only did she wash my hair, which was caked with blood, she massaged by scalp gently combing through my dreads, carefully working out all the knots. Her touch reassured me and put me at ease. (Benbenishty & Hannink 2015, p. 1359)

The use of touch here was both intentional and compassionate. A further interview with JH noted that although the non-verbal communication was not remembered, it was a potent reminder that someone cared for her.

> I had many surgeries, and after each surgery, a doctor told me that JB, a nurse I had developed a relationship with, stood at my head during each

> surgery, stroking my hair. I don't remember the actual event, [but] hearing that a human being was with me throughout the surgery confirmed for me her investment in my wellbeing, not just technical health outcomes. Her investment in me made me feel I should invest more in myself, which was difficult for me,' tearfully explains JH. 'JB is responsible for saving my mind and my spirit.' (Benbenishty & Hannink 2015, p. 1360)

Not all touch is welcomed by all patients in healthcare and should be used sensitively. Some healthcare professionals are wary of touching patients of the opposite gender for fear of being misinterpreted. Many healthcare professionals find that women rather than men are more appreciative of touch (Chan 2013), but once again the need for touch is a personal preference.

Non-vocal forms of non-verbal communication have been the source of intense research and are detailed in Table 2.1. A practical example is then given to exemplify the communication, and where possible comment is made where this non-verbal communication may antagonise people's cultural values.

TABLE 2.1 Non-vocal forms of non-verbal communication

Category	Description	Example
Kinesics	Body movement, particularly the face, hands and arms. There are significant cultural differences.	Finger pointing, smiling. For example, a person from a Mediterranean culture may use extensive hand movements and body gestures as an expression of anger, whereas a Japanese person may appear less excited, but just as angry.
Occulesics	Eye behaviour during conversation. Occulesic research has shown that the gaze of both the speaker and the listener during a one-to-one (or interpersonal) conversation is a powerful form of non-verbal communication with significant cultural variations.	In Western culture, looking into the eyes of the other person is common about 40 per cent of the time while talking and 70 per cent while listening. In Japan, it is more common to look at the throat of the other person. In China and Indonesia, the practice is to lower the eyes because direct eye contact is considered bad manners. In Hispanic culture, direct eye contact is a form of challenge and disrespect. In Arabic culture, it is common for both speakers and listeners to look directly into each others' eyes for long periods of time, indicating keen interest in the conversation.
Proxemics	The social use of space during communication, with research demonstrating significant cultural differences.	The closer a person stands to another communicates to the individuals and those around them a level of intimacy or threat.

Haptics	The use of touch (type and frequency) during communication. Cultures are divided into high, moderate and low touch communicators.	Middle Eastern and Latin American cultures use a lot of social touching during conversation. In North America and Europe, social touch is often limited to handshaking and the occasional shoulder tap. The duration of the handshake will often signal the degree of—or hope for—intimacy between two people.
Vocalics	Use of vocal cues to aid communication.	Use of ummms; aaahs; laughter, crying, coughing, sighing.
Chronemics	The use of time. It can be formal (minutes, hours, etc.) or informal (seasons, lunar cycles, social customs, etc.).	Punctuality; being 'fashionably late', etc. Use of silence, pauses in speech.
Appearance	Relates to the influence that a person's physical appearance has on either facilitating or impeding communication.	Body piercings, hats, face coverings, make-up, tattoos.
Environment	The communicative value of the physical space, such as room size, colour, accessibility and location.	Office space, decor, size of desk, etc.
Artefacts	The communicative value of personal belongings.	Car, plane, boat, jewellery, art collection, stethoscope.
Olfactics	Associated with proxemics: the use of smell to convey a message.	Perfumes, incense, car scents.
Synchrony	The impact of association or similarity in behaviour.	Mirroring and mimicry.

Source: adapted from Hargie 2011

All of these perspectives on interpersonal communication have contributed to our current understanding that communication is 'relational'. The multiple theories and concepts about communication have encouraged an appreciation that it is problematic to ask the question: 'What/where is communication?' and expect a simple answer. The individual parts do not make the whole (see Figure 2.4). Irrespective of whether communication is verbal or non-verbal, communication arises out of a relationship with the world around us, from the micro, unspoken conversations that we have with ourselves to the macro-level communications, such as the language we use. We have all experienced the power of a smile. Similarly, we have observed the persuasive ability of charismatic leaders to mobilise the behaviour of a nation towards a common goal.

FIGURE 2.4 The interdependence of verbal and non-verbal communication

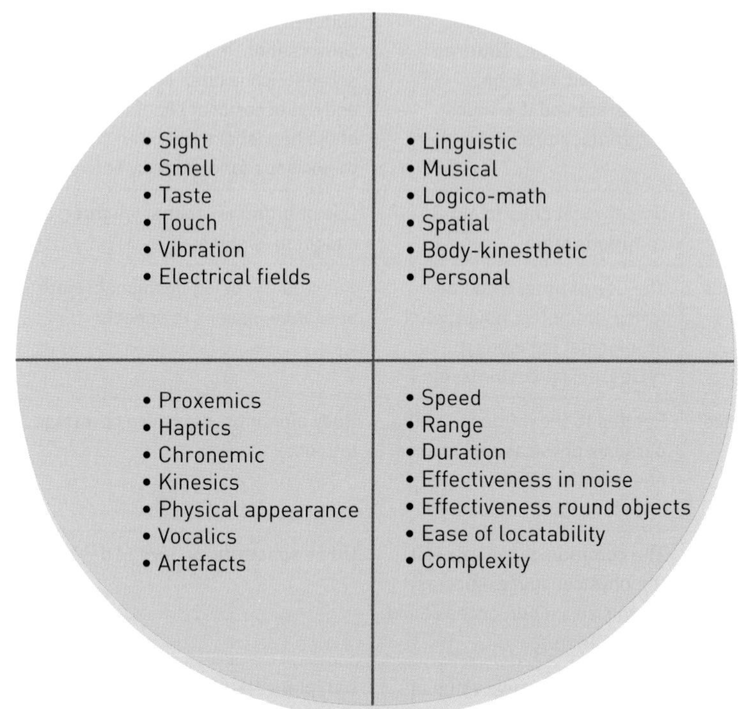

Research in the fields of cognitive science and neuroscience has increased our appreciation that interpersonal communication cannot be 'sanitized' (Petrovici & Dobrescu 2014). As embodied beings, we are continuously communicating with and relating to the world around us through our subconscious and conscious thoughts and feelings. Goleman (1998) popularised these research findings in his seminal work, *Working with Emotional Intelligence.* In Goleman's view, successful communicators have developed skills in interpreting their own and other people's emotional cues. Goleman categorises these skills into five broad groups:

1. self-awareness: knowing personal emotions
2. self-control: managing emotions
3. motivation: self-motivation
4. empathy: awareness and understanding of the emotions of others
5. social skills: interpersonal relationships.

These five dimensions are further divided into 25 different emotional competences, including self-confidence, thoroughness and desire for personal accomplishment. According to Petrovici and Dobrescu:

> Emotional intelligence focuses upon basic human skills inside our being, on the ability to control our feelings and inner potential to create a positive

> interaction. The ability to communicate efficiently for the benefit of a positive interaction may constitute an example of emotional intelligence in action. (2014, p. 1409)

This level of self-awareness is considered by many to be a prerequisite for a healthcare professional to be able to engage in therapeutic communication. Therapeutic communication is a form of interpersonal communication noted for its ability to establish trust and motivation which, in turn, facilitates improved outcomes for that person. Emotional intelligence is an important tool in communicating effectively in a variety of contexts. Emotional intelligence is covered in more detail in the context of managing conflict in Chapter 9 and in the use of self in Chapters 3 and 4.

A person-centred approach to communication

Evidence has shown that effective communication prior to and during healthcare procedures results in decreased anxiety, enhanced coping abilities and adherence to treatment (Lavender 2010). Recognising that the audience in a healthcare professional's daily activities can vary from colleagues, to patients, to family members, and from adults to children, means that the healthcare professional needs to adopt **person-centred communication**, focusing on the person who is the subject of their communication. Awareness of the factors that influence understanding of a message is essential for all healthcare professionals. Such awareness guides appreciation of knowledge and understanding of the audience (O'Toole 2016). Other factors influencing understanding include the age of a person, their intellectual background and their culture or language.

Person-centred communication Communication that empowers others to participate positively.

Therapeutic communication exists when two key qualities are established between the healthcare professional and the person:

1. trust
2. respect.

Mutual trust is considered to be the single most influential factor behind a person's acceptance of a healthcare professional's advice and recommendations (Miles, Mabey, Leggett & Stansfield 2014). A person will engage in positive health-related behaviours when they believe that a healthcare professional has their best interests foremost in their minds. Trust develops in a relationship when each person perceives that their personal beliefs and opinions are valued. Healthcare professionals must always be conscious of the way that different cultures communicate respect; this includes listening to people, acknowledging their preferences, giving choices where possible and treating people with dignity. Genuineness refers to a provider's ability to be open and honest with people. Providers who are genuine are congruent in their verbal and non-verbal communications. There are many verbal and non-verbal strategies that can be used to promote trust and respect. The most used method is active listening.

Active listening

Active listening
An intentional attending skill designed to understand the other.

The complexity of effective listening cannot be underestimated. **Active listening** (also called empathic listening, speaker-listener technique, reflected listening or dialogic listening) is a dynamic, critically reflective process that utilises all the senses, not just sound. Arising from the field of psychoanalysis, active listening is a strategy used by the listener to demonstrate to the messenger an unconditional acceptance and willingness not to judge. This does not mean that the listener does not have an opinion or advice to offer. Rather, the listener adopts a stance of diligent attention to all that is being communicated verbally and non-verbally by the messenger. A core skill of active listening is the ability to observe and supportively respond to a person's body language. In doing so, the listener is being genuinely supportive of the messenger's particular circumstances and needs. When done appropriately, active listening can result in the messenger feeling acknowledged, valued and empowered.

As the name implies, active listening is hard work. Listening with one's whole body requires being fully attentive to the person who is speaking (Stein-Parbury 2018). A wise communicator once said 'if you don't sit down, you won't hear' (Alan Stewart 1994, personal communication). What he was saying is a fundamental principle of active listening—positioning yourself to be on the same level as the person who is speaking.

Although there are several verbal and non-verbal behaviours that can be used to demonstrate and frame active listening (see Table 2.2), it is not something that can be orchestrated. If the messenger perceives any degree of pre-rehearsed, practised responses, trust is lost and communication limited. Research has shown that without full attention and conscious engagement on the listener's behalf, active listening ceases to occur (McKenna et al. 2014). Active listening requires focused time between the healthcare professional and the 'other', whether that be the patient or client, family or a professional colleague. However, this background of 'focused' time can be in conflict with the reality of everyday, chaotic clinical environments.

It is important to note that in healthcare practice in the early 2000s the SOLER acronym prevailed to help people understand how to interact non-verbally with another person in effective communication. Standing for 'sitting squarely, open posture, lean towards the other, eye contact and relax', SOLER was uncritically accepted as a strategy in teaching communication in the health care milieu (Stickley 2011). While this acronym referred to many of the non-verbal skills that are used when interacting, it was somewhat limiting in its approach and by its very nature negated the other processes that influence effective communication. Thus, we propose that you use it sparingly and only as a reminder to yourself of some important aspects as you engage with others. Table 2.2 presents a more exhaustive list of common listening behaviours.

TABLE 2.2 Verbal and non-verbal active listening behaviours

Behaviour	Example
Eye contact	Good eye contact need not mean that the provider is glued to the eye of the person. Rather, good eye contact may be given in spontaneous glances that express interest and a desire to communicate. Poor eye contact consists of never looking at the person, staring at people constantly and blankly, or looking away from people when they look at you.
Posture	Posture includes both body gestures and facial expressions. Being preoccupied and in constant movement that is not related to the person generally communicates distrust. No facial expression, or too much inappropriate smiling, nodding or frowning, can also communicate lack of authenticity.
Verbal quality	These qualities include pleasant, interested intonation that reflects the context of the contact and any particular feeling state that is expressed by the person.
Verbal messages	Messages to the person should be worded to reflect the provider's understanding of the person's perspective. This may include choosing culturally relevant terms; using the person's own words to describe their experience; and analogies or selected clauses paraphrased from the person's perspective.
Paraphrasing	To paraphrase, listen to the speaker and repeat in your own words what they said. Paraphrasing is not 'parroting', which is a mechanical restatement of what another person says. Paraphrasing is used to communicate to the person and give feedback about your understanding of what has been communicated to you, especially the feelings, experiences or behaviours associated with (or underlying) those feelings.
Mirroring	The listener uses mirroring to encourage the person to elaborate further on key words or phrases to increase understanding of what is being said. First, the key word chosen is usually a technical word or phrase with unclear implications. Second, it is used to encourage the person to explore or discuss something at a deeper level; the key word or phrase is usually an emotional label. For example: Person: 'I'm really worried about this.' Professional: 'Worried?' This should be said with an upward inflection of the voice, carefully avoiding an interrogatory tone.

Source: Adapted from Kokavec 2014.

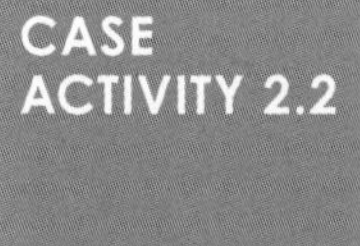

Active listening

Mr Solomon, aged 72, is recovering at home from a recent fall that resulted in him undergoing a hip replacement at his local hospital. He is recovering well and attends the community health centre attached to his local hospital for physiotherapy twice weekly and sees the community nurse for ongoing treatment of his other chronic illnesses, namely, type 2 diabetes and asthma. Jane is his physiotherapist and she makes time in her schedule to nip around to outpatients to see Mr Solomon twice a week. She is impressed by his willingness to try new exercises and is pleased with his mobility improvements.

One particular day Jane is 40 minutes late for her appointment with Mr Solomon. She has been held up by an emergency case that demanded her attention for over an hour. When she arrives at Ambulatory Care, she notes that Mr Solomon looks sad and he is pacing the waiting area. She is eager to see Mr Solomon so she can return to the other patients in the hospital that she has still to see. Mr Solomon tells her he is angry at being kept waiting and Jane offers no explanation; rather, she asks him to demonstrate his walking and stair-climbing abilities without offering any encouragements. Mr Solomon becomes aggressive and the situation begins to escalate.

1. Is there a sense that stopping to 'actively listen' to Mr Solomon could 'get in the way' of the goals of therapy?
2. What strategies might be effective in addressing this situation?
3. In your profession, how would you manage a similar situation?

The final skill of active listening is responding. Although this may seem surprising, Tamparo and Lindh (2017) suggest it is listening with the third ear—that is, being aware of what is *not said* or picking up cues that assist us in responding to clients about what we have heard, seen or felt from their conversation. In responding, we observe clients' physical and emotional states; acknowledge their feelings; clarify and validate so that we know we are sharing *the same meaning* from the conversations; and reflect and paraphrase what the person has said so we can gain insight into the meaning behind the message.

Skills in practice

Active listening and responding

Mrs Bolan is 64 years old and is in hospital to be treated for an infection that has invaded her body. She is quite ill and has to be isolated in her own room. All healthcare professionals have to wash their hands and don masks, gowns and gloves on entering her room and remove them as they exit. One day nurse Veronica Blue was assigned to care for Mrs Bolan—Veronica was new to the ward, so she had not encountered Mrs Bolan beforehand.

Nurse Blue: (donned in gown, gloves and mask) 'Good morning Mrs Bolan. How are you today? I am nurse Veronica Blue; you can call me Veronica if you like. What would you like me to call you?'

Mrs Bolan: (shocked that someone had asked her how she was) 'I am feeling a little flat today, I don't know when I will be going home.'

Nurse Blue: (sits down beside the bed) 'Okay so you're not feeling the best and you want to go home. I will ask the sister in charge when you are due to be discharged, if you like? I want to know all about you as I have not worked on this ward before and after that we can talk about your care today.'

Mrs Bolan: (tells Nurse Blue about her condition and adds) 'No one has ever asked me what I want to do. People come in and out of here without any conversation. You are the first person to sit down in my room with me.'

Nurse Blue: 'Well Mrs Bolan, I will be caring for you all day so it is important to me that I get to know your likes and dislikes and for us to establish how we will communicate with each other.'

Mrs Bolan: (smiles) 'I feel so much better. Someone is actually talking with me and not treating me like a leper.'

At the end of Nurse Blue's shift, she pops in to see Mrs Bolan and say goodbye. Mrs Bolan has tears in her eyes. When Nurse Blue asks why she is teary, Mrs Bolan tells her that Nurse Blue's kindness had made such a difference to her stay in hospital, and that she will miss her until she returns on another shift.

What's happening here?

Nurse Blue has built a good rapport with Mrs Bolan. She has focused on the person behind the disease and given her respect. She has used excellent communication skills—active listening, responding and congruent body language. She does not focus on what went on beforehand (negative interaction); rather, she encourages Mrs Bolan to experience a better form of communication and focus on the positive.

There are multiple situations in the daily life of a healthcare professional where punctuality is at a premium and time is of the essence. Attending to the many requirements of each patient—such as bathing, giving injections or assisting with feeding—can all be performed more speedily if communication is kept to a minimum (Lovell, Lee & Brotheridge 2012). The literature is replete with stories of patients' experiences of such task-orientated care. Patients often find these 'fleeting encounters' unsatisfactory; they lead to a sense of alienation and complaints that care is perfunctory or inhumane (Crawford & Brown 2011, p. 5). Nevertheless, no matter how brisk the encounter, there is still room in the communication to be respectful, interested in the person and their story.

Poor communication in clinical settings is the largest source of patient dissatisfaction and adverse events in healthcare systems across the globe (Kahn et al. 2018; WHO 2012). This conflict between theory and practice has encouraged researchers to investigate the skill set needed for therapeutic communication to occur in brief, episodic encounters (Crawford & Brown 2011; Kahn et al. 2018). A key skill proposed from this research is 'self-awareness', especially observing the triggers that a patient or colleague is stimulating in the healthcare professional, often within the first seconds of an encounter. 'Trigger' is used here to convey the 'lightning-speed' reaction to the person's verbal or non-verbal communication. Interpersonal **communication triggers** can stimulate both positive and negative responses. For example, a particular look with the eyes combined with the tone of voice can communicate a message of misery or joy within seconds. Contemporary communication theorists argue that developing the ability to identify these triggers is critical to improving the overall quality of interpersonal communication (Frederickx & Mechelen 2012; Wood, Chaboyer & Carr 2019).

Communication triggers
Words, facial expressions and voice intonation or behaviour that stimulates a response in another (usually a negative response).

These interpersonal communication triggers are linked to our psychosocial histories and are continuously being developed, and subconsciously registered as our personal likes and dislikes. Each of these personal likes and dislikes affects the way we communicate with the 'other': they colour our verbal and non-verbal communication. Because we are continuously relating to the world around us, these likes and dislikes are either reinforced or modified. When the interpersonal communication in a workplace setting has to involve a particular kind of emotional tone, healthcare professionals often struggle to maintain this standard. Hochschild (1983) first conceptualised this experience as 'emotional labour', in a study of aircraft cabin crew who had to maintain a polite and pleasant demeanour even on long and arduous flights. The everyday clinical environment demands the healthcare professional master these emotions and modify their emotions according to the needs of the patient or family (Bagdasarov & Connelly 2013; Lazanyi 2010).

There are many positive and negative tensions arising from the verbal and non-verbal communication associated with 'managing' emotions when working under the socio-political expectations placed on healthcare professional (Pandey & Singh 2016; Riley & Weiss 2016). In dealing with difficult moments, such as death and dying, controlling tears and the surrounding environment can give healthcare professionals the necessary distance to cope. However, emotional labour requires constant attention and can become psychologically exhausting, resulting in its strong association with workplace burnout (Sheppard, Williams & Klein 2013). One of the ways of showing a caring attitude towards self and others is to couch communication using a compassionate intention.

Compassionate intention

The rapid increase in use of information technology in healthcare has resulted in the information essential for person-centred care being available at the point of decision making. With this abundance of information being readily available, there is an unspoken expectation that the person's care decisions can be made quicker, and therefore that healthcare systems and processes can become more efficient (Smith et al. 2015). The average time for a clinical consultation is 10 to 15 minutes, and is double that in some settings if the consultation is for a new person. Debate exists as to the quality, effectiveness and therapeutic value of the communication that takes place in such time-pressured environments (Blackburn, Ousey & Goodwin 2019). Quality in communication does not necessarily mean that more time needs to be spent with a person; quality refers to the value of the communication as perceived by the person and this quality is achieved by delivering the communication with **compassionate intention**. Compassionate intention signals that the communicator is showing respect and care for the person and has their welfare as a priority in the communication process.

Compassionate intention
Genuine care, consideration and attention to others; these are the goals of communication.

Understanding communication as 'relational' is beneficial for the healthcare professional, who is required to deliver 'person-centred care'. Given that we have no control over how our verbal and non-verbal communication is going to be interpreted by the 'other', the only factor we can control is our intention. For example, is our intention to communicate with a person one of genuine attention and care? Or is our communication predominately unconscious and self-protective? The International Charter for Human Values in Healthcare is an international, multidisciplinary effort to restore the human dimensions of care (see Table 2.3). Research has demonstrated that effective communication, grounded in the core values of care and compassion, can positively impact upon the quality of a person's experience and overall healthcare outcomes (Durkin, Usher & Jackson 2019; Weingartner, Sawning, Shaw & Klein 2019). The work of this international collaboration of healthcare professionals was underpinned by a collective belief that the nature and quality of communication in healthcare is fundamentally influenced by the values held by the individuals relating to each other. Despite the collaboration of members coming from diverse cultures and backgrounds, they quickly learnt that they shared core values (Rider et al. 2014). The charter was published in 2013 following three years of rigorous research and details five fundamental categories of human values that should be present in every healthcare interaction (Rider et al. 2014):

1. compassion
2. respect for persons
3. commitment to integrity and ethical practice
4. commitment to excellence
5. justice in healthcare.

The International Charter for Human Values in Healthcare purposefully includes the essential role of skilled communication in the demonstration of values. The emphasis is on 'skilled communication', as individuals need structured learning opportunities and time to practise these therapeutic communication techniques. According to Rider et al. (2014, p. 276):

> ...effective and caring communication is essential to restoring human values in healthcare. Values are realised by the manifestation in language

> and the interaction process [the relation]. Skilled communication underpins healthcare interactions and relationships and plays an essential role in making values visible.

Our intentions become visible in both our verbal and non-verbal modes of communication. For example, if we start our day at work not really wanting to be there, just hoping to get through the day so that we can have time to do what we really want to do, then this lack of interest will be communicated to everyone we encounter.

TABLE 2.3 The International Charter for Human Values in Healthcare: fundamental values and sub-values

Five fundamental values	Values within each category
Compassion	
Compassion should be central to human relationships. Compassion means to understand the condition of others, and to commit oneself to the healing and caring necessary to enhance health and relieve suffering. These values underlie our efforts to be compassionate.	Capacity for caring Capacity for empathy Capacity for self-awareness Motivation to help and heal Capacity for kindness Capacity for genuineness Capacity for generosity Capacity for flexibility and adaptability in relationships Capacity for acceptance Capacity for curiosity Capacity for altruism Capacity for mindfulness
Respect for persons	
Respect should form the basis of all of our relationships.	Respect for the person and their significant others' viewpoints, opinions, wishes and beliefs Respect for cultural, social, gender, class, spiritual and linguistic differences Respect for autonomy Respect for privacy and confidentiality Respect for all colleagues of the interprofessional team Humility
Commitment to integrity and ethical practice	
The healing professions are built around integrity and ethical practice. These must underlie and permeate all actions in the health professions.	Commitment to honesty and trustworthiness Commitment to reliability Commitment to accountability and responsibility Commitment to the person's well-being Commitment to doing no harm Capacity to acknowledge own limits and seek guidance; awareness of own limitations Commitment to tolerance and non-judgmental care

Commitment to excellence	
We must dedicate ourselves to achieving excellence in all aspects of healthcare. Without excellence, no matter how well intentioned, our efforts to heal will fall short.	Commitment to providing the best, most effective care (scientifically and psychosocially) Commitment to communication excellence Commitment to relational excellence Commitment to self-awareness and reflective practice Commitment to life-long learning, expertise and professional development Commitment to serve the person's best interests
Justice in healthcare	
We believe that healthcare professionals should embrace the values of justice in healthcare and commit themselves to putting these values into action.	Right to healthcare (information, access, quality) Right to equality Commitment to advocating for the person Absence of discrimination and prejudice Attention to social factors, constraints, and barriers to care Commitment to social justice

Source: Adapted from Rider et al. 2014, p. 275.

A more recent study by Straughair, Clarke and Machin (2019) noted that compassion should be a central selection criterion for staff in healthcare and educational programs in healthcare, and that mentors and leaders should also role model this quality so that organisational cultures can promulgate and foster compassion in the workplace.

A healthcare professional's capacity to build trust and a rapport with a person and their family will be hindered if they remain 'unconscious' of their communication intention (Lee, Lovell & Brotheridge 2010). The time pressure of modern clinical environments, combined with emotional labour, can lead to burnout. Emotionally exhausted healthcare professionals have less capacity to listen attentively and spend time developing a rapport either with patients or their colleagues. Emotional exhaustion can be communicated as disinterest; if a person or colleague asks for additional assistance, this disinterest can be communicated as annoyance (see Table 2.4).

TABLE 2.4 Verbal and non-verbal behaviours of disinterest

Verbal	Non-verbal
Flat tone of voice	Lack of eye contact
Short, delayed response to questions	Slow in responding to requests
Minimal questions asked	Inattentive listening

Communication is not a static skill. Through research and new developments, we can enrich our own abilities to communicate. Studies into team dynamics have taught us that successful teams comprise individuals who have a genuine commitment to the team's success (Sheppard, Williams &Klein 2013). In turn, such intention influences their communication with the other members of the team. They remain open to continuously changing circumstances and to finding solutions. The International Charter framework outlined in Table 2.3 provides a foundation for defining and thinking more systematically and intentionally about clinical communication and human values, and for understanding the relationships between them. However, without formalised, structured programs of learning at both the undergraduate and continuing professional development level, these important skills will not translate into everyday clinical environments.

Developing the regular practice of keeping a professional journal is an invaluable way for healthcare professionals to remain 'conscious' of their practice intentions. Taking the time to critically analyse decisions and responses to various events can help in identifying themes of behaviour; professionals can then investigate these further to see if they are examples of unconscious 'triggers'. Once brought into conscious awareness, healthcare professionals then have the power to further develop positive attributes and modify less-constructive behaviours.

Conclusion

Interpersonal communication is a complex mix of socio-political influences that remain largely unconscious until we make an effort to bring them to the fore of our everyday consciousness. How our verbal and non-verbal behaviours are interpreted as we attempt to communicate with the world around us is largely beyond our control. The only factor we have control over is our intention. Through continuously engaging in focused programs of learning about interpersonal communication, we can develop the capacity to communicate with compassion—an intention that ultimately nurtures ourselves and others.

SUMMARY POINTS

- Communication is relational. It takes place with two or more people trying to find some common understanding with mutual respect.
- There are three basic models of communication and each has a place in assisting to achieve health. The linear model is a one-way system that is good for information giving; the interactive model allows for feedback and is a good instructional system; and the transactional model is multifaceted and combines conscious and subconscious signals in reaching a mutual understanding.
- Healthcare professionals should be self-aware. Knowing oneself and how some words or actions trigger negative responses can help healthcare professionals pay attention and not allow negative responses to infiltrate positive communication strategies.
- Healthcare professionals need to pay attention to both their verbal and non-verbal interactions. Congruency between verbal and non-verbal language leads to authentic and meaningful communication.

- Communication in healthcare is person-centred. This facilitates empowerment of the other, allowing them to take a central role in their healthcare and determining their health needs and responses to those needs.
- Active listening is a critical skill for healthcare professionals. It is listening not only with the ears but also with the whole body. Active listening also requires knowledge of when not to speak.
- Compassionate intention is the hallmark of effective therapeutic communication. Care, consideration, genuine attention and respect for the other are the core values of compassionate intention.

CRITICAL THINKING QUESTIONS

1. Identify some of the biases you have about society and the people in it. How might these biases intrude on your ability to provide good and effective healthcare? If you have difficulty identifying your own biases, list some of the biases common in society today.
2. The chapter emphasises that we are all products of our environmental contexts. Thinking about your own circumstances, outline who has had the greatest influence on where you are today. Make short notes about how this person (or persons) came into your life. Do you still rely on their influence?
3. Much of our communication is non-verbal. Choose an interaction where your non-verbal communication might be more noticeable, such as a social situation. Consciously try not to use non-verbal communication—for example, keep your hands by your sides, maintain a straight face, and do not nod approvingly or disapprovingly. Reflecting on this event, how difficult was this exercise? How much of your communication patterns are non-verbal? Was your changed behaviour commented upon by those with whom you were communicating?

Group activity

Models of communication

This chapter highlights three models of communication. In your study groups or via your subject discussion site, take turns to discuss situations when you have utilised each of these models. Was the most appropriate model used in each situation? For each model, identify a situation where it would be appropriate to use and one where it would not.

WEBLINKS

Communication in healthcare

Australian Commission on Safety and Quality in Health Care:
www.safetyandquality.gov.au

Institute for Healthcare Communication:
http://healthcarecomm.org/about-us/impact-of-communication-in-healthcare

Principles and theories of communication

Health Knowledge—Principles, theories and methods of effective communication (written and oral) in general, and in a management context:
www.healthknowledge.org.uk/public-health-textbook/organisation-management/5a-understanding-itd/effective-communication

Active listening

Skills You Need—Active listening:
www.skillsyouneed.com/ips/active-listening.html

Compassionate intention

Greater Good Magazine—Six habits of highly compassionate people:
https://greatergood.berkeley.edu/article/item/six_habits_of_highly_compassionate_people

REFERENCES

Airhihenbuwa, C. & Obregon, R. (2000). A critical assessment of theories/models used in health communication for HIV/AIDS. *Journal of Health Communication*, 5 (supplement), 5–15.

Bagdasarov, Z. & Connelly, S. (2013). Emotional labor among healthcare professionals: The effects are undeniable. *Narrative Inquiry in Bioethics*, 3(2), 125–9.

Benbenishty, J.S. & Hannink, J.R. (2015). Non-verbal communication to restore patient–provider trust. *Intensive Care Medicine*, 41, 1359–60. doi:10.1007/s00134-015-3710-8.

Berne, E. (2010). *Games People Play*. London: Penguin Books.

Blackburn, J., Ousey, K. & Goodwin, E. (2019). Information and communication in the emergency department. *International Emergency Nursing*, 42, 30–5. https://doi.org/10.1016/j.jen2018.2018.07.002.

Boyd, C. & Dare, J. (2014). *Communication Skills for Nurses*. Oxford: Wiley-Blackwell.

Chan, Z.C.Y. (2013). A qualitative study on non-verbal sensitivity in nursing students. *Journal of Clinical Nursing*, 22(13–14), 1941–50. doi:10.1111/j.1365-2702.2012.04324.x.

Chung, C., Barnett, G., Kim, K. & Lackaff, D. (2013). An analysis of communication theory and discipline. *Scientometrics*, 95, 989–1002.

Crawford, P. & Brown, B. (2011). Fast healthcare: Brief communication, traps and opportunities. *Patient Education & Counselling*, 82, 3–10.

Durkin, J., Usher, K. & Jackson, D. (2019). Embodying compassion: A systematic review of the views of nurses and patients. *Journal of Clinical Nursing*, 28(9–10), 1380–92.

Frederickx, S. & Mechelen, I. (2012). Identifying the situational triggers underlying avoidance of communication situations and individual differences therein. *Personality and Individual Differences*, 52, 438–43.

Goleman, D. (1998). *Working with Emotional Intelligence*. New York: Bantam.

Hall, J.A., Horgan, T.G. & Murphy, N.A. (2019). Nonverbal communication. *Annual Review of Psychology*, 70(1), 271–94.

Hargie, O. (2011). *Skilled Interpersonal Interaction: Research, Theory and Practice*. London: Routledge.

Hochschild, A. (1983). *The Managed Heart: Commercialisation of Human Feeling*. Berkeley, CA: University of California Press.

Kahn, A., Spector, N. Baird, J., Asland, M. Starmer, A., &... Landrigan, C.P., on behalf of the Patient and Family Centered I-Pass Study Group. (2018). Patient safety after implementation of a coproduced family centered communication programme: Multicentre before and after intervention study. *BMJ*, 388, 1–17. doi:10.1136/bmj.k4764.

Kokavec, A. (2014). *Skills to Promote Understanding of Self and Other. Professional Communication*. Armidale: University of New England.

Lavender, V. (2010). Communication and interpersonal skills. In D. Sellman & P. Snelling (eds), *Becoming a Nurse* (pp. 252–83). Harlow: Pearson.

Lazanyi, K. (2010). Emotional labour and its consequences in health-care setting. *Proceedings of FIKUSZ 10 Symposium for Young Researchers* (pp. 149–56). Hungary: Obuda University.

Lee, R., Lovell, B. & Brotheridge, C. (2010). Tenderness and steadiness: Relating demands and resources to burnout and physical symptom stress in Canadian physicians. *Journal of Applied Social Psychology*, 40(9), 2319–42.

Lovell, B., Lee, R. & Brotheridge, C. (2012). Interpersonal factors affecting communication in clinical consultations: Canadian physician perspectives. *International Journal of Healthcare Quality*, 25(6), 467–82.

Manadal, F. (2014). Nonverbal communication in humans. *Journal of Human Behaviour in the Social Environment*, 24(4), 414–27.

McKenna, L., Brown, T., Boyle, M., Williams, B., Palermo, C. & Molloy, E. (2014). Listening and communication styles in nursing students. *Journal of Nursing Education and Practice*, 4(11), 50–8.

Miles, L., Mabey, L., Leggett, S. & Stansfield, K. (2014). Teaching communication and therapeutic relationship skills to Baccalaureate nursing students: A peer mentorship simulation approach. *Journal of Psychosocial Nursing*, 52(10), 34–41.

Murray, E., Burns, J., See Tai S., Lai, R. & Nazareth, I. (2005). Interactive health communication applications for people with chronic disease, *Cochrane Database of Systematic Reviews* (4), art. no.: CD004274. doi:10.1002/14651858.CD004274.pub4.

O'Toole, G. (2016). *Communication: Core Interpersonal Skills for Health Professionals* (2nd edn). Chatswood: Elsevier.

Pandey, J. & Singh, M. (2016) Donning the mask: Effects of emotional labour strategies on burnout and job satisfaction in community healthcare. *Health Policy and Planning*, 31(5), 551–62.

Parikh, P. (2000). Communication, meaning and interpretation. *Linguistics & Philosophy*, 23, 185–212.

Pelletier, D., Green-Demers, I., Collerette, P. & Heberer, M. (2019) Modelling the communication-satisfaction relationship in hospital patients. *SAGE Open Medicine*, 7, 1–12. https://doi.org/10.1177/2050312119847924.

Petrovici, A. & Dobrescu, T. (2014). The role of emotional intelligence in building interpersonal communication skills. *Procedia: Social and Behavioral Science*, 116, 1405–10.

Rider, E., Kurtz, S., Slade, D., Esterbrook Longmaid, H., Ho, M.-J., Kwok-hung Pun, J., Eggins, S. & Branch Jr, W.T. (2014). The International Charter for Human Values in Healthcare: An interprofessional global collaboration to enhance values and communication in healthcare. *Patient Education and Counseling*, 96(3), 273–80.

Riley, R. & Weiss, M. (2016). A qualitative thematic review: Emotional labour in healthcare settings. *Journal of Advanced Nursing*, 72(1), 6–17. doi:10.1111/jan.12783.

Schaefer, R.S., Beijer, L.J., Seuskens, W., Rietveld, T. & Sadakata, M. (2016). Intuitive visualizations of pitch and loudness in speech. *Psychonomic Bulletin and Review*, 23(2), 548–55.

Schramm, W. (1954). How communication works. In W. Schramm (ed.), *The Process and Effects of Communication* (pp. 3–26). Urbana, IL: University of Illinois Press.

Sheppard, F., Williams, M. & Klein, V. (2013). TeamSTEPPS and patient safety in healthcare. *American Society for Healthcare Risk Management*, 32(3), 5–10.

Smith, A.W., Mitchell, S.A., DeAguiar, C.K., Moy, C., Riley, W.T., Wagster, M.V. & Werner, E.M. (2015). News from the NIH: Person-centered outcomes measurement: HIH-supported measurement systems to evaluate self-assessed health, functional performance, and symptomatic toxicity. *Translational Behavioural Medicine*, 6(3), 470–4.

Stein-Parbury, J. (2018). *Patient and Person* (6th edn). Sydney: Elsevier.

Stickley, T. (2011). From SOLER to SURETY for effective non-verbal communication. *Nurse Education in Practice*, 11(6), 395–8.

Strack, F. & Förster, J. (2015). *Social Cognition—The Basis of Human Interaction*. Hove, East Sussex: Psychology Press.

Straughair, C., Clarke, A. & Machin, A. (2019). A constructivist grounded theory study to explore compassion through the perceptions of individuals who have experienced nursing care. *Journal of Advanced Nursing*, 75, 1527–38.

Tamparo, C.D. & Lindh, W. (2017). *Therapeutic Communications for Health Care* (4th edn). South Melbourne: Delmar Cengage Learning.

Treasure, J. (2014). How to speak so that people want to listen. www.youtube.com/watch?v=eIho2S0ZahI.

Weingartner, L.A., Sawning, S., Shaw, M.A. & Klein, J.B. (2019). Compassion cultivation training promotes medical student wellness and enhanced clinical care. *BMC Medical Education*, 19(1), 139.

Wood, C., Chaboyer, W. & Carr, P. (2019). How do nurses use early warning scoring systems to detect and act on patient deterioration to ensure patient safety? A scoping review. *International Journal of Nursing Studies*, 94, 166–78. doi.org/10.1016/j.ijnurstu.2019.03.012.

World Health Organization [WHO]. (2012). *Patient Safety Research: A Guide for Developing Training Programmes*. Geneva: WHO Press.

CHAPTER 3

COMMUNICATION AND SELF

JULIE SHEPHERD AND NARELLE BIEDERMANN

CHAPTER FOCUS

After reading this chapter and completing the activities, you will be able to:

- discuss the importance and benefits of self-awareness and identify some of your own values, beliefs, characteristics and abilities
- define concepts relating to the development of your own professional identity to promote professional and therapeutic communication
- outline the important role that mindfulness and emotional intelligence have in developing self-awareness
- discuss the importance and benefits of self-care and identify your own strategies to care for self.

KEY TERMS

Emotional intelligence
Empathy
Identity
Mindfulness
Professional presence
Self-awareness
Self-care

Introduction

Effective therapeutic and professional communication in healthcare are recognised as essential to the delivery of high-quality and safe patient care. As healthcare professionals, we continuously communicate, both verbally and non-verbally, with a diverse amount of people in perpetually changing contexts. This activity can be demanding, challenging and exhausting. Every episode of communication we engage in includes a very important, yet often neglected, element: ourselves. This chapter explores communication through an introspective lens, considering the ways in which we present ourselves and the influence that we have on the process of communication. In order to understand ourselves in communication, we need to understand our 'self' in the first place. We will explore the awareness of self that is paramount as part of effective communication, touching on emotional intelligence, empathy and mindfulness as important strategies in the communication toolkit. We also discuss the role that our sense of professional identity has on effective communication and consider the need to remain reflective practitioners, with an exploration of the importance of self-care in the therapeutic relationship. Without this understanding of our 'self' in communication, we risk unsuccessful and ineffective communication, which can have a detrimental impact on all our professional relationships and place those in our care in a vulnerable position.

Self-awareness

Creating a conscious awareness of our emotions, thoughts, feelings, capabilities, along with our personal strengths and limitations, is the first step towards ensuring that as healthcare professionals we engage in more effective therapeutic and professional communication and relationships. Levett-Jones (2018, p. 485) describes **self-awareness** as 'being consciously aware of your own self, such as your thoughts, feelings, beliefs, biases, prejudices, behaviours and values'. Knowing yourself is to be mindful of how you impact on others. So, self-awareness can be defined as a state of being mindful of your thoughts and motivations, how you engage with others and the effect you have on them.

Self-awareness
A state of being mindful of one's thoughts and motivations, including how one engages with others, and the effect this has on them.

Reflect and apply

Take a moment to think about the impact you have on those around you. They can be those closest to you, professional relationships or even strangers. What effect do you have on them? How might they see you?

Your words, behaviours, actions and, importantly, your attitude, affect those with whom you interact and will impact on your ability to communicate effectively and develop relationships with others. Having a good awareness of self will help you to ensure these relationships are positive ones, built on effective, rewarding and, perhaps, inspiring interactions.

Let's look at self-awareness from the aspect of our professional roles and responsibilities. Self-awareness is discussed widely throughout health professional literature, as it is recognised as being a fundamental attribute for the healthcare professional to demonstrate effective communication skills in the healthcare setting. The effectiveness of communication skills has a direct relationship with patient safety, which is now emerging as a critical issue in healthcare. Research shows that when there is good communication between patients and the healthcare professional, there are fewer errors and better treatment outcomes (World Health Organization 2011). The healthcare professional who is highly self-aware will develop effective communication skills, resulting in therapeutic and professional relationships with others that are built on mutual trust and respect, while offering greater connectedness.

The importance of the professional relationship is central to any discussion of self-awareness. A strong awareness of the professional role, along with feelings and emotions when entering a therapeutic relationship, will help to prevent the healthcare professional from engaging in dangerous patient relationship boundary violations. Healthcare professional codes of conduct and standards of practice endorse this view.

Reflect and apply

Locate your professional codes of conduct and standards for practice (Nursing and Midwifery Board of Australia 2018). Read through these and find the appropriate sections that relate to professional and therapeutic relationships.

While we have codes of conduct and standards of practice that guide us professionally, we also know that a lack of self-awareness will result in poor relationships, ineffective communication skills and the repeat of poor behaviours. So, how do we practice, or '*do*' self-awareness?

Learning about self can be achieved by examining the Johari window, a model that helps people to better understand themselves and their relationships with others. The Johari window was developed by Joseph Luft and Harrington Ingham in 1955 (Luft & Ingham 1955). The 'window' is represented by four window panes or quadrants, which signify four areas of self (see Figure 3.1). Each quadrant represents information that is either known or unknown by the person and/or others. The Johari window is an effective tool that helps people to map their self-awareness so that can evaluate their behaviours, feelings and motivations.

Quadrant 1 is the optimum quadrant to be in. It is the open self, whereby information is open and public to self and others. Quadrant 2, the blind self, is a dangerous quadrant to be in, as it is here that people are unaware of their behaviours, feelings and motivations. For example, if a person's behaviour or body language does not match the verbal message they are sending, this would be considered incongruent communication, which can result in poor communication and mistrust within the relationship. Quadrant 3 is known as the 'hidden self' and relates to a person's private self, hiding the things they are unwilling to convey to others. Finally, quadrant 4 is the 'unknown self', an area where the knowledge about oneself is not apparent to the self or others.

Many people find using the Johari window helpful for developing their awareness of self. By exploring those things we don't see—or perhaps choose not to see—in ourselves, we have the opportunity to acknowledge them, name them and create strategies to eliminate them. This can be a confronting exercise, as we usually can only discover these things about ourselves by being informed by another person. While nobody likes to hear critical feedback about who they are and how they portray themselves publicly, it is a vital step in creating deeper self-awareness while also helping to develop emotional intelligence (discussed later in this chapter).

FIGURE 3.1 Johari window

	Known to self	Not known to self
Known to others	Open	Blind spot
Not known to others	Hidden	Unknown

Source: Luft & Ingham 1955.

Using the Johari window as a reflection tool can help us to learn about our 'self' and to discover previously unknown biases, judgmental stances or stereotyping tendencies that otherwise may impede our therapeutic relationships and even become a patient safety issue. Being aware of how your communication impacts on another is of vital importance in healthcare as it will enhance your therapeutic presence and enable you to use yourself as a therapeutic tool.

Another step towards practising self-awareness is to clarify your personal values and beliefs. Doing this will help you to understand why you behave and think about things the way you do. Acknowledging your values and understanding how they influence your behaviours and thinking can help you to empathise with the values, beliefs and behaviours of others, those close to you, those you work beside and, in particular, the people in your care. Exploring your values and beliefs can also reveal previously hidden or unconscious barriers to therapeutic communication. Biases, stereotyping, making assumptions or taking a judgmental stance are harmful within the healthcare setting as these, if active and are hidden (remember the Johari window!), will affect the way you interact with another and obstruct your ability to connect and empathise with them.

Reflect and apply

Think about a time when you may have been engaged in communication with a group of colleagues—for example, during a break—and the communication style of one person was not what you would consider appropriate for the workplace. Perhaps they were talking loudly, swearing or sharing personal information that you had no interest in.

Reflect on what you think about this person. Do you think of them as someone you could trust? Are they someone you would want to spend a lot of time with? Now think of them in a professional role. How do you think patients or healthcare consumers might view them if they were to behave like that in their presence? Do you think they would be mindful in their practice? Do you think they would make a good listener?

Revealing your 'unknowns', challenging these biases and assumptions and eliminating them or putting them aside, will improve not only your awareness of self but, importantly, your ability to connect openly and authentically with others. Conversely, not revealing your 'unknowns' will result in harm within the healthcare setting where labelling, making assumptions or being blind to the patient's cues can result in critical incidents, resulting in poor patient outcomes.

Practising self-awareness can bring illuminating benefits to individuals, such as developing emotional intelligence, acquiring more leadership style qualities and gaining a better understanding of why they do the things they do. This knowledge will ultimately support you to practice using a more mindful approach in your care. As a healthcare professional, this will help you to experience more profound relationships, with a greater optimistic outlook and attitude, and enable you to present yourself as a caring and empathetic professional as you use a mindful approach in all that you do. This means you can become a therapeutic tool within your practice, something that can achieved through developing emotional intelligence. This is explored in the following section.

Emotional intelligence

Emotional intelligence is a term heard more and more frequently in business contexts. It can be defined as the awareness of one's own emotions and those of others. Emotional intelligence includes having the aptitude to manage these emotions to enhance personal feelings and interactions with others. The concept was first popularised in the early 1990s by psychologists Peter Salovey and John Mayer (Salovey & Mayer, 1990), and five years later became a part of the vernacular when psychologist Daniel Goleman published his book, *Emotional Intelligence: Why It Can Matter More Than IQ* (Goleman 1995).

Emotional intelligence
The awareness of one's own emotions and those of others. Includes having the aptitude to manage these emotions to enhance interactions with others.

As demonstrated throughout this textbook, the ways in which we communicate with others are closely governed by our emotions, and they are also closely tied to the emotions of the person with whom we are communicating. Salovey and

Mayer's model (1990) identified four levels of emotional intelligence: perceiving emotions; reasoning with emotions; understanding emotions; and, finally, managing emotions. The table that follows explores these four levels in relation to their relationship with communication.

TABLE 3.1 Four levels of emotional intelligence

Level	Description	Examples in communication
Perceiving emotions	When we communicate, we need to be aware of our own emotions and of those with whom we are communicating. At this level, we need to notice and understand non-verbal cues, such as facial expressions and body language, as a guide to the emotions of the other person.	*Your colleague is flushed and glaring at you with closed fists and a rigid stance in the doorway to your office.*
Reasoning with emotions	When we communicate, we need to be able to use our emotions to activate our cognitive activities. This level helps us to prioritise what we pay attention to. As humans, we tend to respond emotionally to things that gain our attention.	*You stop what you are doing on your computer and swivel in your chair to face your colleague because you can sense they are feeling angry.*
Understanding emotions	Once we have recognised the emotions involved, we need to interpret the cause of the emotion and what this could mean. Some basic emotions, like happiness, surprise or pride, are generally easy for most people to recognise. Other emotions, such as anger, sadness, shame and disgust, can be a little more difficult to recognise.	*Your colleague could be angry because you have done something to upset them, or perhaps they had a bad morning at home getting the kids ready for school.*
Managing emotions	In this final level, you are engaging in high level conscious reflection of emotions and its regulation. Someone with high emotional intelligence is able to regulate or control their own emotions and respond appropriately to the situation, not the emotions in the situation.	*You invite your colleague to sit down and ask if they want to talk about what has made them so angry. You listen attentively and calmly, nodding sympathetically as they tell you about the speeding ticket they received coming into the office this morning.*

In healthcare, we are ourselves surrounded by all kinds of people with often unique and dynamic needs at any given moment. One of the most significant components of emotional intelligence is the ability to experience and demonstrate empathy (Mosca 2019), a critical element of the most basic relationships we have in healthcare—with patients, their families and other members of the healthcare team. Without empathy, we cannot truly have the necessary emotional intelligence required to provide effective therapeutic care.

Additionally, the healthcare professional with high emotional intelligence is considerably more likely to understand the emotions and behaviours of others. In the therapeutic relationship with a patient, the healthcare professional with high emotional intelligence will understand why a patient is behaving in a particular way, and not rush to judgment or react adversely to the behaviours. For example, a patient may be angry, shouting, not making eye contact and refusing to answer questions. A person with a low emotional intelligence may want to respond by yelling at the patient, mirroring their anger, or simply refusing to speak to them any further. However, through the application of the levels of emotional intelligence, it is possible to understand that the patient's behaviour is not personal; rather, these behaviours are symptomatic of something else, whether it is fear, anxiety, illness, medications or altered cognition. With this understanding, the healthcare professional is able to remain calm and empathic towards the patient, attempt to de-escalate the situation and continue the therapeutic relationship.

Emotional intelligence is now seen as an essential and fundamental attribute in healthcare, helping to resolve challenging communication and conflict situations. The healthcare professional with high emotional intelligence can be seen as trustworthy, calm, competent and less stressed (Stein-Parbury 2017).

Empathy

Demonstrating **empathy** enables the person receiving your care to feel valued and safe, which will directly relate to their healthcare experience as one of quality. When you bring yourself into your practice, you bring not only your knowledge and clinical skills but also your empathy for the person you are caring for. The International Charter for Human Values in Healthcare (2011) reminds us that the 'capacity for empathy is recognised as a core human value and should be present in and inform every healthcare interaction' (p. 276).

Empathy
A conscious awareness of another person's perspective, feelings and behaviours.

TABLE 3.2 Empathy vs sympathy

Description	Examples in communication		
Empathy	*Feeling with*	How do they feel about what is happening to them? Keeps a focus on the person's suffering without losing one's own perspective.	*'I can see you are experiencing considerable distress. Would you like me to sit with you and we could talk a little about how you are feeling?'*
Sympathy	*Feeling for*	How would I feel if I was in their position? Feeling pity or sorrow, thereby shifting the focus onto oneself and away from the person.	*'I am feeling your pain.'* *'I understand what you must be feeling.'*

Empathy can be defined as a conscious sense of understanding and awareness of another person's perspective, feelings and behaviours. Rousseau (2008) describes empathy as 'the ability to understand the thoughts and emotions of another person' (p. 261). In other words, it is the ability to observe the person's current experience and imagining how it must feel to be living that experience. It is important to note here that sympathy is not the same as empathy.

Stein-Parbury (2017) tells us that when we reach out to the person and seek to understand their perspective and their experience, we demonstrate empathy, whereas when we express sympathy we are moved by their distress, which urges us to act to alleviate their suffering. Jeffrey (2016) importantly notes that sympathy takes a 'self-orientated' stance whereby in order to relieve our own sympathetic distress, we are motivated by our ego to help the other person. Importantly, taking a sympathetic approach in healthcare can put the healthcare professional at risk of being distressed or overwhelmed, particularly if their own practise of self-awareness is reduced.

Of particular interest is the strong connection between self-awareness, mindfulness, empathy and emotional intelligence. McCormack and McCance (2017) describe how Daniel Goleman, who is widely known for his research on leadership, argues that it is not a person's skill or intelligence that sees them succeed, but rather it is their emotional intelligence, and the characteristics that contribute to their emotional intelligence.

BOX 3.1

CHARACTERISTICS OF EMOTIONAL INTELLIGENCE

- *Self-awareness:* the ability to recognise one's moods, emotions and drives as well as their effect on others.
- *Self-regulation:* the ability to control or redirect disruptive impulses and moods and the ability to suspend judgment and to think before acting.
- *Motivation:* a passion to work for reasons that go beyond money or status and a propensity to pursue goals with energy and persistence.
- *Empathy:* the ability to understand the emotional make-up of other people and skill in treating people according to their emotional reactions.
- *Social skills:* proficiency in managing relationships and building networks and an ability to find common ground and build rapport.

Source: Goleman (1999, as cited in Archee, Gurney & Mohan 2013, p. 182).

Genuine and heartfelt empathy has many benefits for the patient, when it gives them a sense of being genuinely cared for, being valued as an individual, and feeling safe. The benefits extend beyond the patient, as the caregiver can experience the rewarding feeling of providing genuine care with the knowledge they are helping another—this is known as compassion satisfaction. Compassion satisfaction can be defined as the feeling of pleasure one gains when caring at a high level for patients.

Rousseau (2008), further in his discussion on empathy, describes Anatole Broyard's book (1992), *Intoxicated By My Illness: And Other Writings on Life and Death*, while he was living with metastatic prostate cancer, where he so eloquently wrote:

> To the typical physician, my illness is a routine incident in his rounds while for me it's the crisis of my life. I would feel better if I had a doctor who at least perceived this incongruity... I just wish he would... give me his whole mind just once, be bonded with me for a brief space, survey my soul as well as my flesh, to get at my illness, for each man is ill in his own way. (p. 262)

Rousseau (2008, p. 262) concludes by stating: 'therein lies our duty as healthcare professionals: to survey our patient's soul and flesh so that we may understand their illness in their own personal way'.

Mindfulness

According to Langer (1989), **mindfulness** can be described as a state of having complete awareness of oneself in the present moment. In other words, the conscious and collective awareness of one's thoughts, feelings, emotions, bodily sensations, and the surrounding environment for a sustained period of time, with the implicit intent to understand the uniqueness and 'newness' of the moment.

Mindfulness
A state of having complete awareness of oneself in the present moment.

What, then, is mindful communication? An interesting observation by Stephen Covey suggests we do not listen in order to understand what is being said to us, but rather we listen in order to reply (Covey 2013). If we think about this, we can see how by listening simply to reply means we are not consciously listening, for we are forming the dialogue that will make up our response in our minds, rather than just taking time in the moment to 'hear' what is being said.

Reflect and apply

Think about a recent conversation you had, perhaps with a colleague or classmate. Cast your mind back to what you were thinking and doing in this conversation. How much of a role did you play in the conversation? How much can you remember of what was happening around you during this conversation? Do you remember the facial expressions of the person with whom you were talking? What was going through your mind during the conversation?

A mindful listener will not just 'hear' what is being said—they will also become aware of what they are thinking about what is being said, what they are feeling about what is being said, what their body is doing in response to what is being said, as well as what is going on around them at the time. In mindful communication, our response is not necessarily the most important part of the communication event.

When we are mindful in our communication in healthcare, it helps to remind us that we sometimes don't know the experience as well as we think we do. For example, a clinical nurse is admitting a patient into the surgical ward for surgery that afternoon. For the nurse, admitting a patient is a routine task. It involves asking a series of questions, checking that the patient has consented to the procedure, and that they are prepared for the procedure. However, for the patient, this is not routine. Through mindful listening, the nurse will learn new things about this patient as part of their admission that will help them realise that this is not routine. Rather, they will start to notice the uniqueness of that patient—their story, their experiences, their emotions and feelings, their lives, as well as becoming more aware of their own story, experiences and emotions. Through this mindfulness, the nurse can develop a greater sense of empathy towards the patient as an individual and adjust their care accordingly.

Reflect and apply

Hold an apple in your hands. Pretend this is the first time you have ever seen an apple. As you hold the apple, take notice of the way your apple looks—the flecks and imperfections in the apple skin; its colour; the shininess of its skin. Now feel the apple. How does the skin of the apple really feel beneath your fingers? What does the stalk feel like? What does the calyx at the bottom of the fruit feel like? Now lift the fruit to your nose. What does the apple smell like? How would you describe its smell? Place the apple against your cheek. What does it feel like? Is it cool to touch? Smooth against your face? Finally, the best part—take a bite of your apple. Take notice of its taste. What does it taste like? How could you describe its taste? What does the apple piece feel like inside your mouth? Is it crisp? Is it soft?

Focusing on the apple is meant to help you focus your mind on the present moment, to the object in your hand. Throughout the exercise, did you notice anything else going on around you? Did you momentarily forget any worries or problems you had while you were concentrating on the apple?

When we are deeply mindful, we can connect solely with what is happening in front of us at that moment in time. This is the art of mindfulness, and we can apply this focus on the person with whom we are communicating, giving them our complete and undivided attention for that moment.

Professional presence
A combination of communication, professional etiquette, behaviour, attitude and appearance to produce the optimal version of oneself in a professional context.

Professional presence

As a healthcare professional, it is important that you present yourself in a manner that espouses all the attributes expected of your profession. **Professional presence** can be defined as a combination of communication, professional etiquette, behaviour, attitude and appearance to produce the optimal version of oneself in a professional context. As you have read in this chapter, self-awareness, emotional intelligence and mindfulness significantly contribute to your effectiveness as a therapeutic and professional communicator. Likewise, your ability to *think* like a professional will go a long way to enhance your communication skills. For example, Code 3 of the Australian Medical Association's (AMA) *Code of Ethics* (2016, p. 4) states the medical professional must build a professional reputation based on integrity and ability. When this is the case, those who are receiving medical care will feel safe, well cared for, and confident in the doctor's abilities. For you to present yourself as a professional, you need to think and behave like a professional. This in turn will promote your 'self' as the epitome of professionalism and enhance your overall therapeutic and professional presence. It is this unique blending of both professional and therapeutic presence that can afford you the ability to use yourself as a therapeutic tool.

The formation of identity in healthcare is not linear in any sense, with peaks and troughs in the development of the professional 'self' as learning and growth occur. One tool used to help educators and learners understand their level of professional knowledge is known as Miller's pyramid (Cruess et al. 2016). Miller used this pyramid as a framework to guide assessment practices in a variety of health education areas. The structure of the pyramid represents different levels against which clinical competence is assessed: *Knows*, *Knows how*, *Shows how*, *Does* and *Is*. Interestingly, Miller's pyramid has also been used to assist in the assessment of professionalism. It is the last level, *Is*, that is most relevant in the context of therapeutic communication. It was added to reflect the values and beliefs and the level of professional identity of the individual—that is, where the person's role comes to represent their personality or identity, whereby they think, act and feel like the professional that they have trained to become (Cruess et al. 2016).

FIGURE 3.2 Miller's Pyramid

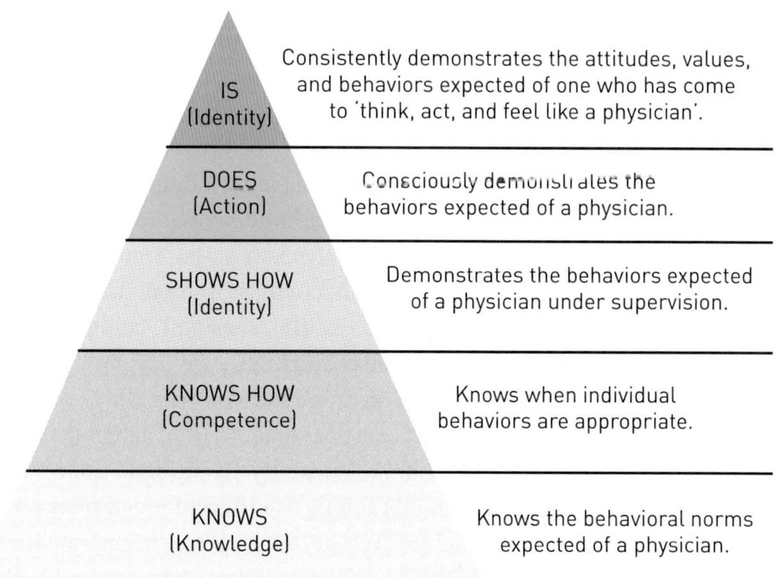

Your professional presence can also be endorsed by your profession's codes of ethics. For example, in the nursing profession the International Council of Nurses code of ethics (2012) states 'the nurse demonstrates professional values such as respectfulness, responsiveness, compassion, trustworthiness and integrity' (p. 2).

As a learner or a novice in your profession, how do you identify as a professional? The best approach is to start now. Discover the attributes and qualities of the profession. Read the standards of practice, codes of ethics and conduct, and other professional competency standards. Think about the relationships and conversations you have with those in your care. Now embrace your awareness of self, including all your values, beliefs, attitudes and actions—it is these that will help you identify your professional self. You have an obligation to represent the profession, and therefore to think, act, speak and feel like a professional. Over time, your therapeutic and professional communication will become natural, as it will become part of *who* you are as well as *how* you are.

Self-care in communication

As healthcare professionals, the care and concern we provide is a key tenet of our role. We often don't question this, because it is simply part of who we are as providers of healthcare. However, caring and compassion can come at a personal cost. We must learn to also provide such care and compassion to ourselves, in other words, to ensure our own **self-care**. Unfortunately, few students in healthcare are explicitly taught how to do this in their undergraduate programs. Throughout this chapter, we have reinforced our belief that effective and safe communication is not just about understanding how the other person thinks and feels; who you are, or your identity, in the communication is equally as important. **Identity** can be defined as a conscious awareness of how a person's individual characteristics and culture combine to form a realisation of how they see themselves.

Self-care
A conscious practice of undertaking purposeful actions to sustain and maintain one's own holistic well-being.

Identity
A conscious awareness of how a person's individual characteristics and culture combine to form a realisation of how they see themselves.

Self-care begins with self-compassion and self-kindness. Compassion is a central tenet of healthcare, and goes hand-in-hand with the concept of caring. We can understand compassion as being driven to assist another by a sense of emotional, spiritual or psychological connectedness (Lown, Dunne, Muncer & Chadwick 2017). Self-compassion, then, is the sense of being compelled to help ourselves by connecting emotionally, spiritually or psychologically to our experience or experiences. Following on from self-compassion is self-kindness. When you speak to yourself, do you use the same style of language as you use when you talk to a friend or loved one, especially in difficult times? For many people, the answer is 'no'. We often talk to our friends and loved ones with much kinder language than we do ourselves. When our patients, friends or loved ones are hurting or suffering our language is generally compassionate and loving, and free from judgment or harshness. Imagine how comforting it would be to speak to yourself in the same way.

If you find this difficult to do, try writing yourself a compassionate letter, or imagine you are a friend writing the letter to you. What would this compassionate and caring friend say to you in your moment of distress and pain? What would your friend want you to know about you? What would your friend want to say about the harsh way you are describing yourself right now? What might your friend want to remind you about how they and the rest of the world see you? After the letter is written, put it away for a while. Then, at a later time, take it out and reflect on the kindness and compassion you have shown yourself in the letter.

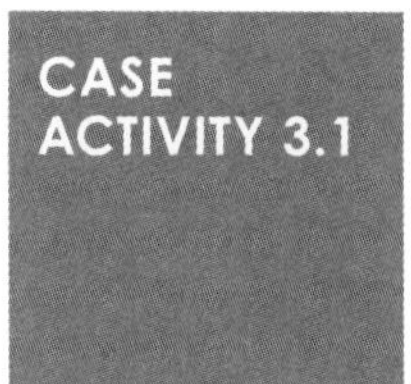

Self-compassion

Nina has had a difficult day on placement. She made some minor mistakes and has spent the last couple of hours berating herself. Read through the following examples and write down examples of how Nina might practise self-compassion and how self-kindness could be expressed. We have given you one example to help with your thinking.

- 'I am so stupid' becomes 'This is hard for me right now'.
- 'I can't believe I did that' becomes...
- 'Everyone is so much smarter than me' becomes...
- 'I am the worst midwife ever' becomes...
- 'I hate myself. I am a total fake' becomes...

Caring for yourself should become normal practice for you, a part of your daily routine. This will help to limit the impact of the stresses and challenges you face within the healthcare environment. Your self-care routine should involve regular activities and practices to reduce and manage your stress while maintaining and enhancing your health and well-being. By practising consistent self-care, you will be better equipped to identify and manage challenges, be aware of your own vulnerabilities, reduce the chance of burnout or compassion fatigue and maintain an appropriate balance between your personal and professional life. It is important to remember that self-care is not just about managing professional stress but also about promoting well-being in all areas of your life.

What self-care means to each of us and how we employ self-care practices will vary. A good way to commence your own self-care is to undertake a stress and well-being self-assessment prior to developing a self-care plan. See the weblinks at the end of this chapter for some guidance on how to do this.

Conclusion

This chapter has described how communication skills are a core component that directly affects the level of quality and safety in patient care delivery. Healthcare roles are demanding and healthcare professionals can be under extraordinary workload pressure as they communicate with a diverse amount of people in ever-changing contexts. It will be the healthcare professional's ability to maintain self-awareness, develop emotional intelligence and build resilience through practising mindfully and reflectively that will enhance their ability to be an effective communicator, one who demonstrates empathy and thinks like a professional.

SUMMARY POINTS

- Self-awareness is seen as a fundamental attribute for the healthcare professional as the level of effectiveness in communication skills directly impacts on patient safety.
- Demonstrating empathy for another provides the person receiving care to feel valued and cared for, and this will directly relate to their healthcare experience as one of being quality care with a positive experience.
- Therapeutic relationships are more effective when the healthcare professional has a high emotional intelligence, as they will understand why those in their care behave in a particular way, and not rush to judgment or react adversely to patient behaviours.
- There is a strong connection between self-awareness, mindfulness, empathy and emotional intelligence, all attributes that are favourable in the healthcare professional.
- The healthcare professional can provide comfort and aid the healing process through developing and blending their professional and therapeutic presence experience.
- Self-care enables the healthcare professional to care for themselves and maintain their caring practice by connecting emotionally, spiritually and psychologically to their experiences.

Group activity

Professional behaviours

In your study groups or via your subject discussion site, compile a list of behaviours that you consider important for the health professional to demonstrate. Discuss what values and beliefs drive these behaviours. Explore strategies within the group that are, or could be, used to enhance your professional presence.

WEBLINKS

Self-awareness

Communication Theory:
www.communicationtheory.org/the-johari-window-model

Very Well Mind:
www.verywellmind.com/what-is-self-awareness-2795023

Emotional intelligence

Psychology Today:
www.psychologytoday.com/au/basics/emotional-intelligence

The Emotional Intelligence Institute:
www.theeiinstitute.com

Mindfulness

Mindful.org:
www.mindful.org/meditation/mindfulness-getting-started

Smiling Mind:
www.smilingmind.com.au

Self-care

Black Dog Institute:
www.blackdoginstitute.org.au/docs/default-source/default-document-library/my-self-care-plan_black-dog-institute_2018.pdf?sfvrsn=0

Your Ultimate Self-Care Assessment (with resources!):
www.psychologytoday.com/au/blog/living-the-questions/201504/your-ultimate-self-care-assessment-resources

REFERENCES

Archee, R., Gurney, M. & Mohan, T. (2013). *Communicating as Professionals* (3rd edn). South Melbourne: Cengage.

Australian Medical Association. (2016). *AMA Code of Ethics*. Retrieved from https://ama.com.au/sites/default/files/documents/AMA%20Code%20of%20Ethics%202004.%20Editorially%20Revised%202006.%20Revised%202016.pdf.

Broyard, A. (1992). *Intoxicated By My Illness: And Other Writings on Life and Death*. New York: Ballantine.

Covey, S.R. (2013). *The 7 Habits of Highly Effective People: Powerful Lessons in Personal Change*. London, England: Simon & Schuster.

Cruess, R., Cruess, S., Boudreau, J., Snell, L. & Steinert, Y. (2016). Amending Miller's pyramid to include professional identity formation. *Academic Medicine*, 91(2), 180–5. doi:10.1097/ACM.0000000000000913.

Goleman, D. (1995). *Emotional Intelligence: Why It Can Matter More Than IQ*. New York, NY: Bantam Books.

International Collaborative for Communication in Healthcare. (2011). *International Charter for Human Values in Healthcare*. Retrieved from http://charterforhealthcarevalues.org/?page_id=1579.

International Council of Nurses. (2012). *The ICN Code of Ethics for Nurses*. Retrieved from www.icn.ch/sites/default/files/inline-files/2012_ICN_Codeofethicsfornurses_%20eng.pdf.

Jeffrey, D. (2016). Empathy, sympathy and compassion in healthcare: Is there a problem? Is there a difference? Does it matter? *Journal of the Royal Society of Medicine*, 109(12), 446–52.

Langer, E.J. (1989). *Mindfulness*. Reading, MA: Addison-Wesley.

Levett-Jones, T. (2018). Communicating. In *Kozier and Erb's Fundamentals of Nursing: Concepts, Process and Practice* (4th edn). Melbourne: Pearson.

Lown, B.A., Dunne, H., Muncer, S. & Chadwick, R. (2017). How important is compassionate healthcare to you? A comparison of the perceptions of people in the United States and Ireland. *Journal of Research in Nursing*, 22(1), 60–9.

Luft, J. & Ingham, H. (1955). The Johari window: A graphic model of awareness in interpersonal relations. *Proceedings of the Western Training Laboratory in Group Development, UCLA*. Retrieved from https://en.wikipedia.org/wiki/Johari_window.

McCormack, B. & McCance, T. (2017). *Person-centred Practice in Nursing and Health Care: Theory and Practice* (2nd edn). Sussex: Wiley-Blackwell.

Mosca, C.K. (2019). The relationship between emotional intelligence and clinical teaching effectiveness. *Teaching and Learning in Nursing*, 14(2), 97–102.

Nursing and Midwifery Board of Australia. (2018). *Registered Nurse Standards for Practice*. Retrieved from www.nursingmidwiferyboard.gov.au/Codes-Guidelines-Statements/Professional-standards/registered-nurse-standards-for-practice.aspx.

Rousseau, P. (2008). Empathy. *American Journal of Hospice and Palliative Care Medicine*, 25(4), 261–2.

Salovey, P. & Mayer, J. (1990). Emotional intelligence. *Imagination, Cognition and Personality*, 9(5), 185–211.

Stein-Parbury, J. (2017). *Patient and Person: Interpersonal Skills in Nursing* (6th edn). Chatswood: Elsevier.

World Health Organization. (2011). *WHO Patient Safety Curriculum Guide: Multi-Professional Edition*. Geneva: WHO.

CHAPTER 4

REFLECTION AND CLINICAL SUPERVISION

MICHELLE FRANCIS AND AMY SALMON

LEARNING OBJECTIVES

After reading this chapter and completing the activities, you will be able to:

- discuss concepts of professional self-awareness, reflection and supervision
- critically analyse the importance of reflective and supervisory practice
- examine the role of feedback in professional practice
- apply models of reflection and supervision to your clinical situation.

KEY TERMS

Feedback	Resilience
Reflection	Self-efficacy
Reflective practice	Supervision

Introduction

Reflection is about improving practice and drawing links between theory and action. It is an increasingly important exercise for health professionals as many registering authorities in the health professions have reflective practice as a mandatory requirement in their standards of practice (Kolyva 2015). The self-awareness aspect of reflection is important for learning and development and realising that personal beliefs, thoughts and attitudes can influence our work. While much of healthcare work involves building a trusting relationship with others, we need to be able to discern our personal needs from our professional responsibilities. Reflection on our actions will help us to achieve this outcome (Snyder 2014).

This chapter describes reflection and reflective practice and articulates their importance. It explores models and theories of reflective practice, the role of supervision and the advantages and disadvantages of reflective practice in contemporary healthcare. Alongside these concepts, the chapter explores the notion of resilience and the place of self-awareness and self-care in professional life.

Professional self-awareness

In the previous chapter we learnt about the importance of self in the context of communication theories. In this chapter, we consider the place of self-awareness in learning, development and improving the professional self. Self-awareness is essential for professional growth and development. It allows us to monitor our own biases and how these impact on our practice, while also helps us be aware of how we may be perceived by those with whom we are developing therapeutic relationships.

Skills in practice

Professional self-awareness

John is an occupational therapist working in the disability sector. Someone in John's family is affected by mental illness and John spent many years caring for this family member before returning to the workforce. During his time caring for his family member John felt unsupported by the mental health system and developed a view that it was ineffective. As a new practitioner, John comes into professional contact with people experiencing mental illness. John feels pulled towards these clients and feels that he is able to provide them with a higher level of care than his co-workers because of his personal experience.

What's happening here?

John is aware of his biases towards the mental health system more widely. Although he has had a poor experience in his personal life, he is able to realise the benefits of his personal experience and use this in advocacy when explaining his client's needs to workers within the mental health system. If John did not have self-awareness, John may be tempted to become over-involved with his client and believe he could do a better job than the trained mental health professionals.

Reflect and apply

Can you think of a time when you or someone close to you came into contact with the health and/or human services system? How did you feel the system supported you or your loved one? Did you have any feedback that you were not able to provide?

How did this experience shape your perception of the health and/or human services system? How might these perceptions impact on your work with someone experiencing similar needs to your own?

As can be seen from the case activity, being self-aware is important for health professionals as it allows them to ensure their own experiences and perceptions are not impacting negatively on the care they provide to others. One way to build self-awareness is through reflection.

Reflection

Reflection is a process of reviewing and adapting our behaviours, thoughts and ways of working to improve our clinical skills and the care provided to others. As healthcare professionals, we reflect constantly in our day-to-day lives and through this we learn and change our behaviours. For example, one of the authors of this chapter purchased a secondhand car and did not service this car for the first three years. After three years the car engine failed, and the car needed to be repaired and subsequently replaced at a significant cost. On reflection, the author was able to identify several warning signs that the car required a service and that doing so would have avoided catastrophic engine failure and significant cost. This author learnt from this experience and is now careful to service their car regularly.

Reflection
A series of practices that allow a person to look back on events and analyse what happened and what they might do differently next time.

Reflection is a conscious process, and it is only through practice that we become effective in our ability to reflect. Reflection does not happen accidentally; it is a learnt process. Children rely on their parents to learn from their mistakes and adapt their behaviour—for example, to test the bath water to avoid burns, and to share toys so they will have friends to play with. Parents undertake a basic reflective process with children, without which children may maintain a non-functional behaviour with negative impacts.

There are a number of formal models of reflection used in professional practice, and these are discussed below.

Reflective practice
A process of analysing one's experiences to improve the way a person works. It is a continuous professional development activity and assists people to become proactive professionals.

Reflective practice

Terry Borton (1970) was an early thinker on **reflective practice** and suggested practitioners ask themselves: 'What?', 'So what?' and 'Now what?' Through asking these questions, practitioners describe what has occurred (*what*), consider why that is important (*so what*) and how they can improve (*now what*). This model started in the field of education and was later adopted by health professionals who continue to use it as the most basic form of reflective practice.

Kolb and Fry (1975) highlighted the concept of experiential learning and translated information into action. Kolb later built on this work and conceptualised the Kolb Cycle of Learning (1984). The cycle entails four steps:

1. *Doing:* The event or situation that has occurred.
2. *Observing:* Thinking back on the experience, what happened?
3. *Thinking:* Looking at the bigger picture and considering alternative perspectives, including theories and frameworks that might apply.
4. *Planning:* Considering what you have learnt by reflecting on the situation and what you would do next time the situation occurs.

Kolb considers reflective practice to be an ongoing process in which the person builds on existing knowledge and prior experiences.

FIGURE 4.1 The Kolb Cycle of Learning

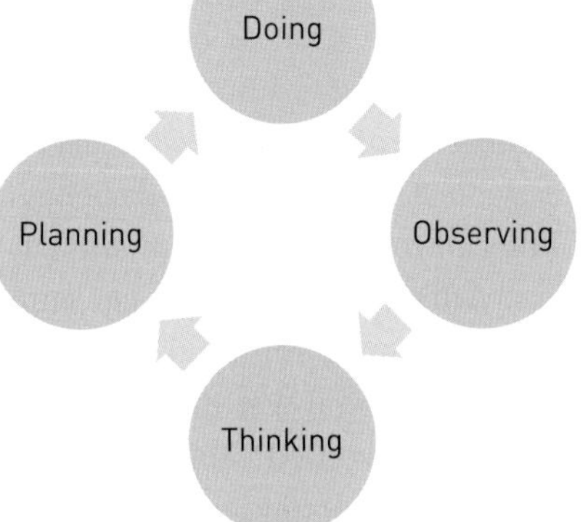

Gibbs (1998) built on the work of Kolb and advocated the use of structured debriefing to promote reflection while including the influence of feelings on actions. The stages of Gibbs' (1998) structured debrief are:

1. description
2. feelings
3. evaluation
4. analysis
5. conclusions
6. personal action plan.

Reflect and apply

Think about a situation that has not ended the way you would have liked it to. This may be in your personal or professional life—for example, an argument or a poor clinical outcome. Use Gibbs' (1998) stages to work through a structured debrief.

- *Description:* What happened? It is important here to only focus on the description of the event, and to exclude any feelings and judgments. When and where did it happen? Why were you there? Who else was there? What happened? What did you do? What did other people do? What was the result?
- *Feelings:* What were your feelings and reactions? What did you feel before, during and after the situation? What do you think other people felt? What do you feel about the situation now?

- *Evaluation:* What went well in the situation? What did not go well? What did you and others do that contributed to the situation, both positively and negatively?
- *Analysis:* What was good about the situation? What was bad about the situation? You can make value judgments here. What sense can you make of the situation? What was really going on? Were other people's experiences similar or different to your own, and in what ways?
- *Conclusion:* How could it have been a more positive experience for people involved? What can be concluded from this situation about your own way of working? If you were faced with the same situation again, what would you do differently? What would you do the same? What skills do you need to develop so you can handle the situation in the future?
- *Action:* What are you going to do differently? What steps are you going to take based on what you have learnt from this reflection?

CASE ACTIVITY 4.1

Reflective practice

Phyllis is an older registered nurse (RN) working alongside Petra, a newly graduated RN. They are working in the dementia unit of a major teaching hospital. Phyllis notices that towards the end of each shift Petra takes her well-worn exercise book into the tearoom where she scribbles down lots of words. Phyllis thinks Petra is wasting time writing in this book and one day asks, 'What are you writing every day in that book of yours?' Petra responds: 'It's my journal, Phyllis. I write in it every day.' The conversation develops and Phyllis learns that Petra uses her journal to write about the significant events of each shift so she can learn from them. Phyllis ends the conversation by saying, 'Well in my day, we didn't do any of that stuff and I've turned out okay'.

If you were in Petra's situation, what might you say next?

Being able to reflect is essential for health professionals as they grow and develop into competent practitioners. The skills you have learnt in this section will help you to reflect on your practice. Supervision also provides an important place to reflect on professional practice in a supported way.

Supervision

Supervision has a long history in the fields of allied health; to engage in supervision completely, we must be willing to reflect and learn. According to Davys and Beddoe (2010, p. 19), supervision 'demonstrates an ongoing professional commitment to reflection, analysis and critique by professional practitioners who take individual responsibility to use supervision to renew and refresh their practice and ensure

Supervision
A process that allows a person an opportunity to discuss and resolve workplace issues and dilemmas.

that they continue to work within the mandate of their work with other people'. Supervision provides health professionals with the opportunity to be involved in a lifelong journey of growth and development that can ensure they provide the highest levels of care.

Supervision can take many forms. It may be provided by line managers or be separate to line management. It may be provided from within the organisation or by a person external to the organisation. Supervision may be undertaken in a group or one-on-one and could be provided face-to-face, via the telephone or via other electronic means. This will depend greatly on the workplace, and most people find over time that they develop a preference for one form of supervision over another.

There are a number of different approaches to supervision within the allied health professions. However, it is generally agreed that all are focused on enhancing the effectiveness of the professional in their helping role. There are no clearly agreed upon set of functions of supervision. However, according to Wonnacott (2012), most theorists agree that supervision functions include an administrative/managerial component and an educative/development function, while other models include supportive and mediation functions. The administrative/managerial function involves monitoring standards, performance and ethical functions. The educative/development function involves identifying and meeting ongoing professional development needs. The supportive function involves personal support and providing a space for people to recharge their energy and discharge emotions. Finally, the mediation function involves providing a space for people to engage with the organisation and resolve any conflict that may be occurring between themselves and the workplace. It is unlikely that one supervision session will encompass all of these functions; however, they are likely to be present at some point in the supervision relationship.

Developmental approaches to supervision were popular from the 1950s to the 1980s and were based on the premise that 'practitioners follow a predictable, staged path or development' (Davys & Beddoe 2010, p. 31). Developmental approaches tend to have a focus on taking a professional from a novice or inexperienced clinician to an expert practitioner through the utilisation of stages of supervision based on supervisee developmental needs.

More recent supervision models focus on a reflective supervision approach. These approaches encourage healthcare professionals to utilise reflective practice to achieve the learning and growth required in high-quality clinical practice.

One reflective model for supervision is that developed by Allyson Davys in 2001, since which time it has been adapted and updated. The Reflective Learning Model for Supervision sees the supervisor as a facilitator, rather than an expert, and allows the healthcare professional, as the supervisee, to define any problems and be responsible for their own learning through exploration with the supervisor. This model combines reflective practice and social learning models to promote supervision as a space for growth, development and learning. The Reflective Learning Model of Supervision describes a four-stage cycle that is used in the supervision relationship: the event, the exploration, the experimentation and the evaluation stages. These align closely with the four stages in Kolb's learning cycle discussed earlier in this chapter: doing, observing, thinking and planning.

The *event stage* of supervision is about discussion of an identified issue and the identification of goals related to this issue. The aim is for you, as the supervisee, to describe and define the issue being discussed, creating clarity for the supervision discussion. The *exploration stage* of supervision is divided into two parts—reflection and conceptualisation. During the reflection, your task is to utilise reflective practice skills to explore the issue from a range of different perspectives. Feelings, beliefs, attitudes, assumptions and intuitions are all valid during this reflective process. The supervision will then move onto a conceptualisation of the issue, when professional values, ethics, policy and theory are explored to gain an understanding of how these impact on the issue. Once you have reached a decision or conclusion about the issue, the supervision will move into the *experimentation stage* where the solution can be tested to see whether it is viable in practice, taking into account the many constraints of working within organisations and communities. The final, *evaluation stage* of the cycle involves evaluating the process of supervision and exploring whether the initially established goals have been met. If not, this should be further explored and perhaps the process repeated. If the goals have been achieved, supervision will either conclude or move on to the next identified issue (Davys & Beddoe 2010).

Another reflective model of supervision is the supervision cycle developed by Morrison in 2005; again, this is based on the Kolb Cycle of Learning. This model involves you, as the supervisee, working with your supervisor to understand your experience as the experience of the service user. The supervision cycle involves considering the experience, reflecting on the experience and analysing the experience to understand the meaning, before moving into an action planning stage. During supervision the discussion may move backward and forward between stages to ensure a comprehensive exploration of the experience. According to Wonnacott (2012), the supervision cycle developed by Morrison allows for complete exploration of the knowledge and skills that are used in the reasoning process, including formal knowledge, values, practice wisdom, emotional wisdom and reasoning skills.

Reflect and apply

Think of an interaction you have had in your professional life that has left you feeling uncomfortable. This might be in your role as a health professional or in a previous role you held. Using the supervision cycle to explore this interaction, answer the following questions as if you were discussing them with your supervisor.

The experience

- Tell me about the interaction. What was your role and who else was involved?
- What was the purpose of the interaction?
- What were the words that were said?
- Were you surprised by anything that was said?
- Did you have access to any other information about the situation?
- What was the other person's demeanour?
- What did you notice about yourself during the interaction?
- Did the interaction go how you planned?

The reflection

- What were your feelings throughout the interaction?
- Did your feelings alter during the interaction? In what way?
- Have you ever had a similar interaction before? What happened on this occasion?
- Were you reminded of anyone else during the interaction?
- Had you had previous interactions with the other person? What were they like? How was this interaction different?
- What might the other person have been feeling during the interaction?
- How did you feel after the interaction?

The analysis

- How might you explain the interaction to another professional?
- Did the interaction confirm or challenge your previously held thoughts?
- Is there any research or theories that you believe might be relevant to the interaction? In what way?
- What don't we know about the interaction? What else do we need to explore?
- What were your employer's expectations in relation to your work with this person or the interaction?
- Is there any training that would have assisted you in the interaction?

The action planning

- What outcome would you like to achieve with the person?
- What did they want to achieve?
- In light of this review, what would be your idea about what needed to happen next?
- What is a desirable outcome?
- What would you do next time?

Supervision is an essential part of professional practice and finding the right supervisor is important. Some workplaces offer professional supervision; however, if yours does not, or you are finding that the workplace-provided supervision is not beneficial, you can seek external supervision. When considering who might be a beneficial supervisor, it is important to recognise that supervision is a space in which you may feel challenged while also being supported. A good supervisor will be able to both challenge and support you at the same time.

CASE ACTIVITY 4.2

Supervision

Sarah is a newly graduated social worker. She has recently started working for a local area health network. Sarah has begun to look for a supervisor to assist her in developing her skills as a professional social worker. She begins by speaking to her social work colleagues about their own supervision and gains their recommendations. Sarah decides to meet with three separate potential supervisors to determine who might be a good fit.

Imagine you are in Sarah's shoes.

1. What questions might you ask potential supervisors?
2. How might you know who will be beneficial for your practice moving forward?

Supervision forms an essential part of professional practice. High-quality supervision will allow you to reflect on your practice in a safe and supported way. Through ongoing supervision, you will build resilience as a practitioner and provide the highest possible level of service to those you care for.

Giving and receiving feedback

An important attribute of a professional is their ability to give **feedback** and, more importantly, to receive it. In healthcare we are often asked to comment on another person's work or performance. This action is called feedback. Feedback might occur as part of formal supervision or informal professional interactions.

Feedback Constructive information in response to a specific work activity or overall performance.

Sometimes it can be difficult for the giver to give effective responses and also difficult for the receiver to listen to what they perceive as unwanted feedback. The ability to receive feedback, however, is a critical element of reflection and an important professional characteristic. We will examine how we give and how we receive feedback, starting with why we need feedback.

You may recall a situation where you were told you were doing something incorrectly, even though you have been doing it that way for years. Your immediate response might be: 'I've always done it that way!' For this reason, early feedback is most effective. Feedback is essential to bring attention to something that is incorrect. Feedback is a mechanism by which others perceive us, and it lets others know how we perceive ourselves.

Skills in practice

Giving and receiving feedback

Robin is a student in health administration, and he is asked to complete several tasks by his supervisor. The instructions are brief and Robin does not understand how to complete the tasks. Robin provides feedback to his supervisor that he does not understand the instructions.

What's happening here?

The feedback Robin provides is valuable for the supervisor, who now takes more time and care in giving instructions. She is able to provide Robin with valuable feedback as well, as she now has a better understanding of his needs and capabilities.

BOX 4.1

CHARACTERISTICS OF FEEDBACK

Matua, Seshan, Akintola and Thanka (2014) suggest effective feedback needs to be:

- prompt—given at the time of the action
- neutral—without malice or judgment of character
- objective—based on observation, not emotion or assumption
- thoughtful of the receiver—recognises the needs of the receiver rather than the giver
- specific—focused on the action
- usable—allows the receiver to develop achievable and better performance
- checked for understanding—clarification is sought that the message has been understood.

Feedback should not about being right or wrong; it is about quality progression. Feedback comes from a position of care.

CASE ACTIVITY 4.3

Giving feedback

Natasha, a good friend of yours in the same class, has just delivered an in-class presentation. You knew how nervous she was and know that she could improve her presentation by slowing down her delivery and speaking loudly and more clearly. Many people in the class feel sorry for Natasha and tell her that her presentation was great. You, however, as a good friend who cares about her, provide feedback that her content was excellent and offer some tips on slowing down and speaking louder and more clearly. Without your feedback, Natasha may never have the opportunity to improve her oral presentation skills.

1. How might you have structured your feedback to Natasha?
2. What do you think might happen to Natasha's presentation skills if she had never received that feedback?

BOX 4.2

TIPS FOR RECEIVING FEEDBACK

- Listen—be attentive to the message being delivered.
- Don't take it personally—feedback is about improving communication and performance; it is not a character attack.
- See it as an opportunity—it is a chance to understand how we are seen in the world and how we can improve.
- Clarify—tell the person your understanding of their feedback.
- Reflect—take a moment to use your reflective skills.
- Action—decide what practical steps you will take to implement the feedback.

Reflect and apply

In your next classroom situation when you are asked to give and/or receive feedback, how might you prepare yourself?

Resilience

Working in healthcare settings can be challenging. Healthcare personnel are frontline workers with people in often difficult times, when people are experiencing crisis and despair. Often outcomes are positive, but sometimes they are not. The political climate places much pressure on the healthcare system and its workers to provide high levels of care within limited resources. Innovative solutions to an overloaded healthcare system include online and telehealth services, based on the idea that many people may be able to help themselves or avoid entering the healthcare system. This has led to higher acuity in patients accessing services and higher demands on healthcare workers for their time. The competing needs of complex care, higher acuity, discharges and outcomes can lead to overload and burnout. These responses to workplace challenges are negative; however, developing resilience enables more positive responses. **Resilience** is the ability to bounce back in a difficult situation. It is essential that healthcare workers look after themselves and develop resilience in the face of adversity. Developing skills such as **self-efficacy** can help health professionals to adapt to challenges in the workplace, leading to improved confidence in dealing with changes and challenges and ultimately providing improved patient care.

Resilience
Refers to the ability to adapt or bounce back in difficult situations.

Self-efficacy
Belief in oneself to meet challenges or complete a task.

Resilience can be associated with certain personality traits; however, even people who have lower resilience or less adaptability can increase their resilience.

Davis-Laack (2014) explains that strong connections and relationships with others build resilience. Fundamental to strong relationships is good communication, using active listening skills and being responsive to others' emotions. Being connected and part of a team helps to protect people from feelings of isolation. Having purpose in one's work and focusing on the importance of what they do also helps people to maintain focus in difficult times. In their study, Maddi and Khoshaba (2005) found that resilience has three core components: commitment, control and challenge. An example of commitment is staying connected to your team and the people you are involved with rather than pulling away during hard times. Control is to keep trying to positively influence the work you are involved in rather than disengage; and challenge refers to using the opportunity to see how you can grow and develop rather than give up.

Skills in practice

Resilience

Helen and Paul are nurses working in the emergency department. They are informed that they must reduce their triage time by three minutes per patient to improve the patient flow. Paul immediately feels overwhelmed and states: 'It's just too much, I can't do it'. Helen says, 'Wow that's a challenge. I'm not sure how we are going to do it, but we got it done last time, so let's find out if there's more information on how to cut back the time'. These are two different responses. Paul has automatically gone to a place of hopelessness and negativity. Helen has remembered that she and the team have worked through challenges before and it's been okay.

What's happening here?

Helen's resilience is a result of the hard work she has been doing with her supervisor during her supervision sessions. Each fortnight Helen and her supervisor identify a couple of small skills that Helen can practise for the following fortnight, when they meet again, and reflect on the process, skill development, what went well and areas for improvement. Helen and her supervisor have set achievable tasks. By practising and reviewing these skills and engaging in reflection, Helen is developing her self-efficacy, her belief that she can meet future challenges. She is also increasing her resilience in the workplace; she is bouncing back from challenges by being able to reflect in a neutral way.

Conclusion

Healthcare professional practice is both challenging and rewarding. Reflection and supervision are important processes for healthcare professionals. These processes help professionals to engage in continuous lifelong learning and development, and they improve practice and ultimately the patient experience. Healthcare professionals are often at the forefront of complex and demanding situations. In this environment, self-efficacy and reflection are vital skills and practices that help build resilience and promote well-being.

SUMMARY POINTS

- Professional self-awareness is essential for growth and development as a healthcare professional.
- Reflection and reflective practice are key skills to improve practice and develop resilience.
- Supervision is an important workplace process and people must be willing to learn and reflect to get the most out of the process.
- The ability to give and receive feedback is an important element of both reflection and supervision.
- Healthcare workers often face stressful situations. Self-efficacy and resilience are vital skills and practices that promote well-being, health and wellness in healthcare workers.

CRITICAL THINKING QUESTIONS

1. Do you agree that reflective practice is an essential skill for healthcare professionals? Why, or why not?
2. What do you consider are the most important aspects of professional supervision?
3. What does the concept of resilience mean to you? What do you believe are the characteristics of a resilient professional?

Group activity

Reflection and supervision

In your study groups or via your subject discussion site, review the features of the Johari window discussed in the previous chapter. Discuss how the practices presented in this chapter (professional self-awareness, reflection, supervision, giving and receiving feedback) assist professionals to better understand themselves and their relationships in the context of that framework.

WEBLINKS

Workplace wellbeing

At-Ease Professionals:
https://at-ease.dva.gov.au/professionals/professional-development/online-resources

Black Dog Institute:
www.blackdoginstitute.org.au/clinical-resources/wellness/workplace-wellbeing

Clinical supervision

Australian Clinical Supervision Association:
http://clinicalsupervision.org.au

REFERENCES

Borton, T. (1970). *Reach, Touch and Teach*. London: Hutchinson.

Davis-Laack, P. (2014). Seven things resilient employees do differently. *Psychology Today*. Retrieved from www.psychologytoday.com/us/blog/pressure-proof/201410/seven-things-resilient-employees-do-differently.

Davys, A. & Beddoe, L. (2010). *Best Practice in Professional Supervision*. London: Jessica Kingsley Publishers.

Gibbs, G. (1998). *Learning by Doing: A Guide to Teaching and Learning Methods*. Oxford: Oxford Brooks University.

Kolb, D.A. (1984). *Experiential Learning: Experience as the Source of Learning and Development (vol. 1)*. Englewood Cliffs, NJ: Prentice-Hall.

Kolb, D.A. & Fry, R.E. (1975). *Toward an Applied Theory of Experiential Learning*. Cambridge, MA: MIT Alfred P. Sloan School of Management.

Kolyva, K. (2015). Casting a new light on reflection. *Primary Health Care*, 25(2), 13.

Maddi, S.R. & Khoshaba, D.M. (2005). *Resilience at Work: How to Succeed No Matter What Life Throws at You*. New York: AMACOM.

Matua, G.E., Seshan, V., Akintola, A.A. & Thanka, A.N. (2014). Strategies for providing effective feedback during preceptorship: Perspectives from an Omani hospital. *Journal of Nursing Education and Practice*, 4(10), 24–31.

Morrison, T. (2005). *Staff Supervision in Social Care*. Brighton: Pavilion.

Snyder, M. (2014). Emancipatory knowing: Empowering nursing students toward reflection and action. *Journal of Nursing Education*, 53(2), 65–9. doi:10.3928/01484834-20140107-01.

Wonnacott, J. (2012). *Mastering Social Work Supervision*. London: Jessica Kingsley Publishers.

PART 2

PROFESSIONAL AND THERAPEUTIC COMMUNICATION IN CONTEXT

OXFORD UNIVERSITY PRESS

CHAPTER 5

INTERPROFESSIONAL COMMUNICATION

BERYL BUCKBY AND SUSAN GORDON

LEARNING OBJECTIVES

After reading this chapter and completing the activities, you will be able to:

- describe interprofessional communication and its role in the healthcare environment
- identify and critique factors that contribute to effective and ineffective interprofessional communication
- analyse your own beliefs and knowledge in the context of effective interprofessional communication
- devise and implement strategies to improve interprofessional communication.

KEY TERMS

Interprofessional communication
Interprofessional relationships
Liminal space
Professional identity
Respectful communication

What is interprofessional communication?

Interprofessional communication occurs when students or practitioners from different professions communicate with each other in an authentic, collaborative, responsive and responsible manner (Canadian Interprofessional Health

Interprofessional communication
When students or practitioners from different professions are self-aware and communicate effectively with each other in a collaborative, responsive and responsible manner.

Collaborative 2010). Effective interprofessional communication is essential for practice in contemporary healthcare (Frank & Rowett 2018). Respectful interprofessional communication incorporates full disclosure and transparency in all interactions with others, including patients, clients and families, and other members of the healthcare team. Although even clearly defined communication skills, when applied in the education and practice contexts, are affected by individual characteristics that occur automatically and may contribute to miscommunication and tensions. This chapter aims to raise healthcare professionals' awareness of their own communication style when engaging with others in the care team in the contexts in which they work and practice.

Why is interprofessional communication important?

Interprofessional relationships
The interactions between people from different professional groups that incorporate the principles of respectful communication.

Respectful communication
Incorporates full disclosure and transparency in all interactions with others, including patients/clients, families and other members of the healthcare team.

Interprofessional relationships build trust, respect and understanding, and ensure that all knowledge about the patient is shared with others, including patients, families and members of the healthcare team: this leads to better person-centred health outcomes. Regardless of context, respect for the knowledge and skills of people from different professional groups is the cornerstone on which full disclosure and transparency—**respectful communication**—develops, flourishes and ensures that the quality of care and safety of patients remains the key concern in the health environment (Kohn, Corrigan & Donaldson 2000; Watson, Heatley, Gallois & Kruske 2016). Team interdependence developed with such goals in mind is more likely to create a team climate of psychological safety (O'Leary 2016). However, under stressful conditions such as staff shortages, corrosion of trust can lead to rapid staff turnover affecting patient care (Welander, Astvik & Isaksson 2017). Poor communication can lead to inefficiencies in resource use, negative patient and staff experience and, most significantly, risks to patient safety (Vermeir et al. 2015).

What are the elements of effective interprofessional communication?

People unfamiliar with working in an interprofessional environment will always need a period of adjustment before they establish a sense of place in the team. The elements that support adjustment, and are necessary for effective interprofessional communication, include:

- established teamwork communication principles embedded in the group
- effective communication to ensure common understanding of care decisions

- trusting, respectful relationships with patients, families and other healthcare team members
- effective use of information and communication technology to improve interprofessional patient, client or community-centred care (Canadian Interprofessional Health Collaborative 2010)
- organising and communicating information to patients' families and healthcare team members in a form that is understandable, avoiding discipline-specific terminology when possible
- listening actively and encouraging ideas and opinions of other team members, including patients, families and healthcare team members (Interprofessional Education Collaborative Expert Panel 2011)
- recognising how one's uniqueness—including experience level, expertise, culture, power and hierarchy within the healthcare team—contributes to effective communication, conflict resolution and positive interprofessional working relationships (Interprofessional Education Collaborative Expert Panel 2011).

It is clear from these elements that the client and their family are considered part of the healthcare team. Throughout this chapter, however, the emphasis on the interprofessional healthcare team (IPHCT) will refer to all healthcare professionals involved in delivering person-centred healthcare, as communication with patients and their family or caregiver is discussed in detail in other chapters.

Reflect and apply

Before reading further in this chapter, take a minute to reflect on your chosen career and other disciplines within the interprofessional team. What influenced you to pursue your chosen profession? Why didn't you choose to pursue another career path in healthcare? What do you know about other healthcare professions that may have influenced your decision?

What have you noticed about your own style of communication when working with others: your strengths; your weaknesses, how others might perceive you?

Poor interprofessional communication

CASE ACTIVITY 5.1

Iris is an active, 72-year-old female who drives a car and lives alone in a high-set house. She has an unmarried son who is a fly-in, fly-out miner. She was diagnosed with Parkinson's disease three years ago. While her condition has been well controlled with medication, she sometimes forgets to take the medication.

Last week as Iris was leaving the house to go to lawn bowls she fell down the stairs. She remembers nothing of the incident—only that she woke up to find her neighbour was shaking her. An ambulance was called. Paramedics believed Iris fractured her femur (hip) and provided pain relief. She was admitted to the local general hospital. The attending paramedics were very efficient and told the accident and emergency receiving nurse, 'This is Iris, a sweet old lady who forgot her meds. She's had a bit of a fall, haven't you love'. The exchange occurred without making eye contact with Iris.

During healthcare episodes, transition of patients—for example, at the initial point of intervention, hospital admission, when moved to or between wards, when a change in staff occurs between shifts and at discharge—there is a high risk for poor interprofessional communication that decreases the quality of patient care.

1. Standing in the shoes of Iris momentarily, reflect on how you would feel at the initial exchange and why.
2. Document three possible ways that a breakdown in interprofessional communication could happen during Iris's admission and initial assessment in the emergency department. What might be the implications for Iris's care if this does occur?

The follow-up care that Iris received after being admitted to hospital is considered in Case activity 5.2.

CASE ACTIVITY 5.2

Effective use of information

Iris has surgery and is transferred to the ward. During the surgery, theatre staff noted greater bleeding than would normally be expected.

During the first two post-operative days, Iris is slightly confused. She is not sure what happened or why she fell, and is asking for her son, who is expected to arrive home that afternoon. The medical staff are very busy as the ward is nearly full and is 'on-take' for emergencies. The nursing staff are concerned that Iris continues to be confused. The physiotherapist stood Iris beside her bed and noticed that her balance is poor and she is having trouble judging distances even with her glasses on. Iris still requires significant pain medication and continues to use more than four prescribed medications that she was taking before her hospital admission.

1. What might be the outcome of care if other healthcare staff are not made aware that Iris continues to be confused?
2. How can you ensure that you effectively communicate your concerns in notes and discussion? Can you, for example, avoid relying on assumptions and instead rely on evidence and clear expression of your concerns?
3. What might be the outcome if the information about her inability to judge distance is not shared?

Healthcare professionals adopt a scientist–practitioner model of practice and hypothesis-testing approach to assessment. In the case activity, Iris's assessment is founded on a thorough interview that is friendly in approach to develop a strong therapeutic alliance so that Iris feels heard and valued rather than marginalised in her care (Scott, Milioto, Trost & Sullivan 2016). Iris's consent for gathering additional information as well as a thorough exploration of the circumstances of her fall and hospitalisation, as well her lived-experience of Parkinson's disease, are essential to cementing the working alliance. The interview, observations and collateral data then form the basis of a comprehensive assessment such as that recommended by the National Institute of Neurological Disorders and Stroke (Toner et al. 2012; Watson et al. 2013).

Holistic assessment goes beyond a baseline assessment and requires collaboration with other disciplines to capture an individual's lived experience (Koerts et al. 2012; Stuck et al. 2015). It is critically important to discuss all assessment findings with the patient, in plain language, to check understanding, and provide an opportunity for them to openly discuss any concerns and ask questions. The assessment outcomes, when shared and discussed within the team, promote common understanding of the patient's current cognitive, physical, emotional condition and capabilities, risk-mitigation needs and treatment planning.

Collaborative communication

CASE ACTIVITY 5.3

Ten days post-op Iris's confusion has settled, and she is looking forward to going home. A ward team meeting is conducted where each member of the health team reports the findings of their assessments, and a plan is made for Iris to go home based on shared information. Evidence shows that age accelerates Parkinson's disease progression (Hindle 2010), and that cognitive impairment and neuropsychiatric symptoms affect a substantial number of people and such non-motor changes can occur at all stages of the disease (Fields 2017; Kang et al. 2016). These considerations in planning are necessary for risk reduction for Iris to remain safely at home.

The physiotherapist considers that Iris is physically able to cope with stairs and general walking but needs equipment at home to safely shower and use the toilet. Iris has an outpatient appointment scheduled in two weeks' time for progression of balance exercises and gait re-education. An occupational therapist (OT) is booked to visit Iris's home three days before discharge to organise any aides such as a toilet and shower chair that might be required. The OT will also assess Iris's ability to cook her own meals. The pharmacist has reviewed all medications and confirmed they are safe. Nursing staff report that Iris has been independent with hospital equipment when showering and using the toilet for the last three days. The psychologist provides Iris's assessment data to the group for discussion. Iris's age and disease progression, combined with evidence of prospective and recognition memory deficits prior to her hospitalisation, as well as perceptual disturbance and poor balance, suggest that independent living without supports in place leave her vulnerable to repeated hospitalisations. The high likelihood of age-related decline in haptic perception (Konczak et al. 2012; Li, Chu & Pickett 2017) needs further investigation by the OT and social worker, plus a review of Iris's home environment in the light of what the care team now knows. It is important for the team to be inclusive and develop the therapeutic alliance with Iris to discuss her inevitable changes at home as enablers, to empower her ongoing independence.

The doctor has the final decision regarding discharge for Iris, so it is important to have comprehensive information from the whole team. Risk identification and mitigation will ensure that Iris has a smooth transition home and optimal outcomes following her surgery.

1. Iris's son needs to be part of the communication loop and healthcare team in this activity. Who will have the key responsibility for maintaining communication between the team members?
2. Reflect on how you will engage Iris in planning and risk management at home. How can you be sure that Iris has retained what you discussed with her?

For true professional collaboration to be achieved, Nugus et al. (2019) advocate for deliberative democracy among health professionals in different occupational roles. Historically, democracy in interprofessional communication has been transactional and based on the quantity of power of each health professional. Deliberative democracy is transformational and uses broad-based discussion and negotiation for rational deliberation and shared decision making (Nugus et al. 2019). This approach potentially reduces barriers of organisational structuralism and power relationships among health-related professions. At the same time, it promotes understanding of the perspectives of each health professional in the care of the patient and enables effective communication to provide the best possible outcomes. Person-centred care requires this of all practitioners through cross-disciplinary trusting relationships that involve 'power sharing', willingness to respect differences in knowledge and practice, and learning micro-communication, as defined by the Interprofessional Education Collaborative Expert Panel (2016).

Conflict and tensions can occur in interprofessional practice. The sources and consequences are dependent on individual, interpersonal and organisational factors (Kim et al. 2017). Although this conflict can be destructive, it can be constructive if it is directed towards accomplishing group goals and establishing group norms, as outlined in the focus box 'Aims of interprofessional group norms'.

BOX 5.1

AIMS OF INTERPROFESSIONAL GROUP NORMS

- Encourage respect.
- Encourage sensitivity towards others.
- Emphasise the appreciation of differences.
- Encourage assertive (not aggressive) communication.
- Encourage actively listening to each other.
- Encourage members to agree to disagree.
- Emphasise staying on task and completing tasks.
- Support a clear, accepted decision-making process.
- Reinforce member acceptance of group decisions.

Source: Interprofessional Education Consortium 2001. Used with permission.

Strengthening interprofessional practice through communication skills

Effective communication in interprofessional contexts requires skills that transcend professional training. Established habits such as using profession-specific acronyms inhibit translation of meaning with potential consequences within the team and for the patient or client.

Originally described in the early 1970s, communication accommodation theory (CAT) is a theory of intergroup and interpersonal communication premised on the assumption that communication mediates and maintains relationships (Gallois, Ogay & Giles 2005). Since its first description, many additions have been made to the theory (see Figure 5.1). The theory describes people coming from two different backgrounds or groups (A and B) and the factors that may influence the way they communicate. It is suggested that speakers come to interactions and conversations with a point of view that is informed by professional 'cultural' factors such as relevant interpersonal and intergroup histories—in interprofessional settings, this means profession-specific training, as well as the prevailing socio-historical context (Giles & Gasiorek 2014). Similarly, adapting interaction to develop a therapeutic alliance in cross-cultural interactions requires special consideration in verbal and non-verbal communication as the quality of the relationship can significantly affect outcomes for patients and potentially for team cohesiveness (Hays 2016).

FIGURE 5.1 The communication accommodation theory model

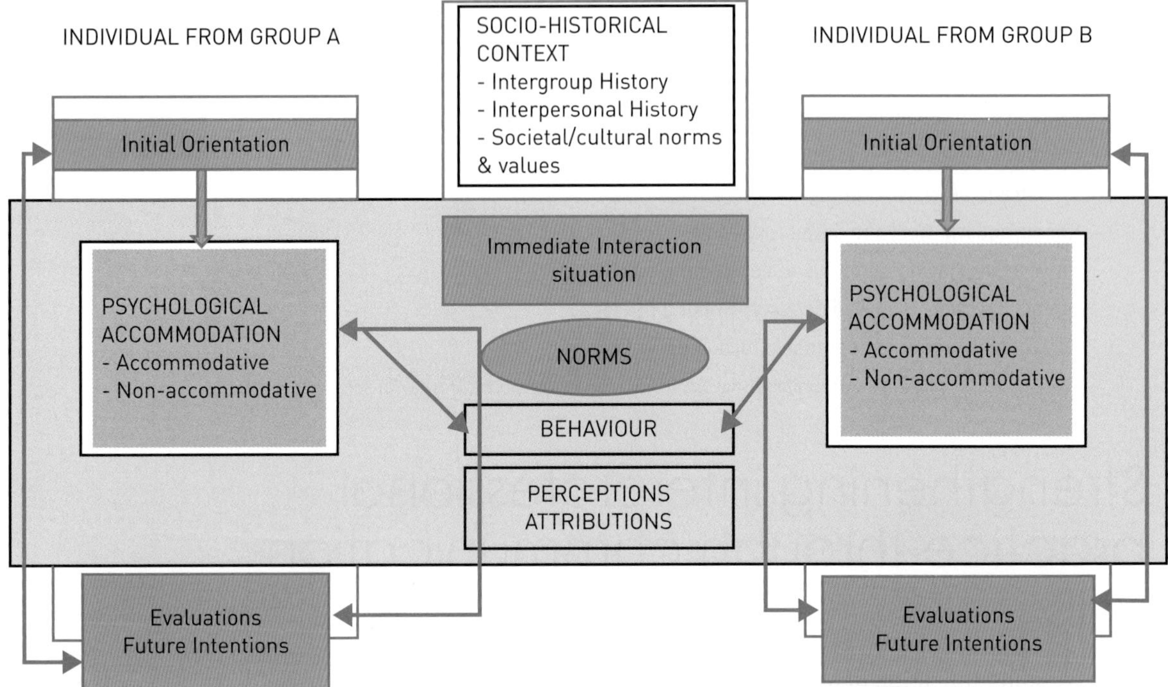

Source: Adapted from Giles & Gasiorek 2014.

During interaction with other speakers in the group, people adjust their behaviour according to their evaluation of other speakers' communicative characteristics in context specific ways (e.g. professional group meetings, debriefings, and individual face-to-face interviews and discussions). Group members bring to the group their desire to establish and maintain a positive personal and social/professional identity and an evaluative mindset and make attributions about the encounter as well as of other speakers on the basis of their *perceptions* of the behaviour of other group members. Such personal attributions and evaluations affect the quality and nature of the conversation and inform the intention to engage now and in future interactions with the other health professional or group.

Sensitive multidisciplinary group members will also choose to adapt the way they present information to make it more comprehensible or interpretable according to their perception of other members' capacities to understand. Such conscious awareness can become automatic through practice (Lineweaver, Hutman, Ketcham & Bohannon 2011). A wisely self-aware practitioner might choose to adjust their manner of speaking to reaffirm or subvert power or status differentials according to the context of interaction (e.g. working with a patient's family or when assuming a leadership role). Intergroup communication is at the heart of interprofessional practice—it is embedded in the word and the reality of practice and provides a higher level of understanding beyond the interpersonal and the societal, relying on the interconnections and mutual influences between groups and individuals

(Gallois, Watson & Giles 2018). In professional and therapeutic communication, it requires willingness to adapt and learn at the personal practitioner level.

When adjustments are made by any speaker to ensure that they use appropriate common language that maximises audience understanding they are using *accommodative communication*, which is generally experienced as helpful, positive and respectful of the diversity of people present (i.e. the speaker and listener converge, which is an adaptive strategy to adjust one's speech—speech rate, pauses, utterance length and non-verbal communication; smiling, eye gaze) to match the interactant/s (Giles & Gasiorek 2014). When a speaker chooses not to, or cannot, make such adjustments, the quality of communication affects the quality of information transmission, and potentially intergroup relationships.

Non-accommodative communication undermines the intention of therapeutic and professional communication and potentially risks patients, families and colleagues feeling alienated, or at worst not understanding the content at all, which has implications for ongoing care. If deliberate, this style of communication is more than just the form of words—*divergence* is a choice to create distance between the speaker and the listener, perhaps to create a power differential, a struggle for control or social/professional identity in intergroup contexts (Farzadnia & Giles 2015; Giles, Reid & Harwood 2010). Or perhaps the person simply lacks the self-awareness to convert professional terminologies to plain language and ensure the intended message is received by the listener. Other logical non-accommodative ways of subverting effective communication include *maintenance*, *over-accommodation* and *under-accommodation*. Maintenance refers to the speaker's usual style of communication without consideration of the characteristics of the patient and/or their family members, colleagues from other professions or non-health professionals within the system. In some cases, maintenance could be driven by social or professional identity concerns in interprofessional and cross-cultural contexts (Aritz & Walker 2010; McEvoy et al. 2017; Pretorius 2018).

Over-accommodation is a patronising form of communicating that is inconsistent with person-centred care and is often associated with the long-term care of older people (hence, it is sometimes termed 'elderspeak'). For frail aged persons, of which approximately 70 per cent are likely to have some cognitive impairment (Bjork et al. 2016), this form of dialogue offers little opportunity for them to engage in conversation. The most-used interpersonal and social skills, also known as soft-skills, by all practitioners in aged care are in communication with residents and their families (Storlie 2015).

While Ruben (2016) calls for a nuanced understanding of communication dynamics with patients, it is equally needed in the interprofessional context, as Giles and Gasiorek (2014) suggest. How a health practitioner understands, translates and applies what is heard into practice will be influenced by their current knowledge and attitudes, as well as their assumptions, predispositions, historical experience and capabilities. Developing interpersonal micro-skills and self-awareness of such influences will ultimately enhance professional communication, and influence client outcomes through more effective communication.

Stereotyping as a shortcut to knowing

What every health practitioner brings to a conversation in practice is informed by their life, personal learning and experience. Although communication does not represent a simplistic linear relationship of 'message sent = message received', the context of professional communication also matters. Under stressful circumstances, each party to a communication brings to it their personal history and physiological responses as well as cognitive, emotional and non-verbal behaviours that might be activated at any time in the exchange. Familiarity induced by prior exposure decreases analytic cognitive processing and increases reliance on past experiences and intuition, including stereotyping; however, this occurs only when a stereotype provides information that fits the context and is reinforced by frequency of exposure to similar situations as occurs in practice (Garcia-Marques, Mackie, Maitner & Claypool 2016). When the situation differs from prior experience, then a slower, more thoughtful analytical thinking process is induced. In practice, the automaticity of routine tasks can subvert such cognitive processing.

In an Australian study (Braithwaite et al. 2016), the authors set out to examine the basis of multidisciplinary teamwork using an experimental design in a controlled setting quite different from the usual workplace and placed students in heterogeneous small groups. Study outcomes showed that tribalism, hierarchical and stereotype behaviours 'dissolved'. The authors concluded that workplace cultures, rather than 'fundamental sociological or psychological differences between individuals in the professions or aggregated group differences' (p. 1), were implicated. In effect, when participants in the experiment were distanced from role-specific clothing and usual workplace settings, stereotyping behaviours were not replicated. In a completely different context, Gupta, Boland and Aron (2017), in a small qualitative study, showed clearly that changing practice behaviours is difficult, as change in established practice disturbs the status quo and that 'unlearning' is difficult. They concluded: 'It's easier to introduce something new than to take out something old' (p. 4). These two examples speak to the same issue, that reversing over-learned behaviours and practices is slow and potentially stressful.

Maximising communication effectiveness

Ruben (2016) argues that when communication concepts are appropriated within healthcare discourse and practice, the complexity and nuance are often glossed over, which can affect accurate translation in the mind of the patient and also in conversion into other arenas of practice. Ruitenberg and Towle (2015), for example, found that healthcare terms provoked learning and reflection on how words commonly used in one health profession are understood quite differently among other health professions and, further, how health professionals' language might be perceived by patients and clients. Checking in with others that there is common understanding in communication helps to highlight the translational gap that is commonly filled intuitively and, in some cases, inaccurately.

In this chapter's ongoing case activity, the various healthcare professionals working with Iris are likely to observe and hear different aspects of her mental and physical state. This could be viewed as a strength of interprofessional practice, as it potentially provides Iris and her transition process with the most informed options and risk analysis for living a relatively independent life at home. The care team, it seems, must be risk-sensitive to the translational gap to ensure the it shares a common understanding. Claramita et al. (2019) designed an interprofessional education (IPE) guide to aid training in collaborative practice for patient safety, arguing that effective teamwork starting with partnership-based communications should begin early in education to establish effective habits from the start.

Observation

Observation is attending explicitly for information about a patient or client, and uses all the senses required for the context in which the observation occurs. More frequently, observation is taken to be a 'watching' experience which, according to the Oxford Dictionary, is an 'act or instance of carefully observing someone or something over a period of time'. In practice, observation free of prior learning, analysing or inference about the meaning of the observation is difficult—if not impossible—to achieve.

Even in an involuntary task such as watching, which is automatic if our eyes are open, prior learning influences what we see. MacKenzie and Westwood (2013) demonstrated the learning influence when occupational therapists made more fixed observations of shorter duration and more rapid movements between points than non-occupational therapists, although the same instructions were given to both groups. This suggests that professional skills shape *how* we observe. Experiential exercises using artworks stimuli with students have also shown that the quality of observation improves through holistic observation and contextualising information (Boudreau, Cassell & Fuks 2009; Jasni & Saks 2013). These studies show that prior learning and reflection improve observation that is notably distinct from inference. Beck, Gaunt and Chiavaroli (2017), in an Australian study, went a step further and found that after a single art-based seminar students retained their observational skills, which was evidenced by more descriptive detail in reports one year later compared with students who did not do the training. In respect of Iris, described in the case activity, her team will inevitably be influenced by prior learning. Mindfulness, as discussed in Chapter 3, can assist in acknowledging and managing the impact of preconceptions and prior learning on interprofessional communication.

Listening

Developing listening skills is a function of systemic social interactions and consistent with the ethos of interprofessional education of 'two or more professions learn about, from and with each other to enable effective collaboration and improve health outcomes' (WHO 2010, p. 7). However, the listening task occurs in cultural and subcultural contexts that affect what a practitioner will attend to (Claramita et al. 2019; Lau & Ng 2014). This could include cultural difference where one might view the specialist training of each practitioner as a 'subcultural' influence that draws attention via prior learning. In the case activity featuring Iris, her slow speech requires practitioner patience for Iris to feel her contributions are valued and respected, while breaking eye contact could trigger thoughts that (a) Iris is hearing something she finds distressing (psychologist) or (b) has hearing loss (speech pathologist). Listening is therefore a more complex task than it seems at first.

It is clear that Iris will want to feel her health concerns have been heard and understood from her point of view, and that the care team has insight into her Parkinson's experience. The IPHCT must understand the perspectives and knowledge that each member contributes to Iris's care. To be an effective listener, a practitioner should first have the intention to understand Iris and her situation, learn something of her experience and provide targeted professional expertise. Learning how to encourage, paraphrase, clarify, provide feedback and listen with empathy, openness and awareness are described in Table 5.1. The concept of active listening was introduced in Chapter 2 and is explored here in the case of Iris and interprofessional communication.

TABLE 5.1 Active listening in interprofessional communication

Description	Outcomes and commentary
Technique: Encouraging	
Minimal verbal and non-verbal prompts; smiling; simple repetition of a few key words; head nods.	Prompts all members of the IPHCT including Iris to continue talking, elaborating and feeling valued.
Technique: Paraphrasing	
Short feedback to and within the team using key words of what the patient/client said immediately prior—e.g. Iris expressed worry about going home by herself, having another fall and not being able to get up without help, and repeated the worry several times: *Iris's biggest worry is falling alone at home.*	Ensures transmission of accurate information and understanding and provides an opportunity for all team members to correct misunderstanding. Iris feels heard. The practitioner remembers more effectively. Paraphrasing prevents interference from listening barriers.

Technique: Clarifying	
While verbally tracking the patient, idiosyncratic use of words that are confusing or unclear are reason to ask a clarifying question of a team member: *You said Iris would be safe enough at home. I am wondering what 'safe enough' means.*	Clarifying ensures that each IPHCT member gets sufficient information to fully understand Iris's situation. Clarifying tells Iris and the team that the practitioner is interested in her and will work to understand her situation and concerns.
Technique: Feedback	
Active listening requires the practitioner to give an honest non-judgmental reaction to what the team has had to say: *I have some concerns about Iris's home situation and I think we need to discuss home-safety further.*	Feedback to the team and Iris helps everyone to understand the effect of her communication and provides a further opportunity for her to correct misunderstandings.
Technique: Listening with empathy	
Listening with empathy requires the practitioner to stand briefly in other team members' and Iris's shoes: *Iris now feels some anxiety and fear after the previous comment.* The practitioner sees the other team members and Iris's anxiety, and can overcome personal discomfort by reflecting on these questions: *'How hard must it be for Iris to hear this?', 'What is Iris afraid might happen now?', 'Why is this team member uncomfortable with the decisions being made?'* and *'What skill can I bring to this situation?'*	Listening with empathy promotes honesty and trustworthiness in the therapeutic and team relationship. Iris feels her fear of what might happen has been heard and understood. The practitioner develops a deeper understanding of how to manage difficult conversations with patients/clients.
Technique: Listening with openness	
Openness requires practitioner naivety, *focused attention* and taking an eyewitness stance, watching and listening for clues. Mackay, Davis and Fanning (2018) recommend becoming the 'anthropologist', by trying to know how other team members see Iris's point of view makes sense for her, and how it fits into their own particular worldview, history and social system. A practitioner's mind, busy on matters other than the team, is deaf to important information about and from Iris.	Listening with openness allows the whole message to be transmitted without deletions—i.e. there will not be any transmission gaps because the practitioner went 'offline'. Openness also prevents making premature evaluations before the information is available on which to make them.

TABLE 5.1 ***Continued***

TABLE 5.1 Continued

Description	Outcomes and commentary
Technique: Listening with awareness	
There are two aspects to consider: *Noticing non-judgmentally:* How the information from the team and Iris fits with the practitioner's known facts. *Listening and observing congruence:* Does the team members'—or Iris's—tone of voice, expressive repetitions and emphases, facial expression and posture match the words they speak—e.g. expressing delight at going home and getting back into social activities is belied by Iris's tears and breaking eye contact.	Observations of congruence promote open dialogue with the team and Iris about her care now and into the future. Observations of incongruence tell the practitioner that the story is incomplete, as is their knowledge about Iris and her situation. The practitioner then asks clarifying questions and gives some feedback to the team member or Iris about the discrepancy.
Technique: Listening for meta-messages	
Meta-messages are statements with two levels of meaning: *Basic level:* Information delivered and received as a series of words that say what is intended and mean what is said. *Secondary level:* *Communicates the speaker's emotional state and attitudes.* *(Iris) 'I am in hospital. Of course, I am JUST fine.'* *(Practitioner) 'Of course she can go home. WHO NEEDS to be able to climb stairs?'*	Observation of the team members, and Iris's tone of voice and emphasis clearly communicates anxiety and resentment. Iris has lived an independent life alone for some time and has some resentment about the direction of the conversation. The emphasis on 'JUST' by Iris and 'WHO NEEDS' by the health professional provides the opportunity to check-in with the interpretation of the comment, provide follow-up information about the direction of care and ask further questions to help manage any anxiety or resentment.
Technique: Listening for verbal modifiers	
Words that modify meaning of a sentence. *(Practitioner)* 'NATURALLY you want to go home ...' (implies 'BUT' will follow) Common modifier words: certainly, slightly, merely, still, sure, again, only, now NOW all we need to do is get you on your feet. Phrases: Of course, I'm sure, I guess (I'M SURE you did your best) Quantity: Little, lot, slightly, always Discharge might be SLIGHTLY delayed.	Practitioner reluctance to be open negatively affects the therapeutic alliance and erodes trust. The practitioner has transmitted a meta-message and communicated to Iris that it is unlikely she will be going home yet, with the emphasis on *naturally; now, I'm sure; slightly.* The way verbal modifiers work in this exchange are more likely to increase Iris's anxiety than to reassure her. A plainly expressed explanation is the most respectful and person-centred method. 'Iris, I know you want to go home and I would like to say you could, unfortunately the assessment shows that you are not ready yet as the falls risk remains too high. Patience now really is the best course. You said plainly that you do not want to be in hospital again. Staying a little longer now should reduce that risk.' (These words combined with person-focused non-verbal behaviour is *accommodative communication*.)

Sources: Ivey, Ivey & Zalaquett 2018; Mackay et al. 2018; O'Toole 2012; Warnock, Buchanan & Tod 2017; Weger, Bell, Minei & Robinson 2014.

Unfortunately, in a busy schedule, many factors can affect the perfect listening scenario. Partial listening while worrying about being late to the next event on a busy daily schedule, listening for one specific piece of information while not paying attention to anything else, or buying time to prepare yourself to deliver bad or disappointing news, are some examples. Environmental factors are also critical. Sitting beside a noisy air-conditioner, or in an open space where others can tune in, inhibit open communications and threaten privacy (Burkell et al. 2014; Morhayim 2019; Sweet & Wilson 2011; Swenne & Skytt 2014).

Some of these barriers are described in Table 5.2.

TABLE 5.2 Barriers to listening (with patients/clients and colleagues)

Barrier	Description
Red flag barriers related to ethical practice	
Comparing	Self-referenced thoughts in comparison to others—e.g. *I could do that better than X can.*
Mind reading	Anticipating what someone will say without actually listening to their response; just knowing what they will say.
Interrupting	Breaking into a patient or client's response—e.g. finishing Iris's sentences as her speech is slow and you have a busy schedule.
Monopolising	Talking too much in a patient or client discussion restricts a practitioner's ability to gather useful information from the interviewee.
Derailing	Changing the topic or introducing irrelevancies—e.g. delaying the moment you might have to disappoint Iris about going home. Using humour to disrupt the flow of discussion.
Rehearsing	Directing attention inwards to rehearse what you want or need to say; this divides the attention available for listening.
Daydreaming	Losing the thread of the discussion, or following a thought association triggered by something in the conversation (occurs more when tired or bored). Sends a clear signal to the patient that the practitioner does not value what they have to say
Advising	Impatience with the process; problem solving and offering suggestions without having all relevant information prevents the practitioner from attending.
Sparring	Arguing or defending a position—e.g. in the interprofessional team. Sparring can also occur when patients or clients are resistant to change, and the practitioner tries to convince them of a different point of view. This strategy increases resistance.
Filtering or partial listening	Being preoccupied; tuning into information the practitioner wants to know about and nothing else.
Barriers related to unmet personal needs	
Being right	Being resistant to criticism, making excuses for mistakes, being resistant to change, having difficulty working collaboratively in teams and receiving feedback. Tends to be self-focused rather than other-focused in practice and with patients/clients.

TABLE 5.2 ***Continued***

TABLE 5.2 Continued

Barrier	Description
Placating or reassuring	Conflict avoidant with colleagues and with patients or clients. Needs approval, and for colleagues and patients or clients to like them.
Identifying	Lacks boundaries with patients or clients. Clients' issues are constantly referred to the personal experience of the practitioner.
Judging	Pre-judging the personality and other attributes of colleagues and patients or clients before hearing their message/story divides attention. Psychologically inflexible.
a. Breaking confidences b. Intimidating c. Interrogating	These barriers individually and together are explicitly contrary to the ethical standards and guidelines of all professions and organisational codes of practice; there is a risk of disciplinary action for any practitioner who behaves in such a manner.
Barriers to effective multi-system care	
One-sidedness	The patient as a singular source in some 'stigmatised' conditions has recently been identified as a risk to effective communication and treatment adherence. Secondary sources—e.g. other health providers/family help to ameliorate risk.

Sources: Mackay et al. 2018; O'Toole 2012; Sublette et al. 2018.

Sharing, translating and integrating knowledge bases

Learning continues after students leave university and expand their practice experience. Interprofessional education aims to bridge the transition from the learning environment into practice. The effectiveness of interprofessional training and practice is complex and difficult (Stone 2010). Factors that are considered important to assess are set out in the following focus box.

The basic premise of interprofessional practice teams is that two or more professions learning and working together will produce better outcomes overall. However, research into the effectiveness of interprofessional teams in the workplace has been inconsistent; more importantly, knowing what effectiveness is and how it should be measured is poorly defined. Many practice studies rely on qualitative research, and weak evidence and impact, which limit their generalisability (WHO 2010; 2013), inference from self-reports of team effectiveness (Korner 2010; Mitchell, Parker & Giles 2011; Schentrup et al. 2018), evidence-based practice change (Moyers, Finch Guthrie, Swan & Sathe 2014), and ethics (Brown, Garber, Lash & Schnurman-Crook 2014; Machin et al. 2018; Wilhelm, Poirier, Otsuka & Wagner 2014). Alternatively, evidence of effective interprofessional education (IPE) abounds, although research often lacks generalisability, along with an over-reliance on self-reporting that encourages socially desirable responses (Hale & DiLollo 2016; Lapkin, Levett-Jones & Gilligan 2013; Ravet 2012). A notable difference in the IPE studies cited here was the immersive experience of two hours weekly over a semester in the

Hale and DiLollo study, which required a higher level of interaction where students demonstrated teamwork. It is very likely that the soft skills of relationship, respect and trust were an important unmeasured by-product of this immersion experience.

BOX 5.1

ASSESSMENT CRITERIA FOR INTERPROFESSIONAL EDUCATION AND INTERPROFESSIONAL PRACTICE EFFECTIVENESS

- *Personal capability domains:* Communication, collaborative working, professional relationship, reflective practice, ethics, professionalism, leadership, cultural competence.
- *Evidence-based practice:* Improved patient safety and quality, audit and evaluation, health service accreditation.

Source: Stone 2010.

There remains confusion about what terms such as *interprofessional*, *collaboration*, *practice* and *teamwork* actually mean, and it is unclear how to go about getting a common understanding that closes gaps such as how interprofessional practice improves patient outcomes (Holtman et al. 2011; Thistlethwaite, Jackson & Moran 2013). Hale and DiLollo's methodology might provide a way forward; however, Sims, Hewitt and Harris (2015) concluded that the assumptions underpinning interprofessional practice are insufficiently founded on empirical evidence. This standpoint is echoed by an earlier Cochrane review (Reeves et al. 2013), which included 15 studies measuring the effectiveness of IPE interventions compared with no educational intervention that showed some positive outcomes. However, because of the small number of studies and the heterogeneity of interventions and outcome measures, generalisable inferences about the effective key elements of IPE remain elusive. A recent Australian study (Grace et al. 2017) sheds new light on an old topic through a review of competency frameworks of seven professions and found commonalities based on shared values grouped into two core values: the rights of the client and the capacity of a particular profession to serve the healthcare needs of clients, which potentially offers new ways of conceptualising interprofessional practice. The

BOX 5.2

OUTCOMES FOR COMMUNICATION IN INTERPROFESSIONAL EDUCATION

- Communicate effectively with other health professional students and with other professionals.
- Encourage negotiation and conflict resolution.
- Express one's opinions to others involved with care.

- Listens to others/team members.
- Share decision making.
- Ensure communication at the beginning and end of shifts (handover, handoff).
- Be aware of differences in professionals' language.
- Exchange essential clinical information (health records, through electronic media).

Source: Thistlethwaite & Moran 2010.

important factors for communication resulting from research in IPE are shown in the following focus box.

Professional identity The personal and social identity that develops in a professional as a result of their work activities.

From the perspective of Thistlethwaite and Moran's criteria in the focus box, professional respect for specialised knowledge is given to all team members. Yet perceived threats persist in generating anxiety and conflict that impede interprofessional practice and experiential learning (McNeil, Mitchell & Parker 2013). A recent review (Best & Williams 2019) identified 16 publications using mixed methodological approaches and found several themes related to **professional identity** in Australian studies, as listed in Table 5.3.

TABLE 5.3 Professional identity systematic reviews of Australian interprofessional teams

Aim	Key findings
To explore the moderating role of team identity and professional identity threat in interprofessional team performance	Threat to professional identity impacts on performance.
To focus on employees' multiple group memberships and their acceptance of organisational change	Multiple identities; protective role of identity with professional departments during change that threatened group status. Needs care with management.
To explore the influence of power dynamics and trust on collaboration between health professionals involved in the management of diabetes and their impact on patient experiences	Three themes identified: use of power to protect identity, power dynamics between private and public sector providers and reducing dependency on other health professional to maintain power. Role boundaries between and within professional groups and services are changing. The uncertainty and vulnerability associated with these changes created mistrust.
To explore the role of open-minded interaction in professionally diverse teams	Need for open mindedness limited by strong professional identity. A focus on professional differences enhance value of team interaction.
To explore the integrative potential of a single theory (social identity approach) focusing on group level dynamics (Australia, Canada, United Kingdom, United States)	The need to move forward by working with and through social identities.

Source: Best & Williams 2019.

Promoting understanding

In interprofessional communication it is important that everyone understands what is being said. When this does not happen, it can be experienced as a shaming or humiliating experience and people may feel uncomfortable asking to have the unfamiliar and exclusionary term explained or, worse still, stay silent and remain ignorant about potentially important information. To avoid this, speak plainly, without jargon, abbreviations or the specialised terms that can prevent other professional subcultures, patients and families from understanding information about the health and ongoing care (Marshall, Medves, Docherty & Paterson 2011). Assertive, respectful communication helps overcome unhelpful behaviour and learning opportunities can emerge from interprofessional practice itself as different groups come to understand different professional language and priorities.

Skills in practice

Promoting understanding

The following table presents a series of communicative events that demonstrate how understanding can be achieved in different circumstances.

Skill	What's happening here?
Assertive listening: tune in mindfully, listen, acknowledge	
Turn off distractions such as smartphones (prepare to focus). Calm your breathing as stress or anxiety interferes with listening. Tune-in: prepare to fully participate in listening. Give the speaker your full attention without interruptions; mindful listening, being in the moment rather than problem-solving the next crisis. Acknowledge what others have to say to ensure you have heard and interpreted correctly.	Sets the foundations for a productive meeting. Team member (TM) 3 chairs the meeting: *'Thank you all for getting here at short notice. The only thing on our agenda today is to organise Iris's discharge'.* (Attending mindfully) TM4: *'Have I just heard you say Iris is going home? Does she know about that yet?'* (Person-centred response.) TM3: *'My apologies, I have been rushing to get here and what I mean is to plan the steps to discharge.'* (Acknowledging) TM4: *'I am sure we can give you a moment to catch your breath. It is good to know you didn't mean Iris was going today after yesterday's discussion.'*

TABLE **Continued**

TABLE *Continued*

Skill	What's happening here?
Making assertive statements and questions: your perspective, how you feel about it, what you need	
TM1 uses a 'jargon' word. TM2 says directly to TM1 in a conversational tone, '*[Name], I understand "abracadabra" is important in Iris's case from what you just said, but I am confused and I need you to explain what it is before we go on, otherwise I cannot contribute to the discussion.*' Note that the statement to TM1 here is not blaming, angry or aggressive. The words are descriptive of the situation from TM2's perspective.	The situation is defused. TM1 does not feel challenged and responds, '*Oh [Name], I am sorry, I did not realise I was using jargon, abracadabra is...*' TM2 does not feel resentful at the use of an exclusionary jargon word. '*Thank you, that makes it clear for me, and I think that we could consider... in the light of it.*' TM2 now has an opportunity to contribute specialised knowledge and explain what it is important to Iris's case. Possibly increases the potential for Iris to have a better outcome.
Coping with criticism: acknowledging, defusing, clarifying/probing	
Criticism as rejection In the work context, hurtful feelings of rejection are a warning sign of unmet personal needs or echoes from the past. Notice the contrast with the assertive statement above. **Response type 1**: *Becoming aggressive*, e.g. TM5 to TM3: '*What do you mean Iris is going home today? You haven't even given me a chance to get a word in about that yet!*' TM3 to TM5 (looking flustered and bemused by TM5's response): '*[Name] Are you OK? Is something wrong at home?*' **Response type 2**: *Damaging silence*: TM5 looks away and refuses to speak. Constructive criticism/acknowledging **Constructive feedback** is a helpful teaching and learning strategy. TM1 to TM3: '*[Name] I just wanted to bring up something here that I found rather difficult*'. The situation is defused.	**Criticism as rejection outcomes** Everyone in the meeting goes quiet in amazement at TM5's overreaction and speculates about it while feeling uncomfortable with the tension in the room. The focus of the meeting moves away from Iris to an unspoken (personal) agenda. **Response type 2**: *Damaging silence:* TM5 feels more upset and lapses into resentful silence, contributing nothing to the discussion. When extreme, this response to criticism can lead to destructive 'getting even' behaviour. **Constructive criticism outcomes** Leaping to conclusions based on assumptions or personal insecurities damage within-team relationships. When in doubt, a more constructive way to deal with it is to ask a clarifying question or provide additional information. Team harmony depends on team trust, respect and practitioners' self-reflection.

Making a within-team complaint TM2 to TM1: *'Do you remember that day I was assessing Iris?'* TM4 nods: *'You came in and interrupted when I was doing...with her? That really was not helpful because it delayed me getting it done and Iris was too tired to start again. It would have been poor practice anyway. BUT it was more than a day later I got back to it. That is not OK!'* (Note the person-centred focus on Iris's wellness rather than getting the assessment done under less than optimal circumstances.) TM1 to TM2: *'[Name], I had no idea I did that. I am pleased you have told me about it. Can we talk about it again after the meeting so I can get a better grasp on the "whys and wherefores" from your professional perspective and what to do if something like that happens again? Perhaps others would like to stay on for a bit as well.'* **Taking responsibility** TM1 acknowledged and accepted the criticism as a learning experience that they had not encountered in prior training, and that it was a gap in knowledge that needed to be filled. **Criticism that is accurate** **If you did it, own it!** TM4 to TM3: *'[Name] you were late for that meeting with Iris's son, and that left me in a very awkward position as you had most of the information we needed to talk about. Anyway, he wants to air his concerns for Iris going forward as he is away so much. I said I would bring it to the meeting.'* **Response 1**: *Taking responsibility for your own behaviour* TM3: *'[Name], yes I was late, and I apologise for that.'* TM4: *'[Name], spilt milk! I know things can be unpredictable. Please don't leave me in that situation again—a call would be nice.'* (The situation does not escalate into blaming.) TM1: *'I will call Iris's son and ask if he would like to have a chat to fill us in next time he visits.'* **Response 2:** Evading responsibility. Apologising and making excuses. (*This is a meeting personal needs strategy.*) TM3: *'[Name], I am so, so, sorry, my cat died, and then there was an accident at the crossing that held up the rush hour traffic. It was just one of those unavoidable days that happen sometimes.'*	Iris's wellness and capabilities remain at the centre of the team discussion. A learning opportunity was opened up for others to learn about the assessment technique that TM2 was conducting at the time of TM1's interruption. The focus remained on Iris throughout this encounter rather than blaming and aggressively attacking a team member. TM2's concern should be stated as a description of the facts of the situation, said in a conversational tone, looking directly at TM1, making an open assertive statement, not accusatory. **Taking responsibility outcomes** TM1 accepts responsibility. Team harmony is maintained, the focus remains on Iris and her needs. **Intrusive issues** An unexpected learning opportunity occurred to hear from someone outside of the health team (Iris's son) and his concerns and perspectives about Iris's capabilities provides an opportunity to triangulate sources of data to strengthens assessment outcomes and improve ongoing care. In the way it was disclosed by TM4, it is likely to lead to a detour in the meeting agenda. **Taking responsibility outcomes** The meeting focus could have shifted at the complaint about TM3 and derailed the agenda away from Iris and information from her son. TM3's apology defuses the situation. TM4 has personal needs met by externalising fault—e.g. having insufficient information for the meeting. The call to Iris's son redirects the meeting focus back to the patient's needs. **Evading responsibility outcomes** Evasion of responsibility such as shown in this response affects team cohesiveness and trust. It is also likely that respect for TM3 could be affected.

TABLE ***Continued***

TABLE *Continued*

Skill	What's happening here?
Owning up! Sandy the OT Team member Sandy has been listening intently through the meeting, and finally has the courage to open up about his error. *'Look, there is something I need to let you know. I have been so worried about it. I forgot to check Iris's shoes for suitability and safety when we did the home inspection. I just keep thinking about it and what might happen if she falls again. It will be my fault.'* Sandy's focus is on his error and the potential outcome rather than a solution. His catastrophising rather than problem solving has been exacerbated as a consequence of the delay since Iris's home inspection. **Owning up outcome** Delay in opening up about forgetting to check footwear caused Sandy distress in anticipation of an angry response. The team leader used an effective four-step process to clarify the 'error', assess the situation and quickly sum up a solution without blaming and/or demeaning Sandy.	**Team leader response to 'owning up'** *'Sandy, I can hear you are very worried about it!'* State the problem: *'First, you did a reasonably thorough inspection although did not check her footwear. Is that it In a nutshell?'* (Sandy nods) Assessment: *'I can hear that you expect something very bad to happen because you did not check Iris's shoes.'* (Sandy nods again) Way out/resolution: *'Well, the way I see it is this: you can worry and do nothing and nothing will be resolved, or you can go out there today and just check her footwear.'* Closure: *'If you are able to do that today then we can factor what you find into the discharge safety information.'* *(Process guided by Dahan et al. 2017)* **Owning up outcome** Sandy does not experience humiliation or shame and team cohesiveness is maintained.
Defusing These are non-committal statements that neither agree nor disagree and block an unhelpful or argumentative discussion before it begins. TM5 to TM3: *'Look, could you just stop being so pedantic over every little thing so we can get out of here today!'* Agreeing-in-principle: TM3 to TM5: *'Yes, you're right, I do like to dot the Is and cross the Ts.'* Offering probability of agreement: TM3 to TM5: *'You could be right about that.'* Partial agreement: TM3 to TM5: *'I would like to get out of here today too.'*	**Defusing outcomes** These three response types keep the focus on the detail of what is required for Iris's safe return to home (person-centred care). Defuses any insulting or humiliating trigger. Blocks personal needs erupting into the meeting.

Clarifying and probing	**Clarifying and probing outcomes**
These are useful strategies for situations where it is not clear what the criticism is about, or when it seems there are unspoken messages contained in the criticism. TM5 to TM3: *'You are letting these meetings go on and on so you don't have to do any real work.'* TM3 to TM5: *'[Name] what is it about the way I work that upsets you?'* Response 1: Probing TM5 to TM3: *'Well, we could get this one done in half the time if you just stopped messing about with the detail, and now you want to extend to talk about something else.'* Response 2: Clarifying TM3 to TM5: *'[Name], what is it that bothers you about meeting in working time, given you are here anyway?'* TM5 to TM3: *'[Name], things are on a tight schedule for me today. I have to pick up my children from school.'* TM3 to TM5: *'I see. I appreciate you explaining that to me. When do you have to leave?'*	TM5 has competing role demands which TM3 has found through asking probing and clarifying questions. **Managing role conflicts through clarifying/probing** The focus of the meeting moved from Iris to the team member's parenting needs of TM5 only briefly. TM3 moved the focus back to Iris's case by identifying the source of TM5's angst and providing an opportunity for TM5 to express their needs without further disruption to the meeting focus. This strategy also defused the 'different values' trigger. An opportunity within the meeting context to openly communicate about and problem-solve TM5's situation.

Sources: Clark, Gray & Mooney 2013; Dahan, Ducard & Caeymaex 2017; Hayes, Strosahl & Wilson 2012; Mackay et al. 2018.

Interprofessional practice and the liminal space

One of the profound effects of systemic change that interprofessional practice brings to education and healthcare institutions is the uncertainty and anxiety it delivers to individuals who work in such contexts. As the previous discussion showed, practice is often changing before there is sound evidence of effectiveness. Practice in this respect is in the **liminal space** of 'not knowing via education'.

Liminal space
A space of transition or uncertainty where knowledge is tacit and transformational.

Polanyi and Sen's (2009) basic idea is that subsidiary skill or sense perception is tacit because our attention is elsewhere, on a point of active focal awareness, or ahead of it (p. 256)—that is, *we know more than we can tell* (p. 255).

In the interprofessional team, the liminal space learning with and about other professions occurs in a transformational way that expands and is applied without necessarily recognising the source, or how one knows, into practice (Land 2014). This might explain why it becomes so difficult to translate research into practice, according to Scott et al. (2012). The spaces where information is shared and learning occurs are inherent in interprofessional collaboration, and in the shared physical space where discussions that are of mutual interest occur. In such conversational spaces, learning from others is more subliminal than deliberative (Morris & Matthews 2014; Perrott 2013). In Perrott's study, trust within the team contributed to productive working relationships and knowledge sharing, yet acknowledgment of such learning is neither recognised nor valued overtly.

Garrick and Chan (2017) come to a somewhat similar conclusion: 'Tacit knowledge involves a sense of what is going on and this is not easily measured or codified. Experiential understanding of what is required when engaging with clients, colleagues, senior partners, other contexts in which employees work is central to tacit knowledge' (p. 872). In the context of interprofessional practice, a large of part of learning brought to the team derives from different professional training modalities into a shared person-centred endeavour, which undervalues knowledge and skills acquired tacitly and although unmeasurable, is central to effective practice.

Ways forward

Beyond the published literature on interprofessional education, collaboration and practice, there are some helpful indications of how gaps might be filled. Wagner, Brooks and Urban (2018) found that a workplace intervention involving open discussion between managers and team members as well as structured workplace activities enhanced spirit at work and improved patient care. This might mean adapting current workplace processes without adding to the workload.

The importance of rigorous research was highlighted by Welp and Manser (2016) in their observation that the primary barrier to advancing understanding of causal relationships within teamwork, clinician wellbeing and patient safety is absence of an integrative theory to inform methodologically sound projects. This in line with a large study (Schwartz et al. 2019) that found work–life integration was affected significantly by position and time in a speciality. More importantly, the authors observed that work–life integration appears to operate as a 'climate' associated with better safety culture norms, which supports an evidence-based solution for supportive worker intervention in the workplace. It seems that positive impacts might be achieved by an increased emphasis on a 'climate' (i.e. workplace cultures) (Braithwaite et al. 2016) that indirectly improves safety culture. This seems to integrate seamlessly with Nugus et al.'s (2019) notion of deliberative democracy that uses conscientisation, which is the conscious realisation of power imbalances as a basis for transformation, and deliberation to improve interprofessional practice simultaneously with educational empowerment.

Finally, 'enriched closed-loops' of communication with positive emotional interactions have been found to relate to team effectiveness in emergency situations, whereas incomplete loops of communication involving negative emotional content have a detrimental effect on team effectiveness and therefore potential safety in fire-fighting emergency situations (Jouanne, Charron, Chauvin & Morel 2017). While the context is very different from health and wellbeing workplaces, it seems very likely that effective 'closed-loop' communication has a major role in teamwork, especially in emergency situations. However, before effective communication and positive emotional interactions can develop, trust in the healthcare institution must be established to support worker motivation and team effectiveness.

Reflect and apply

On your own or in a small group, think of a conversation or interaction where you held back some information or provided minimal information assuming that the other person could fill in the blanks (i.e. leave the communication loop incomplete). Did the person you were communicating with catch the intent of your discussion? Reflect on the conversation and what you could have said or done differently to improve and close the communication loop. In terms of your communication style, which mode of the communication accommodation theory styles best described your communication in the interaction?

Conclusion

In this chapter, interprofessional communication has been explored in depth. Couched in terms of developing a 'right' relationship with other professionals, interprofessional communication centres on inclusiveness, trust and respect. For the most part, professionals from other disciplines will concur on what they see or know about a person. However, by refining how one listens, and communicates verbally and non-verbally, it is possible to see and know more than one can tell—that is, tacit knowledge can develop and enrich one's own communication and practice and improve team effectiveness (Jouanne et al. 2017; Welp & Manser 2016).

SUMMARY POINTS

- Effective interprofessional communication occurs when students or practitioners from different professions communicate with each other in a collaborative, responsive and responsible manner.
- Interprofessional communication builds trust and understanding, and ensures in the health setting that all knowledge about the patient is shared, which leads to better person-centred health outcomes.
- Factors that contribute to effective interprofessional communication include observation, active listening, sharing, translating and integrating knowledge bases.
- Actions and values that may trigger professional identity crises include differential treatment, different values, expectations of assimilation, insulting or humiliating actions, and simple contact.
- Assertive communication that embeds respect and trust facilitates effective interprofessional practice.

- Developing assertive communication skills to cope with criticism, including acknowledging, defusing, clarifying and probing, will assist all health professionals to improve patient outcomes and workplace satisfaction.

CRITICAL THINKING QUESTIONS

1. Think about your own situation at university when you were asked to work in teams. Apply the group norms delineated in the focus box 'Aims of interprofessional group norms'. How many of these norms operated within the group? Are there any that did not apply? Are there some norms that were not acted upon? Thinking about the group behaviour, and list ways in which you personally could have improved communication across the group.
2. This chapter delves deeply into active listening. Again reflecting on your university experience, identify situations when active listening skills (see Table 5.1) might have facilitated improvements in the communication processes in and between groups of students.
3. Communication is something that we all think we know about, yet occasionally and unknowingly we might erect barriers to active listening. With reference to Table 5.2, reflect on recent interactions with your student colleagues and identify when you engaged in such behaviours. How might you have prevented these impediments?
4. Reflective practice is a way of studying your own experiences to improve the way you work. After reviewing the chapter and Table 5.4, in particular, critically reflect on and identify your automatic communication traits to enhance your skills for interprofessional practice.

Group activity

Interprofessional communication

In your study groups or via your subject discussion site, discuss how you believe your profession is perceived by other professional groups. How do these perceptions influence interprofessional communication? What are the potential implications for the recipients of healthcare if these perceptions are inaccurate?

WEBLINKS

Interprofessional collaboration

American Interprofessional Health Collaborative:
www.aihc-us.org

Interprofessional education and practice

Australasian Interprofessional Practice and Education network:
https://interprofessional.global/australasia

Centre for the Advancement of Interprofessional Education:
http://caipe.org.uk

WHO Framework for Action on Interprofessional Education and Collaborative Practice:
www.who.int/hrh/resources/framework_action/en/

REFERENCES

Aritz, J. & Walker, R.C. (2010). Cognitive organization and identity maintenance in multicultural teams: A discourse analysis of decision-making meetings. *Journal of Business Communication*, 47(1), 20–41. doi:10.1177/0021943609340669.

Beck, C., Gaunt, H. & Chiavaroli, N. (2017). Improving visual observation skills through the arts to aid radiographic interpretation in veterinary practice: A pilot study. *Veterinary Radiological Ultrasound*, 58, 495–502. doi:10.1111/vru.12517.

Best, S. & Williams, S. (2019). Professional identity in interprofessional teams: Findings from a scoping review. *Journal of Interprofessional Care*, 33(2), 170–81. doi:10.1080/13561820.2018.1536040.

Bjork, S., Juthberg, C., Lindkvist, M., Wimo, A., Sandman, P.-O., Winblad, B. & Edvardsson, D. (2016). Exploring the prevalence and variance of cognitive impairment, pain, neuropsychiatric symptoms and ADL dependency among persons living in nursing homes: A cross-sectional study. *BMS Geriatrics*, 16, 154. doi:10.1186/s12877-016-0328-9.

Boudreau, D.J., Cassell, E. & Fuks, A. (2009). Preparing medical students to become attentive listeners. *Medical Teacher*, 31(1), 22–9. doi:10.1080/01421590802350776.

Braithwaite, J., Clay-Williams, R., Vecellio, E., Marks, D., Hooper, T., Westbrook, M., … Ludlow, K. (2016). The basis of clinical tribalism, hierarchy and stereotyping: A laboratory-controlled teamwork experiment. *BMJ Open*, 6, e012467. doi:10.1136/bmjopen-2016-012467.

Brown, S.S., Garber, J.S., Lash, J. & Schnurman-Crook, A. (2014). A proposed interprofessional oath. *Journal of Interprofessional Care*, 28(5), 471–2. doi:10.3109/13561820.2014.900480.

Burkell, J., Fortier, A., Yeung, L., Wong, C. & Simpson, J.L. (2014). Facebook: Public space, or private space? *Information, Communication & Society*, 17(8), 974–85. doi:10.1080/1369118X.2013.870591.

Canadian Interprofessional Health Collaborative. (2010). *A National Interprofessional Competency Framework*. Vancouver: College of Health Disciplines, University of British Columbia.

Claramita, M., Riskiyana, R., Pratidina-Susilo, A., Huriyati, E., Wahyuningsih, M.S.-H. & Norcini, J.J. (2019). Interprofessional communication in a socio-hierarchical culture: Development of the TRI-O guide. *Journal of Multidisciplinary Healthcare*, 12, 191–204. doi:10.2147/JMDH.S196873.

Clark, M., Gray, M. & Mooney, J. (2013). New graduate occupational therapists' perceptions of near-misses and mistakes in the workplace. *International Journal of Health Care Quality Assurance*, 26(6), 564–76.doi: https://doi-org.elibrary.jcu.edu.au/10.1108/IJHCQA-10-2011-0061.

Dahan, S., Ducard, D. & Caeymaex, L. (2017). Apology in cases of medical error disclosure: Thoughts based on a preliminary study. *PLoS ONE*, 12(7), e0181854. doi:10.1371/journal.pone.0181854.

Farzadnia, S. & Giles, H. (2015). Patient-provider health interactions: A communication accommodation theory perspective. *International Journal of Society, Culture & Language*, 3(2), 18–34.

Fields, J.A. (2017). Cognitive and neuropsychiatric features in Parkinson's and Lewy body dementias. *Archives of Clinical Neuropsychology*, 32, 786–801. doi:10.1093/arclin/acx085.

Frank, O. & Rowett, D. (2018). Facilitating respectful interprofessional communication: How do we get there? *Journal of Pharmacy Practice and Research*, 48(4), 303–5.

Gallois, C.O., Ogay, T.T. & Giles, H. (2005). Communication accommodation theory: A look back and a look ahead. In W. Gudykunst (ed.), *Theorizing about Intercultural Communication*. Thousand Oaks, CA: Sage.

Gallois, C.O., Watson, B.M. & Giles, H. (2018). Intergroup communication: Identities and effective interactions. *Journal of Communication*, 68(2), 309–17. https://doi.org/10.1093/joc/jqx016.

Garcia-Marques, T., Mackie, D.M., Maitner, A.T. & Claypool, H.M. (2016). Moderation of the familiarity-stereotyping effect: The role of stereotype fit. *Social Cognition*, 34(2), 81–96.

Garrick, J. & Chan, A. (2017). Knowledge management and professional experience: The uneasy dynamics between tacit knowledge and performativity in organizations. *Journal of Knowledge Management*, 21(4), 872–84. doi:10.1108/JKM-02-2017-0058.

Giles, H. & Gasiorek, J. (2014). Parameters of nonaccommodation: Refining and elaborating communication accommodation theory. In J.P. Forgas, O. Vincze & J. Laszlo (eds), *Social Cognition and Communication* (pp. 155–72). New York: Psychology Press.

Giles, H., Reid, S.A. & Harwood, J. (eds). (2010). *The Dynamics of Intergroup Communication*. New York: Peter Lang.

Grace, S., Innes, E., Joffe, B., East, L., Coutts, R. & Nancarrow, S. (2017). Identifying common values among seven health professions: An interprofessional analysis. *Journal of Interprofessional Care*, 31(3), 325–34. doi:org/10.1080/13561820.2017.1288091.

Gupta, D.M., Boland, R.J. & Aron, D.C. (2017). The physician's experience of changing clinical practice: A struggle to unlearn. *Implementation Science*, 12, 28. doi:10.1186/s13012-017-0555-2.

Hale, L.S. & DiLollo, A. (2016). Immersive interprofessional education using an evidence-based practice course. *Journal of Physician Assistant Education*, 27(3), 117–25. doi:10.1097/JPA.0000000000000008.

Hays, P.A. (2016). *Addressing Cultural Complexities in Practice: Assessment, Diagnosis and Therapy* (3rd edn). Washington, DC: American Psychological Association.

Hayes, S.C., Strosahl, K.D. & Wilson, K.G. (2012). *Acceptance and Commitment Therapy: The Process and Practice of Mindful Change* (2nd edn). New York: Guilford Press.

Hindle, J.V. (2010). Ageing, neurodegeneration and Parkinson's disease. *Age and Ageing*, 39,156–61. doi:10.1093/ageing/afp223.

Holtman, M.C., Frost, J.S., Hammer, D.P., McGuinn, K. & Nunez, L.M. (2011). Interprofessional professionalism: Linking professionalism and interprofessional care. *Journal of Interprofessional Care*, 25, 383–5. doi:10.3109/13561820.2011.588350.

Interprofessional Education Collaborative. (2016). *Core Competencies for Interprofessional Collaborative Practice: 2016 Update*. Washington, DC: Interprofessional Education Collaborative.

Interprofessional Education Consortium. (2001). *Defining the Knowledge Base for Interprofessional Education* (vol. 1). San Francisco, CA: Stuart Foundation. Retrieved from http://matrixoutcomesmodel.com/MatrixFiles/stuart/Volume1.pdf.

Ivey, A.E., Ivey, M.B. & Zalaquett C.P. (2018). *Intentional Interviewing and Counselling: Facilitating Client Development in a Multicultural Society* (9th edn). Boston, MA: Cengage Learning.

Jasni, S.K. & Saks, N.S. (2013). Using visual art to enhance the clinical observations skills of medical students. *Medical Teacher*, 35, e1327–e1331. doi:10.1080/01421590802331446.

Jouanne, E., Charron, C., Chauvin, C. & Morel G. (2017). Correlates of team effectiveness: An exploratory study of firefighter's operations during emergency situations. *Applied Ergonomics*, 61, 69–77. doi:10.1016/j.apergo.2017.01.005.

Kang, J.H., Mollenhauer, B., Coffey, C.S., Toledo, J.B., Weintraub, D., Galasko, D.R., ... Shaw, L.M. (2016). CSF biomarkers associated with disease heterogeneity in early Parkinson's disease: The Parkinson's Progression Markers Initiative study. *Acta Neuropathologica*, 131, 935–49. doi:10.1007/s00401-016-1552-2.

Kim, S., Bochatay, N., Relyea-Chew, A., Buttrick, E., Amdahl, C., Kim, L., ... Lee, Y.M. (2017). Individual, interpersonal, and organisational factors of healthcare conflict: A scoping review. *Journal of Interprofessional Care*, 31(3), 282–90.

Koerts, J., van Beilen, M., Leenders, K.L., Brouwer, W.H. & Tucha, L. (2012). Complaints about impairments in executive functions in Parkinson's disease: The association with neuropsychological assessment. *Parkinsonism and Related Disorders*, 18, 194–7. doi:10.1016/j.parkreldis.2011.10.002.

Kohn, L., Corrigan, J. & Donaldson, M.S. (2000). *To Err Is Human: Building a Safer Healthcare System*. Washington, DC: National Academy Press.

Konczak, J., Sciutti, A., Avanzino, L., Squeri, V., Gori, M., Masia, L., ... Sandin, G. (2012). Parkinson's disease accelerates age-related decline in haptic perception by altering somatosensory integration. *Brain*, 135, 3371–9. doi:10.1093/brain/aws265.

Korner, M. (2010). Interprofessional teamwork in medical rehabilitation: A comparison of multidisciplinary and interdisciplinary team approach. *Clinical Rehabilitation*, 24, 745–55. doi:10.1177/0269215510367538.

Land, R., Rattray, J. & Vivian, P. (2014). Learning in the liminal space: A semiotic approach to threshold concepts. *Higher Education*, 67, 199–217. doi:10.1007/s10734-013-9705-x.

Li, K., Chu, P. & Pickett, K.A. (2017). The effect of dopaminergic medication on joint kinematics during haptic movements in individuals with Parkinson's disease. *Behavioural Neurology*, article ID 2358386, 8 pages. doi:10.1155/2017/2358386.

Lapkin, S., Levett-Jones, T. & Gilligan, C. (2013). A systematic review of the effectiveness of interprofessional education in health professional programs. *Nurse Education Today*, 33, 90–102. doi:10.1016/j.nedt.2011.11.006.

Lau, L. & Ng, K.-M. (2014). Conceptualizing the counseling training environment using Bronfenbrenner's ecological theory. *International Journal of Advanced Counselling*, 36, 423–39. doi:10.1007/s10447-014-9220-5.

Lineweaver, T.T., Hutman, P., Ketcham, C. & Bohannon, J.N. (2011). The effect of comprehension, feedback and listener age on speech complexity. *Journal of Language and Social Psychology*, 30(1), 46–65. doi:10.1177/0261927X10387101.

Machin, L.L., Bellis, K.M., Dixon, C., Morgan, H., Pye, J., Spencer, P. & Williams, R.A. (2018). Interprofessional education and practice guide: Designing ethics-orientated interprofessional education for health and social care students. *Journal of Interprofessional Care*, doi:10.1080/13561820.2018.1538113.

Mackay, M., Davis, M. & Fanning, P. (2018). *Messages: The Communication Skills Book* (4th edn). Oakland, CA: New Harbinger.

MacKenzie, D.E. & Westwood, D.A. (2013). Occupational therapists and observation: What are you looking at? *OTJR: Occupation, Participation and Health*, 33(1), 4–11. doi:http://dx.doi.org.elibrary.jcu.edu.au/10.3928/15394492-20120928-01.

Marshall, C., Medves, J., Docherty, D. & Paterson, M. (2011). Interprofessional jargon: How is it exclusionary? Cultural determinants of language use in healthcare practice. *Journal of Interprofessional Care*, 25(6), 452–3. doi:10.3109/13561820.2011.597891.

McEvoy, P., Williamson, T., Kada, R., Frazer, D., Dhliwayo, C. & Gask, L. (2017). Improving access to mental health care in an Orthodox Jewish community: A critical reflection upon the accommodation of others. *BMC Health Services Research*, 17, 557. doi:10.1186/s12913-017-2509-4.

McNeil, K.A., Mitchell, R.J. & Parker, V. (2013). Interprofessional practice and professional identity threat. *Health Sociology Review*, 22(3), 291–307.

Mitchell, R.J., Parker, V. & Giles, M. (2011). When do interprofessional teams succeed? Investigating the moderating roles of team and professional identity in interprofessional effectiveness. *Human Relations*, 64(10), 1321–43. doi:10.1177/0018726711416872.

Morhayim, L. (2019). Visitors' use of corridors in internal medicine wards: Modalities of territoriality, proxemics, and privacy while waiting. *Facilities*, 37(5/6), 313–29. doi.org/10.1108/F-01-2018-0024.

Morris, D. & Matthews, J. (2014). Communication, respect, and leadership: Interprofessional collaboration in hospitals of rural Ontario. *Canadian Journal of Dietary Practice Research*, 75,173–9. doi:10.3148/cjdpr-2014-020.

Moyers, P.A., Finch Guthrie, P.L., Swan, A.R. & Sathe, L.A. (2014). Interprofessional evidence-based clinical scholar program: Learning to work together. *American Journal of Occupational Therapy*, 68, S23–S31. http://dx.doi.org/10.5014/ajot.2014.012609.

Nugus, P., Ranmuthugala, G., Travaglia, J., Greenfield, D., Lamonthe, J., Hogden, A., Kolne, K. & Braithwaite, J. (2019). Advancing interprofessional theory: Deliberative democracy as a participatory research antidote to power differentials in aged care. *Journal of Interprofessional Education & Practice*, 15, 100–11. https://doi.org/10.1016/j.xjep.2018.09.005.

O'Leary, D.F. (2016). Exploring the importance of team psychological safety in the development of two interprofessional teams. *Journal of Interprofessional Care*, 30(1), 29–34. doi:10.3109/13561820.2015.1072142.

O'Toole, G. (2012). *Communication: Core Interpersonal Skills for Health Professionals*. Chatswood: Churchill Livingstone.

Perrott, B.E. (2013). Knowledge flows in health communities of practice. *Health Marketing Quarterly*, 30, 319–33. doi:10.1080/07359683.2013.844017.

Polanyi, M. & Sen, A. (2009). *The Tacit Dimension*. Chicago, IL: University of Chicago Press.

Pretorius, M. (2018). Communication accommodation theory analysis of nurse–patient interactions: Implications for course design. *International Journal of Applied Linguistics*, 28, 71–85. doi.https://doi.org/10.1111/ijal.12184.

Ravet, J. (2012). From interprofessional education to interprofessional practice: Exploring the implementation gap. *Professional Development in Education*, 38(1), 49–64, doi:10.1080/19415257.2011.576263.

Reeves, S., Perrier, L., Goldman, J., Freeth, D. & Zwarenstein, M. (2013). Interprofessional education: Effects on professional practice and healthcare outcomes. *Cochrane Database of Systematic Reviews*, art. no.: CD002213. doi:10.1002/14651858.CD002213.pub3.

Ruben, B.D. (2016). Communication theory and health communication practice: The more things change, the more they stay the same. *Health Communication*, 31, 1–11. doi:10.1080/10410236.2014.923086.

Ruitenberg, C.W. & Towle, A. (2015). 'How to do things with words' in health professions education. *Advances in Health Science Education*, 20, 857–72. doi:10.1007/s10459-014-9568-7.

Schentrup, D., Walen, K., Black, E., Blue, A. & Chacko, L. (2018). Building interprofessional team effectiveness in a nurse-led rural health center. *Journal of Interprofessional Education & Practice*, 12, 86–90. doi:10.1016/j.xjep.2018.05.008.

Schwartz, S.P., Adair, K.C., Bae, J., Rehder, K.J., Shanafelt, T.D., Profit, J. & Sexton, J.B. (2019). Work–life balance behaviours cluster in work settings and relate to burnout and safety culture: A cross-sectional survey analysis. *BMJ Quality and Safety*, 28, 142–50. doi:10.1136/bmjqs-2018-007933.

Scott, S., Albrecht, L., O'Leary, K., Ball, G., Hartling, L., Hofmeyer, A., … Dryden, D.M. (2012). Systematic review of knowledge translation strategies in the allied health professions. *Implementation Science*, 7, 70. Retrieved from www.implementationscience.com/content/7/1/70.

Scott, W., Milioto, M., Trost, Z. & Sullivan, M.J.L. (2016). The relationship between perceived injustice and the working alliance: A cross-sectional study of patients with persistent pain attending multidisciplinary rehabilitation. *Disability and Rehabilitation*, 38(24), 2365–73. doi:10.3109/09638288.2015.1129444.

Sims, S., Hewitt, G. & Harris, R. (2015). Evidence of collaboration, pooling of resources, learning and role blurring in interprofessional healthcare teams: A realist synthesis. *Journal of Interprofessional Care*, 29(1), 20–5. doi:10.3109/13561820.2014.939745.

Stone, J. (2010). Moving interprofessional learning forward through formal assessment. *Medical Education*, 44(4), 396–403. doi:10.1111/j.1365-2923.2009.03607.x.

Storlie, T.A. (2015). *Person-centered Communication with Older Adults: The Professional Provider's Guide*. London: Academic Press.

Stuck, A.E., Moser, A., Morf, U., Wirz, U., Wyser, J., Gillman, G., et al. (2015). Effect of health risk assessment and counselling on health behaviour and survival in older people: A pragmatic randomised trial. *PLoS Medicine*, 12(10), e1001889. doi:10.1371/journal.pmed.1001889.

Sublette, V.A., Smith, S.K., George, J., McCaffery, K. & Douglas, M.W. (2018). Listening to both sides: A qualitative comparison between patients with hepatitis C and their healthcare professionals' perceptions of the facilitators and barriers to hepatitis C treatment adherence and completion. *Journal of Health Psychology*, 23(13), 1720–31. doi.10.1177/1359105316669858.

Sweet, G.H. & Wilson, H.J. (2011). A patient's experience of ward rounds. *Patient Education and Counseling*, 84, 150–1. doi:10.1016/j.pec.2010.08.016.

Swenne, C.L. & Skytt, B. (2014). The ward round–patient experiences and barriers to participation. *Scandinavian Journal of Caring Sciences*, 28, 297–304. doi:10.1111/scs.12059.

Thistlethwaite, J., Jackson, A. & Moran, M. (2013). Interprofessional collaborative practice: A deconstruction. *Journal of Interprofessional Care*, 27, 50–6. doi:10.3109/13561820.2012.730075.

Thistlethwaite, J., Moran, M., on behalf of the World Health Organization Study Group on Interprofessional Education and Collaborative Practice. (2010). Learning outcomes for interprofessional education (IPE): Literature review and synthesis. *Journal of Interprofessional Care*, 24(5), 503–13. doi:10.3109/13561820.2010.483366.

Toner, C.K., Reese, B.E., Neargarder, S., Riedel, T.M. Gilmore, G.C. & Cronin-Golomb, A. (2012). Vision-fair neuropsychological assessment in normal aging, Parkinson's disease and Alzheimer's disease. *Psychology and Aging*, 27(3), 785–90. doi:10.1037/a0026368.

Vermeir, P., Vandijck, D., Degroote, S., Peleman, R., Verhaeghe, R., Mortier, E., ... Vogelaers, D. (2015). Communication in healthcare: A narrative review of the literature and practical recommendations. *International Journal of Clinical Practice*, 69(11), 1257–67.

Wagner, J.I.J., Brooks, D. & Urban, A.-M. (2018). Health care providers' spirit at work within a restructured workplace. *Western Journal of Nursing Research*, 40(1) 20–36. doi:10.1177/0193945916678418.

Warnock, C., Buchanan, J. & Tod, A.M. (2017). The difficulties experienced by nurses and healthcare staff involved in the process of breaking bad news. *Journal of Advanced Nursing*, 73(7), 1632–45. doi:10.1111/jan.13252.

Watson, B.M., Heatley, M.L., Gallois, C. & Kruske, S. (2016). The importance of effective communication in interprofessional practice: Perspectives of maternity clinicians. *Health Communication*, 31(4), 400–7.

Watson, S.G., Cholerton, B.A., Gross, R.G., Weintraub, D., Zabetiand, C.P., Trojanowskig, J.Q., ... Leverenz, J.B. (2013). Neuropsychologic assessment in collaborative Parkinson's disease research: A proposal from the National Institute of Neurological Disorders and Stroke, Morris K. Udall Centers of Excellence for Parkinson's Disease Research at the University of Pennsylvania and the University of Washington. *Alzheimer's & Dementia*, 9, 609–61. http://dx.doi.org/10.1016/j.jalz.2012.07.006.

Weger, H., Bell, G.C., Minei, E.M. & Robinson, M.C. (2014). The relative effectiveness of active listening in initial interactions. *International Journal of Listening*, 28(1), 13–31. doi:10.1080/10904018.2013.813234.

Welander, J., Astvik, W. & Isaksson, K. (2017). Corrosion of trust: Violation of psychological contracts as a reason for turnover amongst social workers. *Nordic Social Work Research*, 7(1), 67–79m. doi:10.1080/2156857X.2016.1203814.

Welp, A. & Manser, T. (2016). Integrating teamwork, clinician occupational well-being and patient safety: Development of a conceptual framework based on a systematic review. *BMC Health Services Research*, 16, 281. doi:10.1186/s12913-016-1535-y.

Wilhelm, M., Poirier, T., Otsuka, A. & Wagner, S. (2014). Interprofessional ethics learning between schools of pharmacy and dental medicine. *Journal of Interprofessional Care*, 28(5), 478–80. doi:10.3109/13561820.2014.911722.

World Health Organization. (2010). *Framework for Action on Interprofessional Education & Collaborative Practice*. Geneva: WHO. Retrieved from http://whqlibdoc.who.int/hq/2010/WHO_HRH_HPN_10.3_eng.pdf.

World Health Organization. (2013). *Interprofessional Collaborative Practice in Primary Health Care: Nursing and Midwifery Perspectives, Six Case Studies, Observer Issue 13*. Retrieved from www.who.int/hrh/resources/IPE_SixCaseStudies.pdf?ua=1.

CHAPTER 6

COMMUNICATING IN CULTURALLY DIVERSE CONTEXTS

SUE LIM, ANNETTE MORTENSEN AND MARIA CARBINES

CHAPTER FOCUS

After reading this chapter and completing the activities, you will be able to:

- define concepts of culture, cultural diversity and communication in health settings
- describe the cross-cultural dimensions of communication
- critically examine how cultural dimensions influence communication
- evaluate strategies that enhance cross-cultural communication.

KEY TERMS

CALD
Cross-cultural communication
Cultural competence
Cultural knowledge
Cultural self-awareness
Cultural sensitivity
Cultural value dimensions
Culturally diverse
Culture
Discrimination
Ethnocentrism
Feminine culture
Masculine culture
Prejudice
Racism
Stereotype

Introduction

Although the simple act of greeting would seem to be straightforward, a greeting between two cultures can be a source of confusion or offence. Consider the following as an example: Rosa greeted her manager with, 'Good morning ma'am', at the start of the day. The manager told a colleague, 'I have reminded Rosa to call me by my first name many times and she still continues to call me ma'am. It's really annoying me and it's disrespectful'. The next day, when Rosa greeted the manager, 'Good morning, ma'am', the manager jokingly told Rosa, 'I'll fine you if you don't call me by my first name'. Rosa was confused. She thought to herself, 'I thought I was just being respectful calling the manager "ma'am". It's really difficult for me as a migrant, coming from a hierarchical culture to adjust to calling my manager by her first name'. As societies such as Australia and New Zealand become increasingly multicultural, so does the potential for cross-cultural misunderstandings to occur in the healthcare team, at the bedside, and in the tearoom.

This chapter provides a framework to help health practitioners understand what is happening in their communication with patients and staff and raises awareness of the underlying causes of misunderstanding. The examples given demonstrate the use of effective cross-cultural communication skills, therapeutic relationships and intercultural teamwork. The foundation for explaining the five key concepts that health workers can use to guide cross-cultural interactions with colleagues and patients are:

1. collectivist and individualist perspectives (individual vs group)
2. power distance (status and authority difference)
3. uncertainty avoidance (tolerance of uncertainty and ambiguity)
4. masculine vs feminine (fixed or more flexible roles)
5. communication styles.

What is culture?

Culture
A cluster of societal elements held in common by a particular group of people.

Betancourt, Green and Carrillo (2018) define **culture** as a system of beliefs, values, rules and customs that are shared by a group and are used to interpret experiences and direct patterns of behaviour. When a clinician interacts with a patient, three cultures are juxtaposed: the patient's, the clinician's, and the culture of Western healthcare. All three cultures influence the outcome of the encounter. To understand patients and colleagues from cultural backgrounds different from our own, it is first necessary to recognise our own cultural beliefs, values and behaviours, and, additionally, to be aware that Western health frameworks have their own particular beliefs, values and customs (e.g. the idea of patient autonomy and the value placed on scientific evidence). Finally, the social and cultural backgrounds of patients and clinicians affect the quality of understanding and communication that occurs in cross-cultural clinical encounters (Betancourt et al. 2018).

Misunderstandings between patients and health providers and between colleagues often reflect inherent differences in cultural values and expectations. These misunderstandings can lead to outcomes ranging from mild discomfort to a major lack of trust that disintegrates the therapeutic or collegial relationship. Differences in styles of communication that can lead to discomfort and miscommunication include both verbal and non-verbal communication such as eye contact, touch and personal space. For example, cues such as direct eye contact may be avoided in some cultures, while in others it is a sign of respect.

Cultures are dynamic in nature (Charmaz 2014), being constantly remodelled in response to changing social influences. Culture is fluid rather than static, which means that culture changes all the time, every day, in subtle and tangible ways. Because humans communicate and express their cultural systems in a variety of ways, it can be hard to pinpoint exactly what cultural dynamics are at play.

The focus in this chapter is on cross-cultural interactions between managers and staff; within healthcare teams; and between health practitioners and patients. The term 'culturally and linguistically diverse' (**CALD**) will be used when referring to groups and individuals who differ from the majority group because of their religious, language or ethnic backgrounds (Office of Multicultural Interests 2009).

CALD
Culturally and linguistically diverse.

Communication and cultural diversity

The twenty-first century is characterised by increasing globalisation and increased population movements both within and between countries. One outcome of these changes is an emerging awareness of cultural variation when people who have been socialised in different ways come to interact in social settings such as healthcare. Health workforces in Western nations are **culturally diverse**. The phenomenon of health workforce migration to OECD countries has dramatically increased over the past three decades as a result of workforce shortages and ageing population dynamics (Aluttis, Bishaw & Frank 2014). Nearly all OECD countries rely on recruiting health workers from abroad to fill their shortages (Aluttis et al. 2014; Ono, Lafortune & Schoenstein 2013). Additionally, health systems and health service delivery models are becoming more complex, characterised by greater teamwork and overlaps in the roles and responsibilities of different health professionals and providers (Ono et al. 2013). In Australia, New Zealand and other parts of the OECD, the health populations served are also ethnically diverse, reflecting their respective migration trends (Australian Bureau of Statistics 2012; Statistics New Zealand 2014).

Culturally diverse
The presence of multiple diverse cultures in a population.

Sociocultural differences between patients and health providers influence communication and clinical decision making. A combination of issues has put the field of cross-cultural care and communication in the spotlight. These are increasingly diverse health populations, recognition of the need for effective communication to achieve quality health care, evidence of the disparity in health care provided to patients from CALD backgrounds (Office of Multicultural Interests 2009), and new accreditation standards and quality measures (Betancourt et al. 2018). Cross-cultural care focuses on the ability to communicate effectively and provide quality healthcare to patients from diverse sociocultural backgrounds. There is strong evidence that educating healthcare providers in cross-cultural care improves knowledge and good evidence that it improves attitudes and skills (Horvat, Horey, Romios & Kis-Rigo 2014; Renzaho, Romios, Crock & Sønderlund 2013).

Cross-cultural communication An exchange of information in a context comprising two or more cultures.

Cultural self-awareness Being conscious of our personal reactions to people who are different from ourselves. We need to recognise our own values and biases as well as the values and biases of colleagues and patients, and be consciously aware of our own reactions and the reactions of others who are from diverse cultures.

There are growing concerns from health practitioners relating to the potential for miscommunication, as differences in language and culture can cause misunderstandings that can have serious impacts on health outcomes and patient safety (Crawford, Candlin & Roger 2017). This chapter addresses frameworks for cross-cultural communication from theoretical and practical perspectives that explain how miscommunication between colleagues, and between health practitioners and patients may occur.

It is often the invisible unstated differences between cultural values, norms and expectations that can cause the most confusion and conflict between people. Individuality, direct communication and assertiveness are valued in the Australian and New Zealand health workplace. In Eastern cultures, however, there may be an avoidance of open conflict and disagreement in order to maintain harmony in the group. To ensure that we use a culturally aware approach in our interactions, it is important to take account of diverse communication styles, remain aware that cultures are dynamic and avoid making cultural assumptions about our colleagues. Good communication also avoids misdiagnosis and misunderstanding between health practitioners and patients.

When working in a culturally diverse context, health workers can promote effective **cross-cultural communication** through the strategies listed in the focus box, 'Ensuring effective cross-cultural communication'.

BOX 6.1

ENSURING EFFECTIVE CROSS-CULTURAL COMMUNICATION

- Have **cultural self-awareness**.
- Acknowledge, appreciate and respect cultural diversity, and understand cultural differences.
- Be aware of cultural variations in communication styles, such as in verbal and non-verbal communication and formal and informal forms of address.
- Be culturally sensitive and have the ability to adjust attitudes and behaviours to accommodate diverse cultural and religious beliefs, practices and behaviours.
- Have skills to accommodate and negotiate cultural conflicts and to communicate effectively with people from cultures different from one's own.

For effective cross-cultural communication to take place in healthcare settings, healthcare professionals also need to learn and practise **cultural competence**. The first step is to become aware that there are multiple ways in which any social interaction can be viewed and interpreted.

Cultural competence
An awareness of cultural diversity and the ability to communicate effectively and respectfully during interactions with people of different cultural backgrounds.

Viewing culture

Culturally based assumptions can contribute to mindsets such as **ethnocentrism**, **stereotypes**, **prejudice**, **racism** and **discrimination** (Salter, Adams & Perez 2018). Taken several steps further, these patterns of thought and action can lead to judgments about deviance and non-compliance; concepts which relate to one person's view that another person is not behaving in a way that is 'good', 'right' or 'appropriate'. In these circumstances, the stage is set for misunderstanding, dissatisfaction and conflict.

Ethnocentrism
Using one's own culture to evaluate another culture; one's own culture is generally considered to be superior.

Stereotype
Fixed and inflexible ideas about a social group.

Prejudice
Preconceived opinions or attitudes held by one group about another; often without basis in fact and often resistant to change despite the availability of new information.

Racism
Prejudice based on the physical characteristics of an ethnic group.

Discrimination
Behaviour that prevents members of one group having access to the opportunities available to others.

Values are the norms within a culture that determine what is acceptable or unacceptable. Although usually unspoken, they are integral to most of our actions, and many are expressed in the ways that we communicate. The hidden nature of values is a common cause of misunderstanding and offence between people of different cultures and traditions. Problems arise when a person acts in ways that are only congruent with the perspective that person holds. In any given interaction, even though people behave appropriately within their own established cultural practices, their own cultural biases do not take anyone else's perspectives into account. The interaction consequently occurs in a context where key ideas have been interpreted—and acted on—differently by the people involved. One health-related example is the use of language, a skill that encapsulates intangible ideas in ways that can be expressed to others. Commonly used words may not necessarily represent exactly the same ideas to the people who are expressing or interpreting them. One example is societal views of the roles of health professionals. Patients from societies where formality and status are important, such as China or India, may view their role in relationship with doctors and nurses differently to people who come from societies like Australia and New Zealand, which value a less formal, non-hierarchical relationship between colleagues and practitioners and patients.

Case activity 6.1 demonstrates some of the difficulties of cross-cultural encounters between staff in the workplace when one group stereotypes another.

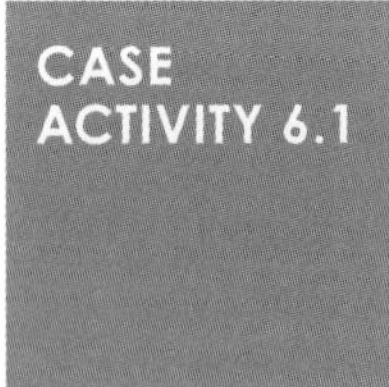

Stereotyping

Ali starts a new job as a social worker at a disability support service. Ali is a Muslim, originally from Ethiopia. He was 'headhunted' from another service, as he has a reputation for good outcomes with families who have children with disabilities. Ali is welcomed into the service and introduced to the wider team and management.

In his second week, Ali attends a team meeting. The meeting goes well and Ali makes a good contribution to the case review process, which is undertaken fortnightly. However, at the end of the meeting, Caroline, the team leader says, 'Some of you have raised concerns that Ali is "different" [meaning that he is an African Muslim man and therefore holds oppressive attitudes towards women], but that has nothing to do with his job and I need the team to work together.' Ali is completely shocked and offended. Ali is the only male social worker in the team. He explains to the team that he grew up with six sisters and that he has the utmost respect for women.

1. Has Caroline managed this situation appropriately?
2. What would you have done differently?
3. What could Caroline do now to address the potential ethnocentricity and stereotyping in this situation?

The journey towards cultural competence begins with questioning our own cultural assumptions.

Cultural competence

Cultural competence is demonstrated in our everyday actions within families, communities and workplaces. Cultural knowledge means a familiarity with, for example, the histories of migrant and refugee peoples, and the customs related to specific cultural groups. **Cultural sensitivity** refers to not assigning values such as 'right' or 'wrong' where there are known cultural differences unless those practices are illegal. As mentioned previously, culture is an integrated pattern of behaviour shared by a particular group of people. Competence implies that a degree of skill and proficiency is demonstrated in a certain field. When phrased together, cultural competence is defined as 'a set of congruent behaviours, attitudes, and policies that come together in a system, agency, or among professionals and enables that system, agency, or those professionals to work effectively in cross-cultural situations' (Cross, Bazron, Dennis & Isaacs 1989, p. 4). The requirement to be culturally competent has implications for individual health practitioners and for the organisations they work in.

Cultural sensitivity Acknowledging the legitimacy of cultural difference and embracing those differences during interactions with people from diverse cultures.

BOX 6.2

DEFINING CULTURAL COMPETENCE

For individuals, cultural competence is the process in which the professional:

> ...continually strives to effectively work within a culturally diverse context.

For organisations, cultural competence is:

> ...the integration and transformation of knowledge about individuals and groups of people into specific standards, policies, practices, and attitudes used in appropriate culturally diverse settings to increase the quality of services, thereby producing better outcomes.

Source: Adapted from Centre for Cultural Competence Australia 2013.

At an individual level, three key elements are commonly identified in the development of cultural competence. They are:

1. developing cultural awareness, including self-awareness about one's own culture and attitudes towards cultural differences
2. knowledge of and sensitivity to different cultural practices
3. the ability to use cross-cultural skills.

Self-awareness and self-examination are starting points for developing effective cultural competence skills. The opposite, a focus on 'the other', tends to perpetuate an 'us and them' way of thinking that is unhelpful (Stangor, Jhangiani & Tarry 2015). Identifying our own internalised beliefs and biases, including those deriving from our organisational and professional cultures, helps with understanding how these might impact on cross-cultural communication and relating. Awareness of our personal worldview paves the way for thinking about the perspectives held by others—people whose viewpoints and socialisation processes may be quite different from our own.

At an organisational level, Cross et al. (1989, p. 8) state five elements they consider essential in the development of cultural competence in a system or organisation. They are:

1. valuing diversity
2. having the capacity for cultural self-assessment
3. being conscious of the dynamics inherent when cultures interact
4. having institutionalised **cultural knowledge**
5. having developed adaptations to service delivery that reflect an understanding of cultural diversity.

Cultural knowledge Familiarity with culture-related evidence and issues.

Evidence of cultural competency in an organisation involves demonstration of these elements throughout the organisational structure and systems of policy-making, administration and services, as well as in the practice and attitudes of employees.

Cross-cultural communication is enhanced by organisational development and workforce development plans; staff recruitment and retention policies; staff orientation and professional development guidelines; and opportunities that are inclusive of cultural diversity in the workplace (Koh, Gracia & Alvarez 2014). Valuing workforce diversity and fostering culturally inclusive workplaces are fundamental to organisational cultural competence strategies.

Cultural competence in practice

Cultural competence in healthcare involves awareness, sensitivity, knowledge, attitudes and skills that support effective communication in the workplace and between health practitioners and patients.

At the interpersonal level, every cross-cultural interaction offers opportunities for learning and self-development. In addition, healthcare professionals can learn from:

- ongoing education about their own cultural values in relation to those of others
- seeking additional information in the literature
- developing therapeutic approaches to care based on cultural considerations
- seeking ongoing mentoring
- seeking or providing supervision of cultural practice.

Mason (1995) devised a continuum to portray the five stages in development of cultural competence identified by Cross et al. (1989). It is useful for organisations, services and healthcare professionals to reflect on this continuum regularly to assess their ongoing cross-cultural proficiency (see Figure 6.1). This self-examination will help individuals and organisations to work towards being proficient in their cross-cultural interactions both as practitioners and team members.

FIGURE 6.1 The cultural competency continuum

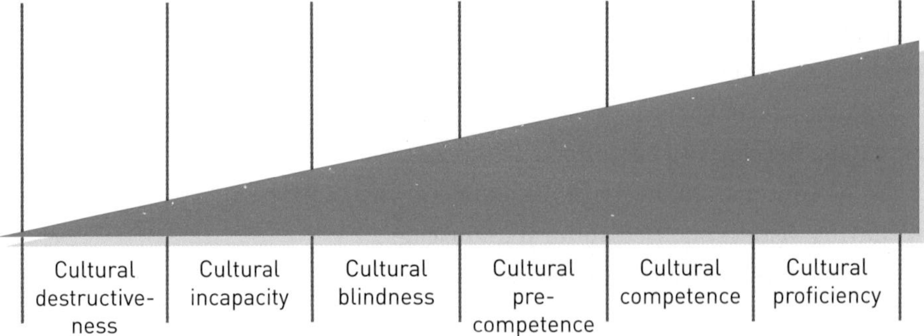

Cultural competence and communication

> ...cultures differ widely in body language, how to show (dis)respect, modesty and privacy concerns, expressions of (dis)agreement, and what constitutes

> courtesy, vary considerably across cultures. It is easy when dealing with someone from another culture to unwittingly give offence or to unintentionally make someone feel awkward, uncomfortable, or confused. (Bacal, Jansen & Smith 2006, p. 306)

Having considered the personal and organisational aspects of cultural competence, it is now important to review cultural influences on communication. An understanding of how context, **cultural value dimensions** and communication styles contribute to the cultural competence of healthcare professionals is essential for developing effective relationships with colleagues, patients and families in a culturally diverse context.

Cultural value dimensions
These include individualism and collectivism; power; distance; uncertainty; avoidance; masculinity; and femininity.

Culture, context and communication

A context is the setting or circumstances in which something occurs. Different rules can apply when relating in different contexts. Cultures incorporate many elements of context into their communication styles.

High-context groups

In high-context groups, people have close connections over a long period of time; cultural norms and values are not made explicit because it is expected that members know the rules due to their interaction within the group. A family is an example of a high-context environment. Characteristics of high-context communication include:

- less verbally explicit communication; less written or formal information
- more internalised understandings of what is communicated
- value placed in long-term relationships
- strong boundaries: who belongs versus who is an 'outsider'
- communication is indirect.

Low-context groups

In low-context groups, people may have many connections, but they are shorter in duration. In these groups, culturally acceptable behaviour may need to be made explicit so that those coming into the cultural environment know how to behave. Workplaces can be low-context places, especially for people coming from cultures that differ from the host or dominant culture of the working environment. Characteristics of low-context communication include:

- rule-oriented; people play by external rules
- more knowledge is contained in published rules that are public, external and accessible

- separation of time, space, activities and relationships
- more interpersonal connections, but of shorter duration
- communication is direct
- task-centred: decisions and activities focus on what needs to be done
- more division of responsibilities.

Cultural value dimensions

Hofstede (1980) identified a range of cultural values in the context of organisational management systems. Four of those dimensions have particular relevance to communication in the healthcare sector: individualism and collectivism, power distance, uncertainty avoidance, and masculine versus feminine cultures.

1 Individualism and collectivism

According to Hofstede (2011), this dimension encompasses the amount of independence a person values.

Traits often found in *individualistic cultures* include:

- Independence is valued.
- Decisions are made without reference to others.
- Personal identity revolves around the 'I'.
- Personal goals and achievement are striven for.
- The rights of the individual are paramount; laws often protect choices and freedom of speech.
- There is free movement between groups.
- Communication is direct and open.
- Assertiveness is valued.

Traits common in *collectivist cultures* include:

- Interdependence and dependence exist within family networks.
- The wellbeing of others is taken into account when making decisions.
- 'We' is more important than 'I'.
- Obedience is expected and considered positively.
- The rights of the family are perceived as important.
- Rules provide security, conformity and harmony.
- There are strong links to one group.
- Communication is more indirect.
- Concern for maintenance of the group is paramount.

Individualism is more common in Western cultures, such as in the United Kingdom, United States, Canada, Australia and New Zealand, while collective cultures are more likely to include those from Africa (e.g. Nigeria, Ethiopia), the Middle East (e.g. Iraq, Iran, Syria), Asia (e.g. China, South Korea, Singapore, Malaysia), Pacific nations (e.g. Fiji), South America (e.g. Brazil, Colombia), much of Mediterranean Europe and the Indigenous cultures of Australia, New Zealand and North America (Hofstede Insights 2019).

2 Power distance

The term 'power distance' refers to the societal importance given to the distance between the position or status of an individual in relation to others in the workplace, community, family or other institutions. Cultures differ in the extent to which they expect, impose and accept hierarchical differences (Hofstede, Hofstede & Minkov 2010). In an organisation, the concept of power distance refers to the acceptance of an unequal distribution of status between members within that organisation (Hofstede 2001). Power distance can be described as *high* or *low* (Hofstede 2011).

High power distance is associated with collectivist cultures and has the following characteristics:

- People in higher or more powerful positions openly demonstrate their rank.
- People of lesser status are not given important work and are expected to get clear guidance from above.
- Arrogance is expressed by authority figures.
- Humility is expressed by those with lower status.
- There is a large gap in status between the powerful and the less powerful, and between employers and employees.
- Politics is prone to dictatorship.
- Societies tend more towards class divisions.

Low power distance is associated with individualistic cultures and has the following characteristics:

- People in higher or more powerful positions treat those with lesser status with respect.
- People of lesser status are entrusted with important assignments.
- There is a smaller gap in status between the powerful and less powerful, and between employers and employees.
- Politics is prone to be more democratic.
- Societies tend more towards equality.

High power distance cultures include many from Asia (e.g. China, India, South Korea), Arabic-speaking nations, much of Latin America, and Russia, while low power cultures include those from the United States, Canada, Australia and New Zealand (Hofstede Insights 2019). These concepts are explored in Case activity 6.2.

CASE ACTIVITY 6.2

Cultural value dimensions

Zahra is a senior social worker. She works for a child disability support service that is contracted to provide care for high-needs children who have been fostered. The work is complex and demanding, involving finding suitable foster care homes for children removed from the care of their families by social services. Zahra, originally from Iraq, is very experienced and is well regarded by her colleagues and the families with whom she works. She receives a phone call from Jane, a foster mother who has in her care a child named Thomas, who has multiple care needs, including overnight cares. Thomas is very settled and happy with Jane and her family. Jane tells Zahra that she has been advised by the disability support service business manager, Hong-Won, that she must now pay tax on her childcare payments. The foster mother's contract with the child disability support service states that the payment for her services (which are modest) are tax-free. If Jane has to pay tax on her payments, she will no longer be able to cover the costs of caring for Thomas.

Zahra takes up the issue with the newly appointed business manager, Hong-Won, politely pointing out that the carer support contract states that the payment is tax-free. Hong-Won is Chinese and has come from the corporate sector. Hong-Won insists that Jane must pay the tax. He does not understand the tax codes that apply to these payments. Zahra adds that it was extremely difficult to find a foster mother of Jane's calibre to undertake the 24/7 care of a very high-needs child and that she does not want to jeopardise the placement. Hong-Won becomes agitated and insists that Jane must pay. Zahra is getting nowhere and decides that it is best to leave Hong-Won's office immediately. When she returns to her desk, Hong-Won follows her and stands over her shouting, 'Who are you to question me?' At this point, colleagues who have overheard the shouting ask Hong-Won to stop shouting at Zahra.

The business manager, Hong-Won, comes from a high-power distance culture. He thinks that Zahra should respect his decisions unquestioningly. In his view, Zahra is being disrespectful to him and therefore he has every right to challenge her in the way he did. This situation has caused him to 'lose face' and is embarrassing, and therefore he has reacted to emphasise his status, which he considers to be at a higher level than Zahra's.

1. What cultural value dimensions are at play in this situation?
2. Has Zahra managed this situation appropriately?
3. What factors need to be considered in effecting a solution?
4. What should Zahra do now?

3 Uncertainty avoidance

The term 'uncertainty avoidance' refers to the extent to which an individual feels threatened by uncertainty, ambiguity and fear of the unknown. It is a cultural measure of the degree to which people tolerate risk and ambiguity (Hofstede et al. 2010).

As is the case with power distance, uncertainty avoidance can be described as *high* or *low* (Hofstede 2011). High-uncertainty avoidance cultures tend to be found in countries with a long history and homogenous rather than multicultural populations. Common traits include:

- Risks (even if calculated) are avoided.
- Introduction or acceptance of changes and new concepts is more difficult.
- Values are clear; there is discomfort with ambiguity.
- People are uncomfortable if rules are unclear.
- Individuals often experience high levels of stress.
- Job stability is valued.

Low-uncertainty avoidance cultures tend to be found in countries with a young history, and where the population is culturally diverse because of migration flows from varied national backgrounds. Common traits include:

- Risks are considered part of business or daily life.
- New concepts are accepted and encouraged.
- Ambiguity is tolerated.
- People are relaxed even when rules are unclear.
- Moving from one job to another is acceptable.

High uncertainty cultures include those from Greece, Portugal, Japan, Israel and Spain, while low uncertainty cultures include the United States, Singapore, Jamaica, Ireland, Sweden and China (Hofstede Insights 2019). These concepts are explored in Case activity 6.3.

CASE ACTIVITY 6.3

High uncertainty avoidance culture

Mrs Cho is a 75-year-old woman who migrated from Seoul, Korea, five years ago with her husband to join their son, a businessman. Mrs Cho does not speak English and her husband has limited English.

Recently, Mrs Cho has been suffering from fatigue, shortness of breath, loss of appetite, weight loss and gradual muscle wasting, along with intermittent fever. The general practitioner (GP) orders several diagnostic tests. The results of the tests are sent to the GP and, although nothing is found, he does not contact Mrs Cho to tell her that the tests are negative. She becomes very anxious about why she has not been contacted about the test results. The GP explains that she would only be contacted if there was a positive result, not a negative result. In Korea, Mrs Cho would have been given a copy of her results. The GP refers Mrs Cho to the gastroenterology clinic at the local hospital for further investigations.

Mrs Cho receives a letter from the hospital, stating: 'You have been referred to the gastroenterology clinic by your general practitioner for further investigations, and you will be receiving an appointment in due course.' Mr and Mrs Cho become very anxious, as there is no time frame for an appointment; in the meantime, Mrs Cho is becoming increasingly unwell. The family attempts to contact the clinic to ask when they can be seen. They are repeatedly put through to people who cannot help. Mr and Mrs Cho decide to fly back to Seoul and seek medical care there.

Mr and Mrs Cho have come from a high-uncertainty avoidance society. What strategies could be employed by the health professional to improve communication and minimise uncertainty in this situation?

4 Masculine versus feminine cultures

Masculinity versus femininity within a cultural context refers to the degree to which the group values and reinforces traditional roles, and the degree to which a culture is focused on tasks or relationships (Hofstede 1998).

Hofstede (2011) outlines a number of common traits found in masculine and feminine cultures. In **masculine cultures**, these include:

Masculine culture Gender-based cultural/societal preference for assertiveness, ambition, control, competition, achievement and technical expertise.

- Societies are more task-focused.
- Achievement, wealth and expansion are priorities in life.
- Settling conflicts in an aggressive manner is acceptable.
- Women and men have different roles in society: there is greater differentiation and discrimination between genders.
- Professionals often 'live to work', meaning longer working hours and short holidays.

Traits found in **feminine cultures** include:

Feminine culture Gender-based cultural/societal preference or focus on nurture, care, sharing, quality of life, people and relationships.

- Societies are more relationship focused.
- Family, relationships and quality of life are prioritised.
- Conflicts are ideally solved through negotiation.
- Men and women tend to share equal positions in society: there is lesser differentiation and discrimination between genders.
- Professionals 'work to live', meaning longer holidays and flexible working hours.

Masculine cultures are found in Japan, the United States, the German-speaking world, Ireland, the United Kingdom, Mexico and Italy, while feminine cultures are found in Sweden, the Netherlands, Spain, Thailand, Korea, Portugal and Iran (Hofstede Insights 2019).

Cultural values and communication styles

The rules that govern communication styles reflect the importance societies give to hierarchies, rank and social class. Communication rules vary between cultures. There are significant differences between the communication styles of high-context and low-context cultures. High-context cultures use *indirect communication* styles, while low-context cultures employ a more *direct communication* style (Hofstede & Bond 1988). Note that these are generalisations and that individuals often combine aspects of different styles.

1 Directness of communication

Direct communicators are forthright. The words they use clearly convey the intended message. No interpretation is expected from the recipient because the communicator takes responsibility for the clarity of what is being expressed. Giving and receiving information is the focus of this style, which is often found in Western countries where context does not have a great influence on communication. In these settings, there tends to be wide cultural variation among the population, and individualistic priorities such as independence and self-reliance dominate. Consequently, assumptions about contextual influences on communication are not generalised. Hofstede and Bond (1988) outline characteristics of direct communicators, suggesting that they:

- assert themselves
- respond with 'No' readily
- use 'I' more often
- value being proactive
- use linear thought processes
- apply directness when making a point or conclusions
- focus on what is said when listening
- do not personalise disagreement
- confront those with higher status directly.

Direct communicators can be misunderstood as aggressive, disrespectful or rude, arrogant, not collaborative, superficial, lacking perceptiveness and as provoking confrontation (Hofstede & Bond 1988).

Indirect communicators are not forthright. The intended message is embedded in a complex, often non-verbal delivery, where recipients need to interpret the meaning being conveyed. Techniques such as pauses and silence, as well as tone of voice, implication and understatement, are clues to guide recipients' understanding of the message. Communicating in this way is used to maintain harmony and to 'save face', so that tension, conflict and uncomfortable situations can be avoided. This style is often found in cultures where context is important and generally understood by a population that tends to be limited in its cultural variation. Such populations are likely to demonstrate collectivist qualities such as prioritising interdependence and social relationships. In cultures where indirect communication predominates, 'people develop deep and often unconscious understandings of what is expected in that culture. Because of shared expectations about behaviour, the context can be altered by the speaker to convey information' (Joyce 2012).

Hofstede and Bond (1998) suggest that indirect communicators:

- tend to not assert themselves
- consider 'No' responses as not permissible, especially when communicating with those in authority
- use 'we' more often
- value following established practices
- use lengthy thought processes
- consider directness in stating points or conclusions as inappropriate
- focus on what is implied when listening
- personalise disagreement
- do not confront those with higher status directly but go through an appropriate channel.

Indirect communicators can be misunderstood as evasive, lacking self-confidence, lacking ability to take control, lacking understanding, not listening, not willing to seek resolutions, ineffective, oversensitive or lacking initiative (Joyce 2012).

2 Formality of communication

Formality and informality in forms of address also reflect how cultures interact. This section is adapted from the Waitemata DHB, eCALD® Service's (2018a) *Toolkit for Working in a Culturally Diverse Workplace*. Again, the following observations are generalised information and not applicable to individuals, because most people have a combination of aspects of different styles.

Formal communicators tend to:

- value formality
- use titles or family names
- value time as cyclical; relationships take precedence over tasks or appointments
- value silence to process information
- tolerate physical proximity more easily (e.g. in queues)
- generally reserve touch for family and close friends—or it is not permitted in public at all
- value soft or no eye contact, or eye contact of short duration
- value control of emotional display, to varying degrees
- control body language
- use less or no facial expression.

Formal communicators can be misunderstood as unfriendly, cold or unwilling to develop a relationship, unwilling to engage or lack initiative, intrusive, rude, evasive, not to be trusted, disinterested or distant.

Informal communicators tend to:

- value informality
- use first names
- value time as linear, and value punctuality
- avoid silences, and can be very verbal
- value physical distance or space
- tolerate touch more readily (e.g. handshakes)
- value direct eye contact
- value expression of emotion, including anger
- readily animate body language
- use more facial expressions.

Informal communicators can be misunderstood as forward, insensitive, rude, disrespectful, lacking wisdom, intrusive, threatening, lacking self-respect and indiscreet.

3 Non-verbal components of communication

As was discussed in Chapter 2, two-thirds of all communication is non-verbal (Hogan & Stubbs 2003). Non-verbal communication can portray a message via the tone, volume and pace of speech. Messages can also be conveyed consciously and unconsciously by a variety of body signals. These include physical features such as facial expressions, eye contact, body positioning, gestures and proximity to others (Ali 2018). For example, cultures vary widely in how they use non-verbal greetings such as:

- a smile or inclination of the head
- a handshake, using one hand or both hands together
- a *hongi*: touching noses
- a kiss on one cheek or both cheeks
- a bow with a slight inclination of the body, or a deep bow
- raising a hat
- a hug
- a salute or wave
- a *namaste:* hands together in prayer position.

In some cultures, the appropriate order to greet individuals, members of a group or a family is a further non-verbal consideration to take into account; this will depend on the group's culturally determined seniority or status.

During interactions in a culturally diverse context, keep in mind cultural norms about non-verbal behaviours, such as eye contact, the use of touch and physical positioning of the people involved. In Western cultures, it is considered polite for people to hold eye contact during verbal communication; however, this is not the case for many Pacific and Asian cultures (Culture Crossing Guide 2014; Government of Canada 2018). Touch can also have a powerful influence on communication. Whereas some Asian and Mediterranean cultures place high priority on touch during interactions, people from a more Western perspective may find this intrusive and threatening. Physical positioning encompasses the relative distance between those who are interacting. Westerners tend to prefer maintaining a reasonable distance from other people, while many other cultures are comfortable being in close proximity.

Some strategies to help avoid making assumptions when working in a culturally diverse environment are outlined in the focus box.

BOX 6.3

AVOIDING ASSUMPTIONS

Considerations for working with colleagues or patients in a culturally diverse context:

- Note that names, appearances and places of birth are unlikely to be sufficient for providing useful information on which to base culturally effective communication. It is best to check how others identify culturally when you are unsure.
- Discuss mutually acceptable ways of showing respect and acknowledgment of potential cultural differences during your interactions.
- If you are unsure about the cultural norms of the person you are communicating with, begin the interaction in a formal manner, then modify your approach as indicated by your subsequent conversations.
- Be aware of generalising about members of a culture. While identifying a group's style of communication alerts us to potential areas of difference, individuals may differ from other members of their group. Many migrants have spent time in different countries, integrating values from host cultures; some live in multicultural families; others may be acculturated to the society in which they live. Some may be the first generation, or their families may have been settled in the country for many generations. Pre-judging people based on visible differences can result in stereotyping. Listening, asking and observing are the keys to good communication and relationships.
- Avoid equating a person's accent or language skills with their level of intelligence or credibility.
- When working with non-English-speaking clients and family members, avoid using colleagues (who may not be fluent in the native language) as interpreters. Also avoid asking colleagues to be cultural advisers when working with patients. You may place your colleague in an awkward position if there are cultural dimensions involved, such as social status or sanctions on men and women interacting, particularly in situations where intimate care or questioning is required. It is also worth remembering that many countries, such as China and India, have multiple ethnic groups, languages and religions within their borders. Your colleague is unlikely to be an expert on all of them.

Skills in practice

Avoiding assumptions

John and Amena have just commenced working as graduate social workers in their local healthcare service. John strikes up a conversation with Amena.

John:	Hi Amena, how are you doing?
Amena:	Good, and you?
John:	Great... You have an unusual name, where is it from?
Amena:	Oh, it's an Afghani name... my parents are from Afghanistan.
John:	*(smiles)* That's cool... so I guess you were born here... you sound like an Aussie?
Amena:	Yeah, I was born here and my sister came with my parents from Afghanistan. And what about you... you sound like an American? *(smiling)*
John:	Haha. No, I'm Canadian. I have been living in Australia for more than 10 years now. I think I'm an Aussie as I love the cricket and rugby league here. So Amena, I was wondering....

What's happening here?

This exchange provides an example of how it is not easy to identify someone's cultural identity by their name, accent and their appearance. From reading this example we learn that when enquiring about culture, it is important to ask a person about their cultural identity rather than making assumptions based on generalised or stereotypical information. It can be offensive to ask someone where they come from because this question assumes someone comes from another country. Instead, showing respect and being open-minded enhances rapport and exchanges of cultural information.

Language barriers and the use of interpreters

Language can be a barrier to cross-cultural communication in healthcare settings. Professional interpreters are essential when communicating with clients who are not proficient in understanding or communicating in English. Professionally trained interpreters provide clients with a safe, private and effective means of communication with healthcare professionals. The right to effective communication is guaranteed for healthcare consumers under human rights legislation, and reinforced through various codes such as the Australian Charter of Healthcare

Rights (Australian Commission on Safety and Quality in Healthcare 2015) and New Zealand's Code of Health and Disability Commissioner's Consumer's Rights (Health and Disability Commissioner 2009).

In the United States, a qualified interpreter is defined as:

> an individual who has been assessed for professional skills, demonstrates a high level of proficiency in at least two languages and has the appropriate training and experience to interpret with skill and accuracy while adhering to the National Code of Ethics and Standards of Practice published by the National Council on Interpreting in Health Care. (National Council on Interpreting in Health Care 2008, p. 7).

An example of such a code in Australasia can be found on the Interpreting New Zealand (2015) website. It is important for healthcare professionals to be familiar with organisational policy about when interpreting services should be used, and how those sessions should be arranged and conducted. All such policies should have a section relating to the 'assessment of need', and particular attention should be paid to this by staff caring for CALD patients. Interpreters provide far more than just a service that translates the words of one language into another. Their cultural knowledge is integral to creating an environment of trust and open communication, which can enhance interactions between CALD patients and healthcare professionals. An interpreter-assisted environment can help non-English-speaking patients feel respected and reassured that they do have a voice (Waitemata DHB, eCALD® Services 2018b). Trained interpreters have been shown to decrease communication errors, increase patient comprehension, improve clinical outcomes, and increase satisfaction with communication and clinical services for those with limited or no English language proficiency (Squires 2017). Failing to use a trained interpreter runs the risk of inadequate communication, which could result in misdiagnosis and inappropriate management and treatment. Untrained interpreters include family members, friends, support persons, volunteers, staff—or anyone who speaks the required language but has not had professional interpreter training. There are some situations in which untrained interpreters may be used, including when patients insist, when the situation is urgent, or when simple or non-medical-related information needs to be communicated. Be very clear, however, that communicating important information, such as that related to consent for surgery, has potential professional, organisational and legal implications if a trained interpreter is not present.

Some important points to consider when planning to work with an interpreter are outlined in the focus box, 'Working with interpreters'.

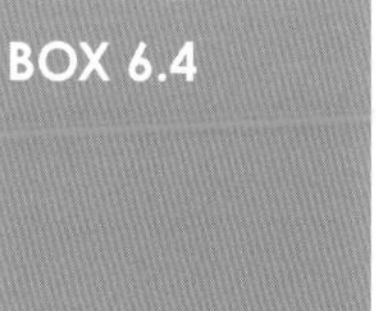

WORKING WITH INTERPRETERS

Examples of questions to ask during pre-briefing

- To improve engagement:
  - Ask about appropriate greetings and gestures.
  - Ask about any customs you should observe (especially for home visits).
- For the assessment process:
  - If using colloquialisms (e.g. 'you've got to take the bull by the horns') to elicit responses from patients, find out if the translated words can create your expected responses. If not, find out if there are there any equivalent terms in the native language.
  - Finding out relevant cultural information and setting ground rules will help you interact effectively with your patient.

Rules of engagement in an interpreting session

While speaking through an interpreter, always engage with your patient directly. Even though you cannot understand what is being said, you can still observe non-verbal communication from the patient (and family members), as well as maintaining eye contact and remaining engaged with them. If you start to converse directly with an interpreter, you are no longer engaging with the patient and may miss a lot of non-verbal information.

Debriefing

Debriefing does not need to be lengthy; however, sufficient time should be made available for this process, especially if the interpreting session becomes very emotional. The purpose of debriefing is to:

- summarise the session, and establish whether objectives were met
- gather further cultural information, if necessary
- clarify any cultural issues and interpretation of words or concepts
- assess whether the interpreter is affected by the content of the session, and address this if necessary
- plan follow-up procedures or appointments as appropriate
- discuss any aspect of the professional relationship, if necessary.

The three main phases in an interpreter-facilitated session with a health professional are pre-briefing, patient interaction and debriefing. For these sessions, it is beneficial to book an additional half-hour per patient beyond the time allocated for an English-speaking patient. This allows sufficient time for all the phases to proceed effectively (Waitemata DHB, eCALD® Services 2018b). The pre-brief allows health workers to establish rapport with interpreters, clarify the type of interpreting method preferred and state the objectives of the session. It is also an opportunity to set ground rules, such as confidentiality, and to arrange seating appropriately.

To engage the patient and ensure an effective interaction, it is important to set up the room well. For a face-to-face meeting, arrange the chairs in a triangle and make sure that your focus stays on the patient, not the interpreter. It is also important to keep your focus on the patient when using a telephone interpreting service. Structuring a session is important for all parties to ensure there are clear expectations about how the interaction will work. This process begins with greeting the patient and family members or support people, directing them to pre-arranged seating, introducing yourself and outlining your role. It also includes assuring the patient of confidentiality, clarifying the mode of interpreting to be used and explaining that everything said will be interpreted. The need for clinicians to demonstrate that confidentiality is the priority cannot be emphasised highly enough. CALD patients are often deeply concerned about the privacy of confidential information related to themselves and their families (Waitemata DHB, eCALD® Services 2018b).

Elements of the debrief session are outlined in the 'Working with interpreters' focus box. Note that it is important to check whether the interpreter has been personally affected by the session and then, if necessary, to arrange for any support that may be required.

Skills in practice

Working with interpreters

Monique is an interpreter who has been engaged to assist Dr Murray to relay information about a diagnosis to his patient Mrs Wong.

Dr Murray: Hi Monique, today we are seeing Mrs Wong and her husband (Mr Wong) and daughter (Jenny) for the results of her breast biopsy. Unfortunately, it's not good news and it may be a difficult session.

Monique: Thank you for letting me know before the session Dr Murray so that I can prepare myself. In the past, I have encountered some Chinese families who get very upset when I've interpreted bad news directly to the patient prior to them knowing. There were instances where some families who understand a little bit of English insist that I do not interpret the bad news to the patient. This is because in their culture they do not expect their loved ones to receive bad news directly for fear that the patient may give up hope. To avoid upsetting the family, could you talk to the family prior to us meeting with the family and patient together, and ask them how they could support the difficult conversation with the patient?

Dr Murray: I am glad you informed me about the potential issue, and I am more than happy to talk to the family first. I will call Mr Wong and Jenny to come in. Can you let me know the protocol for greeting the family, and is there anything else you wanted me to know before I call them in?

Monique: It's important to acknowledge Mrs Wong's husband first. It would be great if you could use the first-person language—e.g. 'I am sorry Mr Wong and Jenny, if only I had better news for you today'—and I will interpret accordingly. Also, if I need to pause to ask you a question, I will use this hand gesture. Another thing is, some families do not understand the role of an interpreter and are not familiar with the interpreting process. Explaining to them my role, assuring confidentiality and that I am required to interpret everything that is said in the session, and to pause for me to interpret at regular intervals after two to three sentences would be most helpful.

Dr Murray: Great. Let's set up the room before I call them in ....

What's happening here?

This exchange reinforces how important it is to understand how to work with interpreters. Such understanding will enable control of the interpreting process and achieve a better outcome for an interpreter-assisted communication. This understanding is especially important when working with families. Interpreters can advise you about greeting protocols to ensure respectful engagement with patients and families from different cultures. Some migrant families may not be familiar with the doctor's legal obligation, treatment consent process, interpreter's role, interpreting process and confidentiality. An interpreter can assist with promoting this understanding. Note how important the pre-brief was in preparing the interpreter for any potential issues, or potentially emotional content. Interpreters should also be informed that, if they are affected by the emotional conversation, there will be time for a debrief at the end of the session to ensure they feel supported.

Bringing it all together

Cultural viewpoints have a significant influence on communication and, ultimately, on relationships. Relationships underpin much of the work involved in healthcare. High-quality care, especially in an increasingly multicultural environment, depends on effective communication between employers and employees; between employees and their colleagues; and between health providers and consumers.

Healthcare professionals who have a clear idea of their own worldviews can look beyond their personal interpretations of a situation to consider the perspectives of others; perspectives that may involve different ideas about issues such as power, respect and the clarity and directness of communication. Healthcare professionals who are culturally aware of their own values, attitudes, beliefs and practices and are able to adjust their communication and behaviours. They can accommodate cultural variance and are well-prepared for effective cross-cultural communication. There are further 'Tips for effective cross-cultural communication' in the focus box. Proficiency in cross-cultural communication is far more a journey than a destination. There is something to be gained from every cross-cultural exchange. Each learning opportunity is a contribution to personal development and to future interactions in the health workforce.

BOX 6.5

TIPS FOR EFFECTIVE CROSS-CULTURAL COMMUNICATION

- If possible, think through the dimensions of a cross-cultural interaction before engaging in it.
- Assess the components that may directly influence your communication, and plan how you might address any potential difficulties.
- Check and use the correct pronunciation of names.
- Check and use the preferred way of addressing a person (e.g. a respectful title; formal or informal manner).
- Speak clearly and avoid speaking quickly.
- Use concrete language rather than abstract terms; avoid terminology such as idioms, irony, sarcasm, slang and jargon.
- Be patient, receptive and listen carefully.
- Ask open-ended questions.
- Be aware that repeated 'yes' answers can mean different things in different cultural contexts; a 'yes' response may not indicate an understanding of what has been communicated.
- Ensure that the other person understands what you have said, and that you understand what they have said. Ask the person to explain what you have said, then paraphrase those comments back to the other person to check that you have understood what has been expressed.
- Use an accredited professional interpreter when working with patients who are unable to communicate effectively in English.
- Reflect on each cross-cultural interaction to identify what went well and where you need to learn more.

Reflect and apply

Think of a cross-cultural situation where you interacted with someone and you perceived awkwardness, or there was evidence of conflict or misunderstanding.

- What was the context of the scenario (Where? When? Who?)
- What roles were involved? (Yours? Other people present?)
- What led to the difficulty you experienced?
- What were you feeling?
- How was the situation resolved?
- What did you do afterwards?
- What would you do if you were faced with the same situation again?

Conclusion

This chapter discussed the broad meaning of culture and the influence of culture on communication. In healthcare settings, health professionals need to be culturally competent to work effectively with cultural groups different from their own, and organisations need to develop the standards, policies and practices that enable quality care and good outcomes for all the cultural groups served. Significant variations in communication occur across cultures. Understanding how language and communication styles vary across cultures leads to knowledge about challenges that can arise. This chapter focused on the skills and attitudes needed by healthcare professionals to enable them to communicate effectively with managers, colleagues, patients and families in a culturally diverse context.

Completing the activities in this chapter will enhance healthcare professionals' knowledge about communicating across cultures, as well as sharpening their culture-focused skills and behaviours. The focus boxes highlight the most important concepts in cross-cultural communication. The authors encourage readers to seek more culture-related information and training opportunities related to their field of practice so that they can improve cross-cultural interactions in the workplace and with clients in clinical and community settings.

SUMMARY POINTS

- Providing high-quality safe and effective healthcare in a culturally diverse environment depends on effective communication between employers and employees; employees and their colleagues; and between healthcare providers and consumers.
- Cultures are comprised of mutually understood, learned behaviours and meanings that are socially transferred among groups of people who have shared

characteristics. Culture is a dynamic process and social rules within various groups continue to change.

- Cultural diversity can apply to a group of any size, ranging from a committee or a multidisciplinary healthcare team through to a residential community, corporation or an entire nation.
- Identifying our own internalised values, beliefs and biases helps us to understand how these might impact on cross-cultural communication and interrelationships between patients and colleagues.
- Perspective refers to seeing and interpreting the world from a particular standpoint.
- The rules that govern communication styles reflect the importance societies give to hierarchies, rank and social class. Communication rules vary between cultures.
- Organisations enable good cross-cultural communication when policies and resources are available to foster a culturally competent workforce. Cultural competency training can assist healthcare professionals to develop the skills, attitudes and behaviours needed to communicate effectively across cultures.

CRITICAL THINKING QUESTIONS

1. Looking beyond your own culture, think of three cultural groups different from your own. For each of them, find out:
   a. how respect is demonstrated to others
   b. how to communicate with authority figures
   c. how to interact with members of the opposite sex
   d. how to work in a team setting
   e. how to express distress and conflict.
2. Write down 10 slang expressions you commonly use when talking to colleagues, friends and family (e.g. 'throw the baby out with the bathwater', 'hang on', 'lose the plot'). Think about how these expressions might be received by someone from a cultural background different to your own. What other ways could you convey the same meaning without using slang?
3. Identify some of the biases you hold about healthcare professionals from cultural backgrounds different from your own. How might these biases make effective teamwork and communication challenging?

Group activity

Cross-cultural interactions

Think about your cross-cultural interactions with patients or with colleagues in the clinical environment. Take turns to discuss these with your study groups or via your subject discussion site. Were you mindful of the way you were communicating? Identify commonalities in the communication exchanges of group members and brainstorm how you may have approached an interaction differently.

WEBLINKS

CALD courses and resources

Enhancing CALD Cultural Competence:
www.ecald.com

Health.Vic (Victorian Government):
www2.health.vic.gov.au/about/populations/cald-health

Hofstede Insights:
www.hofstede-insights.com

Cultural competence

Centre for Culture, Ethnicity and Health:
www.ceh.org.au/culturalcompetence

Cross-cultural Health Resources

EthnoMed:
https://ethnomed.org/cross-cultural-health

Multicultural Health Communication Service (NSW Government):
www.mhcs.health.nsw.gov.au

Queensland Health (Queensland Government):
www.health.qld.gov.au/multicultural/health_workers/support_tools

REFERENCES

Ali, M. (2018). Communication skills 3: Non-verbal communication. *Nursing Times*, 114(2), 41–2.

Aluttis, C., Bishaw, T. & Frank, M.W. (2014). The workforce for health in a globalized context: Global shortages and international migration. *Global Health Action*, 7(1), 23611. http://dx.doi.org/10.3402/gha.v7.23611.

Australian Bureau of Statistics. (2012). *Cultural Diversity in Australia: Reflecting a Nation: Stories from the 2011 Census 2012–2013*. Canberra: Australian Bureau of Statistics. Retrieved from www.abs.gov.au/ausstats/abs@.nsf/lookup/2071.0main+features902012–2013.

Australian Commission on Safety and Quality in Healthcare. (2015). *Australian Charter of Healthcare Rights*. Retrieved from www.safetyandquality.gov.au/national-priorities/charter-of-healthcare-rights.

Bacal, K., Jansen, P. & Smith, K. (2006). Developing cultural competence in accordance with the Health Practitioners Competence Assurance Act. *NZFP*, 33(5), 305–9.

Betancourt, J.R., Green, A.R. & Carrillo, J.E. (2018). Cross-cultural care and communication. *UpToDate*, 26 March. Retrieved from www.uptodate.com/contents/cross-cultural-care-and-communication.

Centre for Cultural Competence Australia. (2013). *Defining Cultural Competence*. Sydney: Centre for Cultural Competence Australia. Retrieved from http://ccca.com.au/Competence-Vs-Awareness.

Charmaz, K. (2014). Grounded theory in global perspective: Reviews by international researchers. *Qualitative Inquiry*, 20(9), 1074–84. doi:10.1177/1077800414545235.

Crawford, T., Candlin, S. & Roger, P. (2017). New perspectives on understanding cultural diversity in nurse–patient communication. *Collegian*, 24(1), 63–9. doi:10.1016/j.colegn.2015.09.001.

Cross, T.L., Bazron, B.J., Dennis, K.W. & Isaacs, M.R. (1989). *Toward a Culturally Competent System of Care (Vol. 1).* Child and Adolescent Service System Program (CASSP) Technical Assistance Center, Georgetown University Child Development Center. Washington, DC: National Institute of Mental Health.

Culture Crossing Guide. (2014). *New Zealand.* Retrieved from http://guide.culturecrossing.net/basics_business_student_details.php?Id=7&CID=148.

Government of Canada. (2018). *Country Insights—Intercultural Issues.* Ottawa: Global Affairs Canada. Retrieved from www.international.gc.ca/cil-cai/country_insights-apercus_pays/countryinsights-apercuspays.aspx?lang=eng.

Health and Disability Commissioner. (2009). *The Code of Rights.* Retrieved from www.hdc.org.nz/your-rights/about-the-code/code-of-health-and-disability-services-consumers-rights.

Hofstede, G. (1980). *Culture's Consequences: International Differences in Work-related Values.* Beverly Hills, CA: Sage Publications.

Hofstede, G. (1998). *Masculinity and Femininity: The Taboo Dimension of National Cultures.* Thousand Oaks, CA: Sage Publications.

Hofstede, G. (2001). *Culture's Consequences: Comparing Values, Behaviours, Institutions and Organisations Across Nations* (2nd edn). Thousand Oaks, CA: Sage Publications.

Hofstede, G. (2011). Dimensionalizing cultures: The Hofstede model in context. *Readings in Psychology and Culture*, 2(1), 5–13. https://doi.org/10.9707/2307-0919.1014.

Hofstede, G. & Bond, M.H. (1988). The Confucius connection: From cultural roots to economic growth. *Organizational Dynamics*, 16, 4–21.

Hofstede, G., Hofstede, G.J. & Minkov, M. (2010). *Cultures and Organizations: Software of the Mind. Intercultural Cooperation and Its Importance for Survival* (3rd edn) (pp. 53–233). New York: McGraw-Hill.

Hofstede Insights. (2019). *Country Comparison Tool.* Retrieved from www.hofstede-insights.com.

Hogan, K. & Stubbs, R. (2003). *Can't Get Through: Eight Barriers to Communication.* Los Angeles, CA: Pelican Publishing Company.

Horvat, L., Horey, D., Romios, P. & Kis-Rigo, J. (2014). Cultural competence education for health professionals. *Cochrane Database of Systematic Reviews*, 5, art. no. CD009405.

Interpreting New Zealand. (2015). *Code of Ethics.* Retrieved from www.interpret.org.nz.

Joyce, C. (2012). The impact of direct and indirect communication. *Independent Voice*, November. Retrieved from https://uiowa.edu/conflictmanagement/sites/uiowa.edu.conflictmanagement/files/Direct%20and%20Indirect%20Communication.pdf.

Koh, H.K., Gracia, J.N. & Alvarez, M.E. (2014). Culturally and linguistically appropriate services—advancing health with CLAS. *New England Journal of Medicine*, 371(3), 108–201.

Mason, J.L. (1995). *Cultural Competence Self-Assessment Questionnaire: A Manual for Users.* Portland, OR: Research and Training Center on Family Support and Children's Mental Health, Portland State University.

National Council on Interpreting in Health Care. (2008). *The Terminology of Healthcare Interpreting: A Glossary of Terms.* Retrieved from www.ncihc.org/assets/documents/NCIHC%20Terms%20Final080408.pdf.

Office of Multicultural Interests. (2009). *Working Definitions of Terms.* Government of Western Australia, Department of Local Government and Communities, Office of Multicultural Interests.

Ono, T., Lafortune, G. & Schoenstein, M. (2013). Health workforce planning in OECD countries: A review of 26 projection models from 18 countries. *OECD Health Working Papers*, no. 62. Paris: OECD Publishing. Retrieved from http://dx.doi.org/10.1787/5k44t787zcwb-en.

Renzaho, A.M.N., Romios, P., Crock, C. & Sønderlund, A.L. (2013). The effectiveness of cultural competence programs in ethnic minority patient centered health care—A systematic review of the literature. *International Journal for Quality in Health Care*, 25(3), 261–9.

Salter, P.S., Adams, G. & Perez, M.J. (2018). Racism in the structure of everyday worlds: A cultural-psychological perspective. *Current Directions in Psychological Science*, 27(3), 150–5.

Squires, A. (2017). Evidence-based approaches to breaking down language barriers. *Nursing*, 47(9), 34–40.

Stangor, C., Jhangiani, R. & Tarry, H. (2015). *Principles of Social Psychology* (1st international edn). Vancouver: Open Textbook Project.

Statistics New Zealand. (2014). *2013 Census QuickStats about Culture and Identity.* Wellington: Statistics NZ. Retrieved from http://archive.stats.govt.nz/Census/2013-census/profile-and-summary-reports/quickstats-culture-identity.aspx.

Waitemata DHB, eCALD® Services (2018a). *Toolkit for Working in a Culturally Diverse Workplace.* Auckland: WDHB eCALD® Services. Retrieved from www.ecald.com/resources/cross-cultural-resources/working-in-a-culturally-diverse-workplace.

Waitemata DHB, eCALD® Services (2018b). *Working with Interpreters.* Auckland: WDHB, eCALD® Services. Retrieved from www.ecald.com/courses/cald-cultural-competency-courses-for-working-with-patients/cald-4-working-with-interpreters.

CHAPTER 7
COMMUNICATION WITHIN THE ORGANISATION

JOHN SOLAS

CHAPTER FOCUS

After reading this chapter and completing the activities, you will be able to:

- discuss the importance of effective communication in healthcare organisations
- examine the flows and dynamics of organisational communication
- identify the barriers to effective communication in healthcare organisations
- describe strategies for improving communication in healthcare organisations.

KEY TERMS

Bureaucracy
Context
Open communication
Organisational communication

Introduction

Effective and efficient healthcare depends on the flow of communication within organisations. Yet organisations are prone to stifle and distort communication, which has the potential to create a toxic environment. The level of toxicity can become lethal if left unchecked. This chapter examines the influence of organisational management, structures and cultures on interpersonal communication, discusses a number of barriers to communicative competence and suggests ways these can be overcome. Organisations are not bricks and mortar. Rather, the building blocks of organisations are the people who staff them and utilise their goods and services. Open, honest, person-centred communication in healthcare organisations strengthens and maintains the vigour and vitality of staff and patients alike.

Straightforward communication?

One of the chief axioms of communication is that we cannot *not* communicate (De Vito 2013). Communication occurs even when it is unintended or when there is silence. We tend to convey more non-verbally, which encompasses anything that is unspoken such as appearance, gesture, proximity, posture, punctuality, scent, touch, intonation, facial expression and even a certain look (see Chapter 2). Not only are most of us in the habit of communicating incessantly, in one way or another, but also few of us would claim not to know how to communicate effectively or deny that we are adept at 'straight talk'. After all, in the transmission model of communication described in the seminal work of Shannon and Weaver (1949), communication appears to be pretty straightforward. This concept is explored further in the focus box 'Straightforward models of communication'.

BOX 7.1

STRAIGHTFORWARD MODELS OF COMMUNICATION

In the simplest of communication models, messages are communicated directly from sender to receiver. Information is sent using a common code, which for many is English, and channelled through audio-visual media. Transmission will be successful provided noise is minimised. While providing a starting point for understanding the process of communication, the linear model (Shannon & Weaver 1949) has been superseded by the interactional model, first described by Weiner (1948), and, subsequently, the transactional model originally put forward by Berlo (1960). These subsequent models retain the basic elements of the simple transmission model, while broadening our understanding of the dynamics, rather than the mechanics, of the communication process. The interactional model highlights the role of feedback in establishing relationships. Information is not simply transmitted; it is processed and fed back. It also introduces the notion of noise to include psychological and semantic (meaning) as well as auditory distortion.

But do we, in fact, know how to communicate effectively? Consider the following well-known snippet:

> There are known knowns; there are things we know we know. We also know there are known unknowns; that is to say we know there are some things we do not know. But there are also unknown unknowns—the ones we don't know we don't know.

The statement was uttered by Donald Rumsfeld while serving as US Secretary of Defense in the George W. Bush administration, in response to a question about the weapons capability of the Iraqi army, and more pointedly, whether Saddam Hussein's arsenal contained weapons of mass destruction (WMD). The question was posed at a press briefing Rumsfeld gave before the beginning of the Iraqi War (Steyn 2003). Rumsfeld's response invoked merciless reaction from all quarters. It was roundly condemned as utter nonsense. Not only was Rumsfeld thoroughly lampooned, but the credibility of George W. Bush's presidency and indeed, the entire war, was also called into question. Despite the international fallout and ensuing blowback, careful examination of the statement reveals that the utterance does make sense. Indeed, talk of the known unknown existed long before Rumsfeld gave it a new audience. The Johari window (see Chapter 3), made famous in many communication texts, is a tool for reflection on and of self. This process embraces what the person knows about themselves, what is shown to others, what is shown to others but not known by the person and is solicited in feedback, and what is unknown to the self and unknown to others. This window, set up in four quadrants, has movable lines so that each pane can be moved to reveal how 'open' or 'closed' a person presents. Also, much scientific progress, including medical progress, is based on discussions about known unknowns. (See Weblinks at the end of the chapter for the Rumsfeld press briefing.)

Context
The physical and psychosocial environment that provides the setting in which communication exchanges occur.

Context is featured in the transactional model. It refers to time and place. Yet there is more to context than its spatial or temporal dimensions. The cultural and historical context in which communication occurs is of equal importance. It is possible to see this by returning once again to Rumsfeld's briefing. Taken out of context, Rumsfeld's statement could hardly be construed as anything more than doubletalk. But it is possible to make sense of Rumsfeld's talk of 'known unknowns' when considered in the context in which it was communicated. At the time the conference was held, there were indications that the George W. Bush administration was anticipating problems in garnering popular support for the planned liberation/invasion of Iraq—especially given America's controversial record of military intervention dating from the Vietnam War—and the government was preparing a range of alternative justifications. Rumsfeld's pronouncement contrived to offer a pretext for war while leaving sufficient room for withdrawal should the invasion go ahead and WMDs were found to be nonexistent. There were, however, increasing signs of a culture of deceit, and Rumsfeld was eventually removed from office.

Reflect and apply

Consider the process of communication between healthcare professionals and clients in the context of a large public hospital. What are the apparent limitations of the linear process model of communication in this instance?

Communication in the organisational context

A highly important context is the organisation. Organisations are as varied as they are pervasive. Indeed, it would be rare to find anyone who is untouched by them. People are born in organisations, most notably hospitals, and many of them spend their lives working for organisations, eating, drinking, learning, playing, praying and residing in them. Organisations are often thought of in physical or symbolic terms, most notably buildings and logos. What springs to mind, for instance, when Coca-Cola or McDonald's are mentioned? However, buildings and brand names are not organisations—they merely accommodate and represent them. Organisations are composed of people, and they are living rather than inanimate systems. Indeed, a corporation has the legal identity and status of a person.

The lifeblood of organisations is communication, whether channelled directly (face-to-face), electronically (email, teleconferencing, videoconferencing) or digitally (blogs, Facebook, Instagram, Twitter, wikis). Communication exerts a profound influence on individual and collective thinking, feeling and behaviour within organisations. The vigour of an organisation depends on its members' willingness and abilities to communicate. While a high level of proficiency will optimise the performance of an organisation, poor communication renders it dysfunctional; this is of particular concern to healthcare organisations where matters of life and death are at stake.

Organisational communication is usually examined in terms of flow. Communication in organisations flows in at least three directions: up, down and across. The structure of most conventional organisations tends to be more or less hierarchical. The larger an organisation, the more likely it is to adopt a hierarchical or bureaucratic structure, and the greater the tendency for communication cascading or escalating within it to be filtered and even impeded. While extolling its many virtues, the earliest proponent of **bureaucracy**, Max Weber (1978), warned of the propensity for it to become an 'iron cage' (p. 975). For Weber, 'bureaucracy develops the more perfectly it dehumanises' (p. 975). Moreover, the more complex an organisation grows, the more internal divisions and strata it creates which, in turn, intensifies the strain on horizontal and vertical communication. Organisations operating in more than one location (multiple suburbs, states or nations) make

Organisational communication
The flow of information between individuals and groups at various levels of hierarchy and across different locations within an organisation.

Bureaucracy
The forms and processes that characterise an organisation and its administration.

the flow of communication even more precarious. Some organisations have attempted to make communication flow more freely by becoming 'flatter' and reducing the number of administrative layers, particularly at middle management level. However, while levelling organisational structures may improve the flow of communication between those at the top and the bottom of the hierarchy, horizontal divisions remain, and may actually multiply. Most organisations use electronic communication networks as a means of integrating units (Heini, Heikki & Marjo 2014). But communication remains fraught, right down to its most common form: the email (Kane 2015). Even the most sophisticated electronic media do not replace communicators, from which distorted messages originate. It seems that whatever structure is adopted, any top-to-bottom and centre-to-periphery configuration will invariably affect the course of communication in an organisation.

Most medium and large healthcare organisations are bureaucratic. While bureaucracies offer both advantages and disadvantages to those who work in or engage with them (Reit & Halevy 2019), most people would agree that the many layers that comprise these often hierarchical organisations impede communication. Indeed, the rank and file of the corporate world, particularly the 'googlites' and 'dot.comers', consider bureaucracy an anathema. In order to succeed in an external environment characterised by unbridled competition and extreme uncertainty, contemporary organisations require the agility, flexibility, inventiveness and enterprise that bureaucracies simply do not have.

Ironically, maladministration and mismanagement are precisely what bureaucracies were designed to eliminate. The bureau sought to supplant the arbitrary and corrupt rule caused by patronage and privilege with legal authority and meritocracy. Thus, despite the bad press it receives, a properly functioning bureaucracy represents the epitome of rational organisation. Even a highly anti-bureaucratic organisation such as Google is unable to avoid the practical and legal necessity of adopting bureaucratic processes, practices and structures as it becomes larger and more diversified. In fact, Google follows a standard functional structure with management positions specialised by value-chain activity. As a multinational corporation, these positions are further divided and grouped into regions of interest that aid the company in managing the breadth of its operations. Within each top-level activity, there is a multidivisional structure where small business units are divided on the basis of geography or product markets.

Some barriers to communicating effectively in the organisational context

Communication in organisations is prone to a number of common barriers that are particularly evident in highly bureaucratic organisations—and are characteristic of most healthcare centres. Among the most significant barriers are the inherent complexity of interpersonal communication, the difficulty of establishing and maintaining open lines of communication, workplace silence, verbal aggression, the repression of emotion in communication and having too little time to communicate.

The complexity of interpersonal communication

Organisations are composed of people and, as such, are full of talk; some organisational theorists consider organisations to be 'discursive constructions' (Putnam & Fairhurst 2015) that are created in and through the process of communication (Vásquez & Cooren 2013). Organisations are not just talk, however. Communication both prompts and inhibits action. Yet, when considering the range of variability possible at each stage in even the most basic interpersonal communication process, it is surprising that there can be any successful discourse between people. Linear models have severe limitations, as they tend to view communication as a clearly defined, step-by-step process, rather than an indefinite simultaneous process and, as a consequence, largely ignore the communication's intrinsic interpersonal dynamics. Linear models have been augmented by sensitivity to the intersubjective nature of communication (interactional model) as well as the overall context (transactional model) in which it takes place. However, common understanding remains difficult to achieve in diverse healthcare organisations. In these organisations, patients seldom share the terminology, assumptions and norms embedded in the culture of the health profession (O'Toole 2012). Moreover, both patients and professionals are encoders and decoders of messages packed with meanings, motives and agenda that may be misconstrued, distorted or undisclosed, but that still shape the process and outcome of communication.

Difficulty in establishing and maintaining open lines of communication

Candour and familiarity have the potential to amplify otherwise distant or obscured voices (Bennis 2014). These redemptive strategies can make communication less inhibited. However, although transparency appears to be highly valued, it rarely occurs in organisations (Bennis 2014), where unfettered openness and informality may generate conflict. There are also occasions when the availability of information is restricted or withheld, even from patients. For instance, discretion can be invoked in instances where disclosure is judged seriously harmful to a patient. The licence to do so in these circumstances is granted under what is known as 'therapeutic privilege' (Hodkinson 2013, p. 106). Bennis (2014) points out that candid communication may not be appreciated or well received, especially by those in positions of power and authority, even if they claim to have an 'open door policy'.

BOX 7.2

AN HONEST ANSWER TO A SIMPLE QUESTION

How differently would US Secretary of Defense Donald Rumsfeld have acted early in 2003 in the face of informed intelligence—that is, 'known knowns'—if he had listened to General Eric Shineski? When asked by a member of the Senate Armed Services Committee how large a force would be needed in postwar Iraq, General Shineski spoke frankly and said, 'Something on the order of several hundred thousand soldiers are probably ... a figure that would be required' (quoted in Reingold 2004). Not only was this the wrong answer, in Rumsfeld's view and that of others in the George W. Bush administration who claimed, incorrectly, that peace could be maintained in Iraq with a minimum of ground forces, but Shineski had, according to some, committed 'candourside' (Bennis 2014). Shineski, who chose a military career despite being seriously wounded in the Vietnam War, had served with distinction for more than 35 years, including a stint as US Army Chief of Staff. As a result, he was publicly criticised by Defense Department officials, and Rumsfeld and other luminaries boycotted his retirement ceremony. Shineski was simply doing his duty in speaking up.

Workplace silence

Where formal, hierarchical communication permeates the healthcare context, there will be censorship, curtailing opportunities to express new ideas, advance alternative viewpoints, have robust discussions and even report malpractice. The latter is highly consequential. There has been growing public recognition in many countries that healthcare facilities are often dangerous places (World Health Organization 2012). Reports published in the United States, United Kingdom, Australia, New Zealand and Canada have focused public and government attention on the safety of patients and highlighted the alarmingly high incidence of errors and adverse events that lead to some kind of harm or injury (World Health Organization 2012). See the focus box 'Incidence of adverse events'.

Most treatment errors are caused by flaws in increasingly complex and overextended healthcare systems, rather than by incompetent individuals (Grube, Piliavin & Turner 2010). Compounding this is a reluctance by healthcare professionals to report errors as a result of barriers such as fear, lack of support, poor reporting systems and varying perceptions of what actually constitutes an error (Soydemir, Intepeler & Mert 2017). While the rate of reported adverse events is over 5 per cent and growing (Australian Institute of Health and Welfare 2018), this figure is likely well below the actual number of errors as a result of this reluctance to report.

BOX 7.3

INCIDENCE OF ADVERSE EVENTS

The World Health Organization (2005, p. 8) defines an adverse event (AE) as:

> An injury related to medical management, in contrast to complications of disease. Medical management includes all aspects of care, including diagnosis and treatment, failure to diagnose or treat, and the systems and equipment used to deliver care. Adverse events may be preventable or non-preventable.

Most current knowledge of AEs is based on reviews of hospital medical records, incident reports by health staff or analysis of administrative databases. The Australian Institute of Health and Welfare reported that in 2015–16, 5.4 per cent of patients admitted to public and private hospitals incurred an AE. In the United States, most recent figures rate medical errors as the third leading cause of death (Makary & Daniel 2016). In a subsequent systematic review of studies conducted across 27 countries, between 2.9 and 21.9 per cent of all patients were reported as experiencing adverse events (Schwendimann et al. 2018).

Reflect and apply

Would you report any medical error you observed, no matter how minor it was? If not, which errors would you not report, and why? How would you go about speaking up against malpractice you personally experienced?

Fear of negative professional and personal repercussions is a major factor in maintaining workplace silence (Manapragada & Bruk-Lee 2016). Noort, Reader and Gillespie (2019) point to research about the concept of 'safety voice', which is the act of speaking up to prevent harm. This concept is particularly relevant in the healthcare setting, where patients are already vulnerable and potentially at risk. Failing to speak out about such matters reduces opportunities for preventative measures that can prove to be lifesaving, particularly in healthcare settings.

Silence also gives free rein to corruption and allows it to become embedded in organisational structures and processes, accepted by organisational members and passed on to new employees (Costas & Grey 2014). The enculturation of corruption is highly destructive. Reticence has caused the downfall of such corporate giants as Enron, and precipitated the global financial crisis of 2008–09 (Solas 2019).

Verbal aggression

While some staff fear voicing their views, especially dissent, others verbalise their aggression (Swain & Gale 2014). Non-physical violence ranges from insensitive and rude remarks to serious verbal abuse. It can be overt, as in bullying, which is 'a repeated pattern of physical and/or psychological violence over time that can be directed at one or more individuals' (Spector, Zhou & Che 2014, p. 73), or covert, as in backstabbing, which involves intentionally spreading rumours, failing to transmit information, belittling opinions or disparaging a person behind his or her back (Malone & Hayes 2012).

Herschcovis and Barling (2010) revealed that the expression of non-physical aggression has a strong negative impact on employees' workplace attitudes towards job satisfaction, commitment and behaviours—for example, lower job performance and higher interpersonal and organisational deviance, which raises general levels of stress, illness and depression. As work standards decline, morale and productivity drop, the intention to quit becomes more prevalent and staff turnover increases. One person targeted by aggression recounted the experience as follows:

> I admit that, before I was bullied, I couldn't understand why employees would shy-away from doing anything about it. When it happened to me, I felt trapped. I felt like either no one believed me or no one cared. This bully was my direct boss and went out of his way to make me look and feel incompetent... I dreaded going to work and cried myself to sleep every night. I was afraid of losing my job because I started to question my abilities and didn't think I'd find work elsewhere.
>
> (Post on a *New York Times* blog, 2008, quoted in Herschcovis and Barling 2010, p. 24)

In a landmark study, deviant employee behaviour and absenteeism were estimated to produce organisational losses of up to $200 billion each year in the United States alone (Murphy 1993). These figures do not take cyberbullying and trolling into account, so estimates could be considerably higher.

Verbal aggression is a major cause of interpersonal conflict in healthcare organisations. It can occur horizontally among healthcare workers (Brinkert 2010), or vertically between workers and management (Birks et al. 2014). Effective communication skills are critical to both preventing and managing aggressive behaviours (Baby, Gale & Swain 2018). Although it is not uncommon for nurses to be physically attacked by patients, nurses were found to be more concerned about verbal aggression from peers (Spector et al. 2014). Spector et al. (2014) point out that persistent conflict among nursing co-workers is a serious issue, and is, according to Croft and Cash (2012), one that continues unabated (strategies for managing conflict are explored in Chapter 9). Bullying, in particular, has been identified as a pervasive culture in the nursing profession, and it is a problem that is increasing (Hartin, Birks & Lindsay 2018).

CASE ACTIVITY 7.1

Verbal aggression

You have just graduated from your studies as a health professional in your particular discipline and have commenced work in your local public hospital. The manager of the unit in which you are working has called an interdisciplinary team meeting. In the following exchange you are staff member 4 (SM4):

SM1: Now we are all here, let's start.

SM2: I'd like to introduce you all to our new team member SM4 [says your name], we are looking forward to learning from her expertise.

SM1: Okay, welcome [says your name]. Let's start with a review of patients.

SM2: Mrs Griffin was admitted yesterday.

SM1: (Tersely) That's Griffith, not Griffin.

SM2: As I was saying Mrs Griffith was admitted yesterday for a biopsy, suspected liver cancer with possible bony mets. She is a lovely lady with lots of family that visit. They are keen to get her home. Next is Mr Wells ...

SM1: That's Wills, can't you get anything right!

SM3: [in a whisper to you] Don't take any notice, he's just showing off.

1. What kind of communication is going on here?
2. How do you think SM1 sees his role in this group?
3. How do you think SM2 is feeling?
4. As a new team member, what are you now feeling about the communication patterns in this unit?
5. What should have been the first thing to happen at the interdisciplinary team meeting?

Repression of emotion in communication

Bureaucratic rationalisation also diminishes the expression of emotion, which is one of the most important distinguishing features of caring professions, and essential for fostering a climate of trust, loyalty, passion and commitment in the workplace. Yet thinking and feeling are typically thought of as polarised in organisations (Goleman & Cherniss 2001). Not only are they considered to be at odds with each other, but conveying emotion at work is generally deemed irrational and counterproductive (Goleman 2006). However, as Daniel Goleman (2006, p. 52) argues, reason and emotion overlap: 'The notion that there is "pure thought," rationality devoid of feeling, is a fiction, an illusion, based on inattention to the subtle moods that follow us through the day. We have feelings about everything we do, think about, imagine, and remember.'

It is important to recognise, therefore, that communication encompasses thinking and feeling dimensions, even in discourses about arcane medical matters. In Chapter 4 we introduced the concept of emotional intelligence. In the organisational context, emotional intelligence is as necessary as technical rationality, based on logic and objectivity, in conversations about how patients will be managed and cared for. Dougherty and Drumheller (2006) contend that emotional ineptitude is a serious liability. They note that 'organizational members would be far more successful at producing rational outcomes if they spent less time and effort trying to shove their emotions into rational norms—this can only happen if the duality is closed and organizations are recognized as both emotional and rational locations' (p. 235).

Emotional intelligence is not the same as the intelligence quotient (IQ). However, emotional intelligence does not oppose IQ. Rather, IQ and emotional intelligence are simply separate and potentially harmonious forms of intelligence. However, unlike IQ, emotional intelligence is not a static faculty and can, through learning, be improved. Furthermore, emotional intelligence does not entail leaving unpleasant feelings aside. There will be times when 'awful truths' have to be talked about. Nor does it license being cavalier with emotions, and letting them run wild. Of course, this does not necessitate becoming a stoic or attaining inner equanimity. Rather, it entails learning to become more adept at managing and expressing emotions appropriately and effectively.

Skills in practice

Heartless communication

Bethany is a graduate nurse working in a palliative care unit. Bethany was told by a preceptor that she should not become 'emotionally involved' with her patients. Bethany is fundamentally a warm and caring person and this approach does not sit well with her, nor is it consistent with why she became a nurse. A patient, Mrs Davidson, confides in Bethany that she is afraid of dying. Bethany's initial reaction is to brush Mrs Davidson off and initially tells her that she is too busy to talk. A few minutes after leaving the room, Bethany returns and sits quietly with Mrs Davidson while she expresses her fears.

What's going on here?

Bethany is keen to provide professional and therapeutic care to her patients. Bethany understands that her preceptor is trying to protect her from the more difficult elements of her role as a nurse, particularly in a palliative care environment. Bethany, however, has the emotional intelligence to realise that this approach is not appropriate for her, nor is it conducive to ensuring the best possible care for Mrs Davidson. While Bethany has limited experience, she knows that by simply being present with Mrs Davidson and listening to her concerns, she is communicating therapeutically.

Too little time to talk

There can be little doubt that the environment in which healthcare is practised is continually stressful and ever-changing. As Wilson and Wilson (2011) observe, no two days are alike. Workload demands seem insatiably high and time diminishingly short, both of which serve to encourage cursory communication. Hemsley, Balandin and Worrall (2011) report that lack of time is an even greater barrier in caring for patients with complex communication needs and developmental disabilities. Nurses were found either to limit conversations or, worse still, walk away out of frustration with these patients. In intensive care units, for example, the approach to communication is often altered depending on whether patients are considered compliant or difficult (Leslie et al. 2017). Communication with patients who identify as lesbian, gay, bisexual, transgender or queer, or for whom English is a second language, also tends to be avoided or dismissive. 'Othering'—or what is more commonly referred to as discrimination—accounts for the lack of communication with these patients no less than time constraints (Chance 2013; Johnson et al. 2004). As one observer noted:

> I find that sometimes the attitude of the professionals in the healthcare system tends to have a tone of racial discrimination. It doesn't come out very verbally so it's hard to pinpoint it and say, 'such and such a person is treating me that way'. But it is just a gut feeling that you have. Especially in a waiting area you will find the nurse will come and be very cordial and polite to a white person when they call them in for a test or to see the specialist. And when they come out and as soon as they realise it's an ethnic person they tend to speak slower to you, they tend to speak loudly to you, and they probably assume that you don't understand the language. (quoted in Johnson et al. 2004, p. 263)

Time will always be important in fast-paced healthcare contexts. However, it need not be an enemy of timely communication. Quality is as important a measure of effective communication as quantity (O'Hagan et al. 2014). While it may not be possible to find or create more time—even if it could be managed with greater efficiency through more careful prioritisation and thorough routinisation of workloads—it is possible to use the limited time available to communicate effectively and productively with colleagues, and caringly with patients. In taking the therapeutic perspective described earlier, attention is directed towards what is communicated and how, rather than how much and how long, particularly since more is conveyed non verbally and para-linguistically than through words alone. This approach is not meant to endorse the expediency so valued by contemporary healthcare organisations (Scott, Matthews & Kirwan 2014). Nor does it suggest that anything more demonstrates genuine professional care. Rather, what counts is perspicacity, receptivity and responsiveness, not verbosity.

Communicate as openly as possible

Open communication Communication that is transparent and accessible; includes the concept of freedom of expression.

Workplace silence is completely indefensible from a moral and legal standpoint. Not only is candour ethical in the context of healthcare, it is also potentially lifesaving. **Open communication** is vital for maintaining the free flow of news and information, and the exchanges of views, ideas, engagement and advocacy necessary for improving organisational performance, productivity, and staff and patient wellbeing. However, there is a risk in committing 'candourside'. Indeed, healthcare practitioners who cared less about either their professional or organisational affiliation were found to be the first to voice their concerns (Grube et al. 2010).

Open communication is equally necessary in stemming conflict, whether it be intraprofessional (among peers, such as aides and nurses), interdisciplinary (between professional groups such as nurses and doctors) or interpersonal (with patients and their families). Conflict and conflict resolution are discussed at length in Chapter 9, which shows how compromise can be effectively reached with a win-win outcome. Although interpersonal conflict is generally viewed as negative, it can be used positively (Brinkert 2010). At the very least, conflict can let vexatious issues and problems surface by getting individuals to acknowledge, clarify and address disparate interests, areas of responsibilities and cross-purposes that impede mutual gains and, ultimately, larger organisational dividends.

While verbal aggression and silence are commonplace in healthcare organisations, most communication usually occurs without force, threat or corruption (Reichertz 2011). Words have no intrinsic power. As the old saying goes, 'sticks and stones may break bones, but words will never hurt me'. Any power words have come directly from relationships between communicators or, more precisely, their relative significance and strength. Reliability is a major factor in developing and maintaining strong, enduring relationships (Reichertz 2011). The parties to a relationship are able to foster reliability by ensuring that their words and deeds match ('congruent' in Rogerian terms) and mutual commitments are honoured (O'Toole 2012). Reichertz (2011) suggests that communication with unreliable people cannot be sustained.

Be vocal without speaking for others

Healthcare organisations have always been diverse. However, there is now greater demand for recognition and appreciation of and respect for the diversity that exists within them. In order to be successful in such contexts, communication requires even greater competence and sensitivity on the part of healthcare practitioners. As discussed in Chapter 6, communicating in culturally diverse contexts entails respecting the values, beliefs and attitudes of others, and becoming attuned to communication cues that signal and transmit important differences. It also means being alert to the notion that heterogeneity exists within all cultures, and not all members identify with their cultural heritage (Johnson et al. 2004).

Johnson et al. (2004) also advise carefully monitoring the language (code) used to communicate with 'others', since it may inadvertently harbour and reproduce divisions between age, class, faith, gender, sexuality, race and ethnicity. To take a simple example, while 'we' seems an innocuous and thoroughly inclusive term, it can suggest alignments, such as 'us', and demarcations, such as 'them'. By the same token, although dialogue is important, it is not always possible to speak with one voice. However, this need not be problematic. Indeed, monologues—that is, speaking for oneself—may be necessary at times, if only to vent frustrations or concerns. What is important is for all voices to be heard without fear or favour. This means listening to, not just hearing, what people say.

Speak from the heart, not just the head

As stated earlier, it is impossible to divorce the affective from the cognitive dimension of communication. Even if this were possible, doing so would be undesirable, as both are indispensable to effective, meaningful communication. Emotional intelligence is not a contradiction in terms. Rather, it involves developing competence in the following areas.

- Knowing your own emotions; being aware of and capable of recognising specific feelings as each is being experienced.
- Managing or regulating your emotions so that they facilitate rather than interfere with self- and mutual understanding.
- Enhancing self-motivation to pursue desires, strive for improvement, and remain resilient following setbacks and frustrations by tapping into emotional reserves.
- Recognising emotions in others by empathising with them.
- Handling relationships by being able to read and influence social situations, particularly those involving testy individuals (adapted from Goleman 2006, p. 318).

The point of learning to become more emotionally intelligent is to facilitate genuine civility and service, not to manipulate communication to serve the irrational ends of the organisation with, for example, command and control (Dougherty & Drumheller 2006).

Conclusion

Healthcare professional practice occurs in an organisational context. An understanding of the impact of this context on effective communication is essential to achieving positive outcomes for clients and patients and enhanced job satisfaction for healthcare professionals. As has been discussed in earlier chapters, verbal and non-verbal communication are influenced by the nature of the exchange and the context in which it occurs. In organisations, the complexity of the environment and competing priorities can exert pressures on the individuals that function within them. These pressures raise challenges for effective communication that can be overcome with attention to a person-centred, empathetic and emotionally intelligent approach in engagement with others.

SUMMARY POINTS

- Communication, both verbal and non-verbal, occurs as inadvertently as it does consciously, and virtually incessantly.
- Though most people communicate on a daily basis, communicating is much less straightforward than it might seem. Even people at the top of an organisation can be inarticulate.
- Models of interpersonal communication, ranging from the transmission through interactive to transactional, invariably fail to capture the full complexity of the communication process.
- Context exerts a profound effect on, and is equally affected by, communication. Organisations are one such context.
- Organisations are built by and for people; the lifeblood of embodied organisations is communication.
- The vitality of an organisation relies on its members' willingness and ability to communicate.
- Authority and power are distributed hierarchically, and communication tends to flow down more readily than up or across organisations.
- Common barriers to effective communication within bureaucratic healthcare organisations are censorship, conflict, expediency, fear, incivility, prejudice, silence and technocracy.
- The prevalence of communication barriers within healthcare organisations can be life-threatening, as they enable corruption to become institutionalised and malpractice to flourish.
- It is possible to counteract barriers to communication by adopting a person-centred approach to communication that emphasises acceptance, congruence and empathy, practising emotional intelligence, and promoting a culture of candour and collaboration that enables all voices to be heard.

CRITICAL THINKING QUESTIONS

1. If you were a sedated or unconscious patient, what would be the first words you would want to hear once conscious from the person assigned to your care?
2. If a doctor shouted abuse at you, would you:
   a. shout back at the doctor?
   b. ignore the doctor?
   c. report the doctor?
   d. How else could you respond?
3. Recall an occasion when you experienced negative discrimination.
   a. What was the basis of discrimination?
   b. How did you feel about being discriminated against?
   c. What did you do in response? What was the result?

4. What do you consider to be the main challenges for you in becoming more accepting of, congruent with and empathic towards others in the work context? What might you do to overcome these challenges?

Group activity

Remaining silent

Refer back to the section in this chapter about open communication. In your study groups or via your subject discussion site, compile a list of times when it would be acceptable to remain silent. What would be the consequences of speaking up on these occasions? What would be the consequences of not speaking up?

WEBLINKS

Organisational communication

Shapiro Communications: What is organisational communication?
http://shapirocommunications.com/organizational-communication-important

SolVibrations:
www.solvibrations.org/organizational-communication

Person-centred therapy

Psychotherapy.net: Carl Rogers on person-centred therapy:
www.psychotherapy.net/video/person-centered-therapy-carl-rogers

The Rumsfeld press briefing

Donald Rumsfeld Unknown Unknowns:
www.youtube.com/watch?v=GiPe1OiKQuk

REFERENCES

Australian Institute of Health and Welfare. (2018). *Australia's Health 2018*. Retrieved from www.aihw.gov.au/reports/australias-health/australias-health-2018/contents/indicators-of-australias-health/adverse-events-treated-in-hospital.

Baby, M., Gale, C. & Swain, N. (2018). Communication skills training in the management of patient aggression and violence in healthcare. *Aggression and Violent Behaviour*, 39, 67–82. doi.org/10.1016/j.avb.2018.02.004.

Berlo, D.K. (1960). *The Process of Communication*. New York: Holt, Rinehart & Winston.

Bennis, W. (2014). Building a culture of candour: A crucial key to leadership. In W.E. Rosenbach, R.L. Taylor & M.A. Youndt, *Contemporary Issues in Leadership* (7th edn) (pp. 279–86). New York: Routledge.

Birks, M., Budden, L.M., Stewart, L. & Chapman, Y. (2014). Turning the tables: The growth of upward bullying in nursing academia. *Journal of Advanced Nursing*, 70, 1685–7.

Brinkert, R. (2010). A literature review of conflict communication causes, costs, benefits, and interventions in nursing. *Journal of Nursing Management*, 18(2), 145–56.

Chance, T.F. (2013). 'Going to pieces' over LGBT health disparities: How an amended affordable care act could cure the discrimination that ails the LGBT community. *Journal of Health Care Law and Policy*, 16(2), 375–402.

Costas, J. & Grey, C. (2014). Bringing secrecy into the open: Towards a theorisation of the social processes of organisational secrecy. *Organization Studies*, 35(10), 1423–47. doi:10.1177/0170840613515470.

Croft, R.K. & Cash, P.A. (2012). Deconstructing contributing factors to bullying and lateral violence in nursing using a postcolonial feminist lens. *Contemporary Nurse*, 42(2), 226–42.

De Vito, J. (2013). *Interpersonal Messages: Communication and Relationship Skills.* Upper Saddle River, NJ: Pearson Longman.

Dougherty, D.S. & Drumheller, K. (2006). Sensemaking and emotions in organizations: Accounting for emotions in a rational(ized) context. *Communication Studies*, 57(2), 215–38.

Goleman, D. (2006). *Working with Emotional Intelligence.* London: Bloomsbury.

Goleman, D. & Cherniss, C. (2001). *The Emotionally Intelligent Workplace: How to Select For, Measure and Improve Emotional Intelligence in Individuals, Groups and Organizations.* San Francisco, CA: Jossey-Bass.

Grube, J.A., Piliavin, J.A. & Turner, J.W. (2010). The courage of one's conviction: When do nurse practitioners report unsafe practices? *Health Communication*, 25(2), 155–64.

Hartin, P., Birks, M. & Lindsay, D. (2018). Bullying and the nursing profession in Australia: An integrative review of the literature. *Collegian*, 25(6), 613–19.

Heini, S.M.L., Heikki, E.K. & Marjo, N. (2014). Digital channels in the internal communication of a multinational corporation. *Corporate Communications: An International Journal*, 19(3), 275–86.

Hemsley, B., Balandin, S. & Worrall, L. (2011). Nursing the patient with complex communication needs: Time as a barrier and a facilitator to successful communication in hospital. *Journal of Advanced Nursing*, 68(1), 116–26.

Herschcovis, S.M. & Barling, J. (2010). Towards a multi-foci approach to workplace aggression: A meta-analytic review of outcomes from different perpetrators. *Journal of Occupational Behavior*, 31(1), 24–44.

Hodkinson, K. (2013). The need to know—therapeutic privilege: A way forward. *Health Care Analysis*, 21(2), 105–29.

Johnson, J.L., Bottorff, J.L., Browne, A.J., Grewal, S., Hilton, B.A. & Clarke, H. (2004). Othering and being othered in the context of healthcare. *Health Communication*, 16(2), 253–71.

Kane, G.C. (2015). Are you part of the email problem? *MIT Sloan Management Review*, 56(4).

Leslie, M., Paradis, E., Gropper, M., Milic, M., Kitto, S., Reeves, S. & Pronovost, P. (2017). A typology of ICU patients and families from the clinician perspective: Towards improving communication, *Health Communication*, 32(6), 777–83. doi:10.1080/10410236.2016.1172290.

Makary, M.A. & Daniel, M. (2016). Medical error—the third leading cause of death in the US. *BMJ Health Services Research*, 18(521). https://doi.org/10.1186/s12913-018-3335-z.

Malone, P. & Hayes, J. (2012). Backstabbing in organizations: Employees' perceptions of incidents, motives, and communicative responses. *Communication Studies*, 63(2), 194–219.

Manapragada, A. & Bruk-Lee, V. (2016). Staying silent about safety issues: Conceptualizing and measuring safety silence motives. *Accident Analysis and Prevention*, 91, 144–56.

Murphy, K.R. (1993). *Honesty in the Workplace*. Belmont, CA: Brooks-Cole.

Noort, M.C., Reader, T.W. & Gillespie, A. (2019). Walking the plank: An experimental paradigm to investigate safety voice. *Frontiers in Psychology*, 10, 668.

O'Hagan, S., Manias, E., Elder, C., Pill, J., Woodward-Kron, R., McNamara, T., ... McColl, G. (2014). What counts as effective communication in nursing? Evidence from nurse educators' and clinicians' feedback on nurse interactions with simulated patients. *Journal of Advanced Nursing*, 70(6), 1344–55.

O'Toole, G. (2012). *Communication: Core Interpersonal Skills for Health Professionals* (2nd edn). Sydney: Churchill Livingstone Elsevier.

Putnam, L.L. & Fairhurst, G.T. (2015). Revisiting 'organisations as discursive constructions': 10 years later. *Communication Theory*, 25(4), 375–92.

Reichertz, J. (2011). Communicative power is power over identity. *Communications*, 36(2), 147–68.

Reingold, J. (2004,). Soldiering on. *Fast Company*. 1 September. Retrieved from www.fastcompany.com/50432/soldiering.

Reit, E. & Halevy, N. (2019). Managing hierarchy's functions and dysfunctions: A relational perspective on leadership and followership. *Current Opinion in Psychology*. https://doi.org/10.1016/j.copsyc.2019.07.017.

Schwendimann, R., Blatter, C., Dhaini, S., Simon, M. & Ausserhofer, D. (2018). The occurrence, types, consequences and preventability of in-hospital adverse events: A scoping review. *BMC Health Services Research*, 18(1), 521.

Scott, P.A., Matthews, A. & Kirwan, M. (2014). What is nursing in the 21st century and what does the 21st century health system require of nursing? *Nursing Philosophy*, 15(1), 23–34.

Shannon, C.E. & Weaver, W. (1949). *The Mathematical Theory of Communication*. Urbana, IL: University of Illinois Press.

Solas, J. (2019). Conscientious objections to corporate wrongdoing. *Business and Society Review*, 124(1), 43–62.

Soydemir, D., Intepeler, S.S. & Mert, H. (2017). Barriers to medical error reporting for physicians and nurses. *Western Journal of Nursing Research*, 39(10), 1348–63.

Spector, P.E., Zhou, Z.E. & Che, X.X. (2014). Nurse exposure to physical and nonphysical violence, bullying, and sexual harassment: A quantitative review. *International Journal of Nursing Studies*, 51(1), 72–84.

Steyn, M. (2003). Rummy talks sense, not gobbledegook. *Daily Telegraph*, 9 December. Retrieved from www.telegraph.co.uk/comment/personal-view/3599959/Rummy-speaks-the-truth-not-gobbledygook.html.

Swain, N. & Gale, C. (2014). A communication skills intervention for community healthcare workers reduces perceived patient aggression: A pretest–posttest study. *International Journal of Nursing Studies*, 51(9), 1241–5.

Vásquez, C. & Cooren, F. (2013) Spacing practices: The communicative configuration of organizing through space-times. *Communication Theory*, 23(1), 25–47.

Weber, M. (1978). *Economy and Society, 2 vols.* Los Angeles, CA: University of California Press.

Weiner, N. (1948). *Cybernetics: Or Control and Communication in the Animal and the Machine.* Cambridge, MA: MIT Press.

Wilson, A. & Wilson, M. (2011). What I wish I knew about nursing. Retrieved from www.whatiwishiknew.com.

World Health Organization. (2005). *World Alliance for Patient Safety: WHO Draft Guidelines for Adverse Event Reporting and Learning Systems from Information to Action.* Geneva: WHO.

World Health Organization. (2012). *Safer Primary Care: A Global Challenge.* Geneva: WHO.Case activity 4.2

CHAPTER 8

COMMUNICATION AND THE COMMUNITY

JANE MILLS AND KAREN FRANCIS

CHAPTER FOCUS

After reading this chapter and completing the activities, you will be able to:

- define the term 'community' and list its core elements
- discuss key factors to be considered when communicating with the community
- describe the process for communicating effectively with community groups
- develop a plan for communicating with a community, including a strategy for evaluating its effectiveness.

KEY TERMS

Burden of disease
Community
Design thinking
Reciprocity
Stakeholder network

Introduction

For health professionals, communicating with individuals, families, whānau (extended family), community groups and organisations forms the basis of their work. In this chapter, we discuss the process of communicating with community groups. The five steps that comprise this process are:

1. identifying the 'why'
2. understanding community boundaries
3. planning for reciprocity
4. developing a communication plan
5. evaluating effectiveness.

Community
A group of individuals who are linked geographically through location, or conceptually through values, beliefs or interests.

A paper published in 2001 provided an empirically grounded definition of **community** for the purpose of public health activities, including research and health promotion. MacQueen and colleagues (2001) identified five core elements of community. These were: locus (physical location), sharing, joint action, social ties and diversity. These researchers found that each of the core elements were present in different communities; however, the level of importance of each was dependent on context. Their definition is the one we will adopt for the purpose of this chapter.

Identifying the 'why'

Healthcare professionals are highly regarded and trusted by society. This trust brings with it weighty responsibility and an inherent power imbalance between healthcare professionals and those they serve. Because of this unequal balance of power, healthcare professionals need to be very clear about *why* they want to communicate with a community group, as it is very likely any group approached will agree with what is suggested to them by professionals.

Communicating with the community is a two-way process requiring commitment, time and energy, so the potential benefits for participants need to be the healthcare professional's priority. The 'why' of communicating with the community could be a problem that has been identified by a community group and brought to the attention of their local health service. It is more likely, however, that a problem has been identified by the health service and a decision made that something needs to be done to improve the problem indicators.

Skills in practice

Identifying the 'why'

Kelly is a final year psychology student who is required to undertake a health promotion project in her community. Kelly has an interest in substance abuse and develops an information session to deliver at the local community health centre. Kelly prepares the session, books the room, disseminates flyers and arranges catering. On the night of the information session, the only people who attend are Kelly's classmates.

What's happening here?

By failing to engage with the community, Kelly has not identified or prioritised their needs. Furthermore, she has failed to promote the benefit of her project to the community. In essence, the 'why' of Kelly's project relates more to her need to complete an assessment task than to provide benefit to the community.

Around the world, countries establish health priorities that guide policy and the subsequent investment of resources. In Australia, national health priorities are guided by the Australian Health Performance Framework (National Health Information and Performance Principal Committee 2017) and reported on biennially in *Australia's Health* (Australian Institute of Health and Welfare 2018). National health priorities are determined by the burden of disease, which is the measurement of loss of years of life related to dying early, or being affected by living with a disease that reduces quality of life. In Australia, coronary heart disease, lung cancer and arthritis cause the greatest **burden of disease** (Australian Institute of Health and Welfare 2018). The AIHW report also indicates that almost two-thirds of Australians are considered obese and that Australians generally do not exercise enough. This is a great example of how health professionals have identified a problem that they could communicate with the community about, and potentially have a positive impact on health and well-being. If every Australian walked briskly for 30 minutes five times a week, the disease burden as a result of physical inactivity would reduce by 26 per cent. However, we know also that it is not that simple, otherwise the problem would not exist in the first place.

Burden of disease
A measurement of the impact of disease and disability on quality and quantity of life.

Reflect and apply

Conduct an internet search to identify the major burden of disease in your community. How effectively is the human and financial cost of this burden communicated with your community? What health promotion programs are available to address the problem and how well is this disseminated to those affected?

Design thinking is a different way of collaboratively identifying problems and coming up with solutions able to be tested over time. We can define design thinking as a 'systematic innovation process that prioritizes deep empathy for end-user desires, needs and challenges to fully understand a problem in hopes of developing more comprehensive and effective solutions' (Roberts, Fisher, Trowbridge & Bent 2016, p. 12). Instead of beginning with a problem that a healthcare professional has defined, using a design thinking process begins with finding out from the affected community what believe their problem to be. Going back to our example of the burden of disease caused by physical inactivity, different communities will think about this problem

Design thinking
A non-traditional, non-linear approach to problem solving that is creative, solutions-focused and human-centred.

in different ways depending on their context. Again the factors of locus (physical location), sharing, joint action, social ties and diversity will affect how the problem is defined, and the potential solutions envisaged (MacQueen et al. 2001, p. 12).

Design thinking, or human-centred design as it is often referred to in health, has four main phases. The first of these is *discovery*—that is, finding out from end-users what they consider the problem to be. This phase might include observation, interviews and/or focus groups, or even a survey of a community. The second phase is *ideation*—that is, working with the community to come up with potential solutions that might be tried as a group. The third phase is *prototyping*—that is, testing the potential solutions. This is an iterative phase, where adjustments are made to improve the end-users' experience. The final phase is the *implementation* of a viable solution with a planned evaluation of the effectiveness of the solution over time (Matheson, Pacione, Shultz & Klügl 2015).

Importantly, adopting this type of participatory co-design approach to communicating and working with communities allows culture to underpin action. A brilliant example of this approach was the development of a mobile phone-delivered healthy lifestyle app for Māori communities in Aotearoa New Zealand (Te Morenga et al. 2018). The Kaupapa Māori co-design process to design health intervention for Māori communities was informed by a set of principles of engagement that provided a touchstone for healthcare professionals and community researchers throughout the process.

BOX 8.1

KAUPAPA MĀORI PRINCIPLES OF ENGAGEMENT

- Trust—building trust with our teams and communities
- Respect—respecting our different worldviews, cultures, and expertise
- Manaakitanga—working, learning, and sharing together and supporting one another
- Empathy—listening and communicating with openness and transparency
- Innovation—thinking outside the square
- Adaptability—open to change and flexible in our approach
- Tika Pono/Aroha—doing what's right and wrapping it up with love

Source: Te Morenga et al. 2018.

These principles of engagement are transferable to communities across the world and can inform healthcare professionals' thinking about the 'why' of communicating with particular community groups.

Understanding community boundaries

The five factors that inform the definition of community used in this chapter (MacQueen et al. 2001) provide a useful framework for scoping a community with which you might want to communicate. Understanding community boundaries is important to identify potential stakeholders. Generally, in a particular community there will be a mix of organisational groups and individuals with whom you will want to communicate. Thinking through the relationships between them, which can also be called the **stakeholder network**, is important in terms of identifying potential influences. There might be a focal organisation that acts as a gatekeeper for the community. This focal organisation might be a community-based organisation, a government agency, or even a media agency or lobby group (Kok, Gurabardhi, Gottlieb & Zijlstra 2015).

Stakeholder network
A set of individuals and organisational groups that are linked together by a common interest.

Reflect and apply

Think about the various organisational groups in your community that have relevance to your healthcare role. Draw a diagram that represents this stakeholder network, identifying the focal organisation.

Once you begin to communicate with the community, it may be that the scope changes to reflect your increased knowledge about who are the members of the community and the role that they play. Valente et al. (2015) suggest that during this initial phase of mapping a stakeholder network and understanding community boundaries, you need to:

1. think about barriers and facilitators to participation
2. identify additional community partners, leaders and gatekeepers
3. identify ecological and delivery system issues
4. gather any benchmark data (such as the rate of obesity or substance use)
5. identify important characteristics (e.g. demographics, resources, culture and context).

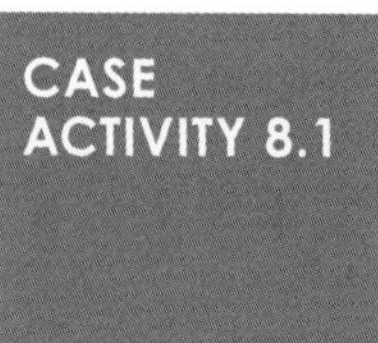

Identifying community boundaries

Your colleague Trisha, an Aboriginal health worker, is discussing with you the problem of diabetes in her community in Far North Queensland. She tells you that many of the indigenous people living with diabetes need to find a way to record their blood sugar levels (BSLs) and food and drink intake. She recalls that there may be a smartphone app that could help, but she does not have the time to look into it.

Trisha would like you to lead a group of Aboriginal health workers working with people with diabetes to find a solution to this problem.

How would you go about identifying community boundaries in this scenario?

Planning for reciprocity

Reciprocity A situation in which each party in a relationship or exchange mutually benefits from the process.

Reciprocity is a significant concept that informs effective communication with the community. Mansfield (2016) defines reciprocity as the give and take in a relationship that has negotiated 'meaning, power and identity' to mutual benefit: 'Reciprocal relationships need to be negotiated and partners need to be respectful and flexible in understanding how relationships are working, in what contexts, and for whom' (p. 723). A recent systematic review and meta-analysis of the literature concerning the effectiveness of community-based initiatives to improve critical health literacy found that establishing reciprocity in relationships was a key characteristic of interventions that improved both co-learning and social support (de Wit et al. 2017). Being conscious of the importance of reciprocity in the development of relationships with community members is the first step to actualising this in practice.

Skills in practice

Ensuring reciprocity

Celia is a physiotherapist with extensive expertise in perinatal health. She has recently relocated to a new town and has limited knowledge about the community. Celia is aware that the community is comprised mainly of young families and there is a need for perinatal education. Before implementing any programs to address this need, Celia makes contact with relevant stakeholders to obtain information to complete a detailed assessment of specific community needs. As a result, she develops a plan for the delivery of information to pregnant women in the community and, with the help of the stakeholder network, successfully implements the program.

What's happening here?

Despite Celia's extensive knowledge of perinatal health, and her evidence-based understanding of the importance of perinatal education, she ensures that she consults broadly with the community before proceeding. As a result, she has ensured that the program will have reciprocal benefits and is therefore be more likely to be successful.

Reciprocity is not guaranteed in relationships of unequal power, so it is important for healthcare professionals to think through what it will take to establish this level of trust. Time, commitment and a willingness to be open to cultural difference are essential to establishing reciprocity in relationships with communities.

Reflect and apply

Consider some of the relationships in your personal and professional life. What part does reciprocity have in this relationships? How is this reciprocity manifested?

Developing a communication plan

The communication plan that you develop will respond to the very first question we addressed in this chapter: answering the 'why'. It is unusual for healthcare professionals to be involved in communicating with the community using one-way communication. There are a number of examples of health promotion campaigns that use evidence-based messaging in this way; however, they are designed by experts in health communication and marketing. Most healthcare professionals will be engaged in a two-way process of communicating with a community and for this they need to develop a plan. The Australian Government has a useful Stakeholder Engagement Framework (Department of Health 2019) that can assist in developing communication plans.

The framework (Figure 8.1) has five key principles. The first is to be purposeful and to begin every engagement with a very clear idea of what needs to be achieved together. This principle aligns with the importance of answering the 'why' question before taking any other steps. The second principle is to be inclusive, identifying key stakeholders and making sure they have the information they need to participate fully in the process. This principle aligns with mapping the stakeholder network and understanding the scope of the community you aim to work with. The third principle is to be timely in the process of communication and consult early with key stakeholders before any decisions are made about action. This principle aligns with the potential design thinking, or human-centred design, has to offer in terms of identifying what problems end-users experience in optimising their health and well-being, and what they think the potential solutions might be. The fourth principle is to be transparent in communicating with communities. This includes setting realistic expectations about what might be achieved together given the available resources. The fifth and final principle is to be respectful when communicating with communities. There is a wealth of intellectual capital available to draw on when developing relationships of trust with community partners. Understanding that relationships have to include elements of reciprocity, or mutual gain, is fundamental to building trust and optimising outcomes for everyone involved.

FIGURE 8.1 Stakeholder Engagement Framework

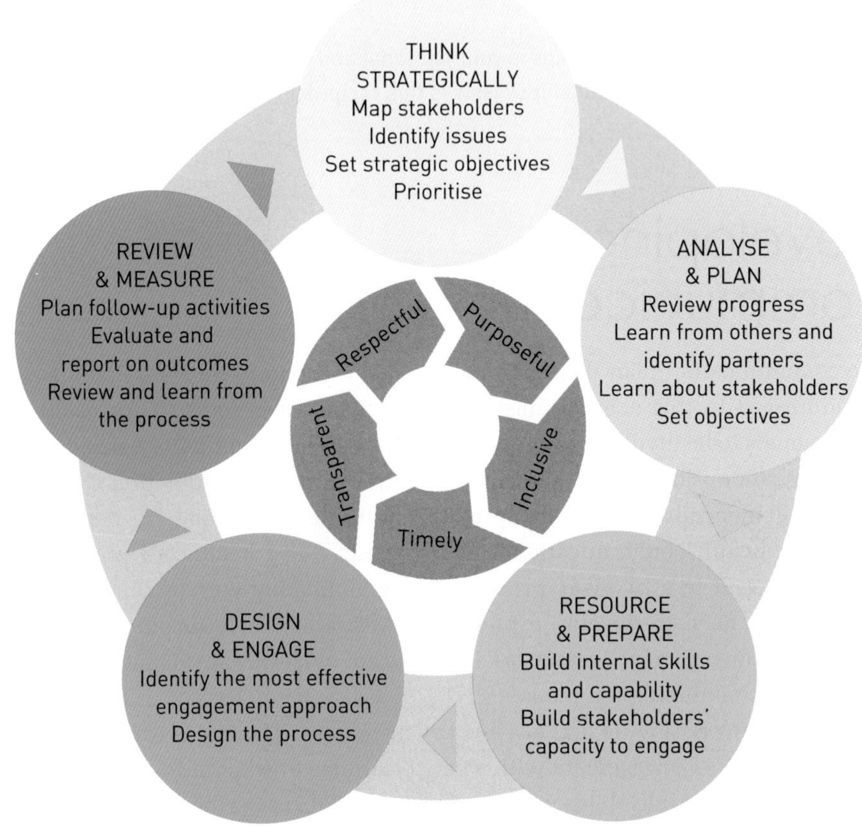

Source: Department of Health 2019.

CASE ACTIVITY 8.2

Applying the Stakeholder Engagement Framework

Review the five principles of the Stakeholder Engagement Framework described above. How would you incorporate these principles into your communication plan for working with the Aboriginal health workers and their clients to improve their care?

As well as five principles for engagement, the framework includes a five-step model of engagement that can form the basis for a communication plan (Department of Health 2019, p. 3).

Using this five-step model will provide opportunities to organise and gather information in different ways depending on the 'why'. Once you have mapped your stakeholder network, and identified the issue you want to address, you can then work out how you want to proceed. If the best solution potentially lies in a co-design process, then the analyse and plan step will look very different than if you have an already formulated solution you want to test. Regardless, each of the five principles that underpin the model—to be purposeful, inclusive, timely, transparent and respectful—all contribute to developing a reciprocal relationship with key community stakeholders.

Finally, the Stakeholder Engagement Framework provides very useful guidance about the different levels of engagement that can result from a variety of strategies. Table 8.1 was adapted from the IAP Spectrum for Public Participation, which is considered an international standard (International Association for Public Participation 2014).

TABLE 8.1 Levels of engagement with the community

Inform	Consult	Involve	Collaborate	Empower
To inform or educate stakeholders in one-way communication. There is no invitation to respond.	To gain information and feedback from stakeholders to inform decisions made internally. Limited two-way communication—ask questions, stakeholder provides answers.	To work directly with stakeholders throughout the process to ensure that issues and concerns are understood and considered. Two-way or multi-way communication where learning takes place on both sides.	To partner with stakeholder and/or stakeholder groups for the development of mutually agreed solutions and joint plan of action. Two-way/multi-way communication where learning, negotiation and decision making take place on both sides. Stakeholders work together to take action.	To delegate decision making in the hands of the stakeholders on a particular issue. Stakeholders are enabled/equipped to actively contribute to the achievement of outcomes.
'We will keep you informed.'	'We will keep you informed, listen to your concerns, consider your insights, and provide feedback on our decisions.'	'We will work with you so that your concerns and issues are directly reflected in alternatives developed and provide feedback on how input influenced the outcome.'	'We will work together to agree on what we will implement and incorporate your advice and recommendations into the outcomes to the maximum extent possible.'	'We will implement what you decide and we will support and complement your actions.'

In terms of changing health behaviours, the most effective communication strategies will focus on the right-hand side of the spectrum, where the aim is to involve, collaborate with and empower community stakeholders in relation to their health and well-being.

CASE ACTIVITY 8.3

Levels of engagement

As you develop your strategy for working with Aboriginal health workers and their clients, what levels of engagement will you aim for as you pull together a strategy for end-users to better record their BSL and food intake?

Evaluating effectiveness

Evaluating the effectiveness of solutions to identified problems is very important as it develops the evidence base about what actually works in practice. Evaluating for effectiveness requires a 'conceptualisation of what constitutes success'(Salmon & Murray-Johnson 2013, p. 100). Effectiveness can be evaluated against a broad range of outcomes, including definitional, ideological, political, contextual, cost-effective and programmatic (Salmon & Murray-Johnson 2013). These authors also point out that effectiveness should not be confused with effects. Although both terms are often used interchangeably and both represent interpretations of communication, they differ in their intentionality. Evaluating the effectiveness of a solution relates to the intended goals, objectives and expectations. In reality, the effects of trialling a solution may be intended or unintended and it is important to understand these effects in order to understand the impact they might have had. This impact could be positive or negative, either of which can form the basis for future action.

The design of an effective evaluation strategy is included from the very first brainstorm about 'why' communication should be made with a particular community. How will we know something has worked? This question has to be posed at the same time as deciding that there is potential benefit in working with a particular group of key community stakeholders. The process of evaluation needs to comply with the relevant standards in the country in which you practice (ANZEA/SUPERU 2014; National Health and Medical Research Council 2014). It is important to understand that ethical integrity is fundamental to all levels of evaluation and that above all else healthcare professionals must demonstrate respect and ensure the safety of those with whom they practice.

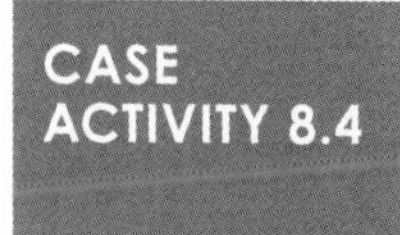

Developing an evaluation strategy

As part of developing your strategy for assisting Aboriginal health workers to assist people living with diabetes to record the BSLs and food and drink intake, you need to develop an approach to evaluation. How will you know which strategies will be most effective for this group?

Conclusion

Communicating with the community is a complex and often time-consuming process. It is also a very rewarding process that, if done well, can facilitate an exchange of knowledge that benefits both healthcare professionals and community stakeholders. Understanding the cultural context in which you are practising is fundamental to answering the 'why' communicate question. Being prepared to be surprised about the problem as it is perceived by end-users, and understanding that the potential solutions to be trialled might not be those that you originally imagined, is all part of effective communication. Respecting that not all wisdom is found in books, and understanding that there is a wealth of intellectual capital in communities, will help healthcare professionals move to a more equal footing with community members. Above all, cultivating an appetite for risk will allow you to prototype solutions and work in an iterative way to finding the most effective and impactful outcome for those whom you serve.

SUMMARY POINTS

- A community is a group of individuals who are linked geographically through location, or conceptually through values, beliefs or interests.
- The process for communicating effectively with community groups involves:
  - identifying the 'why'
  - understanding community boundaries
  - planning for reciprocity
  - developing a communication plan
  - evaluating effectiveness.
- A number of principles, frameworks and innovative approaches to thinking are available that can assist in developing a plan for communicating with the community.

CRITICAL THINKING QUESTIONS

1. A group of refugees living in the centre of your city want information about immunisations for their school-aged children. As a community healthcare worker, what is your role in advising this group?

2. In your town there is a very robust Greek community that is active in health promotion programs and helping assist new immigrants to settle into the community. You are approached by a senior member of this community seeking information on preventing teenage pregnancy. As a healthcare professional, how might you proceed to provide this assistance?

Group activity

Communicating with the community

In your study groups or via your subject discussion site, compile a list of all the communities to which you belong. How are these groups delineated (e.g. by geography or shared values, beliefs and interests)? In what ways does the process of communication differ within these communities?

WEBLINKS

Communication and health promotion

Australian Government:
www.australia.gov.au/information-and-services/health/health-promotion

Health Promotion Agency (Te Hiringa Hauora) (New Zealand Government):
www.hpa.org.nz

VicHealth (Victorian Government):
www.vichealth.vic.gov.au

Design thinking and communities

Design Online:
http://designonline.org.au/design-thinking-community-led-innovation-in-a-regional-context

Stakeholder networks

Australian Health Promotion Association:
www.healthpromotion.org.au

NZ Ministry of Health—Manatū Hauora: NGO Health and Disability Network:
https://ngo.health.govt.nz/home

REFERENCES

ANZEA/SUPERU. (2014). *Evaluation Standards for Aotearoa New Zealand.* Wellington: New Zealand Government. Retrieved from www.anzea.org.nz/app/uploads/2019/04/ANZEA-Superu-Evaluation-standards-final-020415.pdf.

Australian Institute of Health and Welfare. (2018). *Australia's Health 2018.* Canberra: AIHW. Retrieved from www.aihw.gov.au/reports/australias-health/australias-health-2018/contents/table-of-contents.

de Wit, L., Fenenga, C., Giammarchi, C., di Furia, L., Hutter, I., de Winter, A. & Meijering, L. (2017). Community-based initiatives improving critical health literacy: A systematic review and meta-synthesis of qualitative evidence. *BMC Public Health*, 18(1), 40. doi:10.1186/s12889-017-4570-7.

Department of Health. (2019). *Stakeholder Engagement Framework*. Canberra: Australian Government. Retrieved from www.health.gov.au/sites/default/files/stakeholder-engagement-framework_0.pdf.

International Association for Public Participation. (2014). *IAP2'S Public Participation Spectrum*. Retrieved from www.iap2.org.au/Tenant/C0000004/00000001/files/IAP2_Public_Participation_Spectrum.pdf.

Kok, G., Gurabardhi, Z., Gottlieb, N.H. & Zijlstra, F.R.H. (2015). Influencing organizations to promote health: Applying stakeholder theory. *Health Education & Behavior*, 42(1 suppl), 123S–132S. doi:10.1177/1090198115571363.

MacQueen, K.M., McLellan, E., Metzger, D.S., Kegeles, S., Strauss, R.P., Scotti, R., ... Trotter, R.T. (2001). What is community? An evidence-based definition for participatory public health. *American Journal of Public Health*, 91(12), 1929–38. doi:10.2105/AJPH.91.12.1929.

Mansfield, L. (2016). Resourcefulness, reciprocity and reflexivity: The three Rs of partnership in sport for public health research. *International Journal of Sport Policy and Politics*, 8(4), 713–29. doi:10.1080/19406940.2016.1220409.

Matheson, G.O., Pacione, C., Shultz, R.K. & Klügl, M. (2015). Leveraging human-centered design in chronic disease prevention. *American Journal of Preventive Medicine*, 48(4), 472–9. doi:https://doi.org/10.1016/j.amepre.2014.10.014.

National Health and Medical Research Council. (2014). *Ethical Considerations in Quality Assurance and Evaluation Activities*. Canberra: Australian Government. Retrieved from https://www.nhmrc.gov.au/sites/default/files/documents/attachments/ethical-considerations-in-quality-assurance-and-evaluation-activites.pdf.

National Health Information and Performance Principal Committee. (2017). *The Australian Health Performance Framework*. Canberra: Australian Health Ministers' Advisory Council. Retrieved from www.coaghealthcouncil.gov.au/Portals/0/OOS318_Attachment%201.pdf.

Roberts, J.P., Fisher, T.R., Trowbridge, M.J. & Bent, C. (2016). A design thinking framework for healthcare management and innovation. *Healthcare*, 4(1), 11–14. doi:10.1010/j.hjdsi.2015.12.002.

Salmon, C. & Murray-Johnson, L. (2013). Communication campaign effectiveness and effects: Some critical distinctions. In R. Rice & C. Aitken (eds), *Public Communication Campaigns* (4th edn) (pp. 99–112). Thousand Oaks, CA: Sage Publications.

Te Morenga, L., Pekepo, C., Corrigan, C., Matoe, L., Mules, R., Goodwin, D., ... Ni Mhurchu, C. (2018). Co-designing an mHealth tool in the New Zealand Māori community with a 'Kaupapa Māori' approach. *AlterNative: An International Journal of Indigenous Peoples*, 14(1), 90–9. doi:10.1177/1177180117753169.

Valente, T.W., Palinkas, L.A., Czaja, S., Chu, K.-H. & Brown, C.H. (2015). Social network analysis for program implementation. *PLOS ONE*, 10(6), e0131712. doi:10.1371/journal.pone.0131712.

OXFORD UNIVERSITY PRESS

PART 3

ETHICAL AND SUPPORTIVE COMMUNICATION

OXFORD UNIVERSITY PRESS

CHAPTER 9

SAFETY AND QUALITY IN CLINICAL COMMUNICATION

NICHOLAS RALPH, CLINT MOLONEY AND JENNY DAVIS

CHAPTER FOCUS

After reading this chapter and completing the activities, you will be able to:

- discuss concepts of safety and quality in communication
- describe evidence-based approaches to safe, high-quality communication in the clinical setting
- explore inherent risks to safety and quality in clinical communication
- identify and apply evidence-based approaches and strategies in clinical communication.

KEY TERMS

AIDET
Clinical handover
Quality
Safety
SBAR
SOAP
Transitions of care

Introduction

Safety
Awareness, planning and performance of conscious acts to eliminate or minimise the potential for harm to individuals.

Quality
The systematic application of continuous improvement processes and procedures that mitigate a recognised or perceived risk to enable a high standard of care.

Safety and **quality** should define the characteristics and impact of communication in the healthcare environment. Although safety and quality may be seen as interchangeable terms, there is broad evidence in the literature of a general intent to improve communication in modern healthcare to a level of quality beyond a minimum standard of safety (Beckett & Kipnis 2009). The notion of quality in communication stems from proactive approaches to recognised or perceived risks, rather than reactions to failures. While safety is the primary objective, the inherent risk attached to human-oriented systems usually results in the introduction of fail-safe mechanisms. These fail-safe mechanisms elevate the quality of systems to a level in which the risks and impacts of failure are actively or passively mitigated or prevented.

Effective communication in clinical settings is fundamental to the safety and quality of healthcare. There is an expansive body of evidence demonstrating clear links between poor communication and adverse outcomes for patients (Bakon, Wirihana, Christensen & Craft 2017). The Australian Commission on Safety and Quality in Health Care (ACSQHC) states that effective communication is an essential element of patient care and identifies high-risk situations when effective communication is even more critical for patient safety (ACSQHC 2019b). High risk healthcare communication situations include clinical handover, transitions of care, patient identification and clinical documentation. The ACSQHC Communicating for Safety Standard requires that leaders of health service organisations set up and maintain systems and processes to support effective communication with patients, carers and families; between multidisciplinary teams and clinicians; and across health service organisations and workforce to effectively communicate to ensure safety (ACSQHC 2019b).

Beyond healthcare, many other sectors have worked to embed safety and quality in ways that improve the quality of communication, and further reduce the presence of risks and the occurrence of failures. Aviation is one industry that has established exacting standards of quality in communication, introducing sterile cockpit situations to ensure that only relevant communication occurs during critical periods of flying (Pape 2003). Similarly, in healthcare, the introduction of structured and standardised models of communication (communication mnemonics, surgical and other checklists) has worked to reduce human error and improve the flow of information to enhance patient outcomes (Beckett & Kipnis 2009).

Structured models of communication can still be implemented in ways that reflect a caring, compassionate and collegial quality, while still ensuring patient safety (Brewster & Waxman 2018). In this chapter, we explore the notion of safety as the principal focus and purpose of clinical communication. We define the concepts of safety and quality in communication, discuss why a person-centred approach to communication is important for safety, and outline recognised strategies in communication that enhance the safety and quality of processes and outcomes in the healthcare environment.

Safety in communication

The basic premise of safety in communication is to ensure that the potential for patient harm to occur is eliminated or minimised (Halligan & Zecevic 2011). Whether written or verbal, interpersonal or team-based, standardised models of communication exist to improve the safety and quality of care delivery and patient outcomes. The ACSQHC describes the principle of communicating for safety to encompass the systems and strategies for effective communication between patients, carers and families, multidisciplinary teams and clinicians, and across healthcare organisations (ACSQHC 2019b, p.16).

Clinical handover

Clinical handover (or handoff) involves the functional transfer of patient information between clinicians and includes the handover of professional authority and responsibility for care to another, occurring at a point in time and/or transition of care (Smeulers, Lucas & Vermeulen 2014). The intent of clinical handover is to promote continuity of care and reduce miscommunication (Beament, Ewens, Wilcox & Reid 2018).

Clinical handover The transfer of professional responsibility and accountability for some or all aspects of care for a patient, or group of patients, to another person or professional group on a temporary or permanent basis (ACSQHCS 2012).

Handover can vary in location, style, quality and focus and commonly involves nursing, medical and/or multidisciplinary teams (Mardis et al. 2017). No one type of handover is identified as the most effective or efficient (Bakon et al. 2017; Mardis et al. 2017; Sharp, Dahlén & Bergenmar 2019; Smeulers et al. 2014).

Historically, handover occurred away from the patient in the nurses' station and without direct patient involvement (Sharp et al. 2019). Handover now commonly occurs at the bedside and aims to minimise the risk of miscommunication, and to promote patient-centred care and shared decision making (Tobiano et al. 2018). Ideally, bedside handover should include face-to-face communication, active patient participation, the use of structured communication tools (written and verbal) and be supported with information technology (Forde, Coffey & Hegarty 2018; Smeulers et al. 2014; Wong, Tung, Peck & Goh. 2019).

Transitions of care have been identified as times when patient safety risk in communication is increased (ACSQHC 2019b). Transitions of care where clinical handover occurs include: patient transfers (e.g. another ward, facility, to/from community); patient transfers (e.g. operating theatre, tests/appointments); shift to shift changeover; team handover (including multidisciplinary team or specialty teams); admission/discharge; and change in patient condition (e.g. escalation of deteriorating patient).

Transitions of care The process of transferring all or part of a patient's care delivery transferred between healthcare providers or care locations.

Strategies, including bedside handover and use of structured tools, increase patient safety—for example, a multi-site study of the i-PASS handoff tool reported a 23 per cent reduction in medical errors (Starmer et al. 2014). Tools not considered acceptable for clinical handover include recording devices (video and voice), SMS and other social media platforms. Other transition of care examples involve information transfer at discharge, where information and responsibility for care is transferred to the patient and/or carers/families or to care providers in other settings (e.g. aged care).

Skills in practice

Clinical handover

Sandra is the registered nurse in charge of the night shift on a surgical unit. One morning she is conducting handover at the bedside. Sandra is tired after a gruelling shift and just wants to get home. She is standing next to the bedside of Mr Argus, a 75-year-old man who has dementia. Sandra tells the staff assembled for the handover that Mr Argus was 'a nightmare last night. He pulled out his IV three times and was incontinent twice'. Clare, who is in charge of the morning shift, suggests to Sandra that they continue to handover in the Unit Manager's office.

What's happening here?

Sandra's communication lacked professionalism. She appeared more interested in debriefing her experiences of the night shift rather than presenting information that could promote quality of care for her patient. Clare's intervention was effective in reducing the impact of the poor communication in that instant.

Models for safety in communication

Standardised models of communication offer frameworks for identifying and communicating the minimum (critical) information content that will promote patient safety (Fealy et al. 2019). These models feature extensively throughout the healthcare environment, particularly in clinical handover (e.g. SBAR: situation, background, assessment and recommendation); documentation (e.g. SOAP: subjective, objective, assessment and plan); and care delivery (e.g. six rights of drug administration).

Strong evidence exists for the integration of standardised models of communication in healthcare, as these can:

- improve the perception of interprofessional communication (Randmaa, Mårtensson, Swenne & Engström 2014)
- help prioritise specific clinical situations or problems (Blair & Smith 2012)
- decrease clinical errors (Starmer et al. 2014)
- reduce the incidence of unexpected mortality (De Meester, Verspuy, Monsieurs & Van Bogaert 2013).

Models of communication work by:

- improving situational awareness (Leonard, Graham & Bonacum 2004)
- preventing communication breakdown (Randmaa et al. 2014)
- establishing a level of hierarchy for communication to occur (Haig, Sutton & Whittington 2006)
- improving the timeliness of communication (Randmaa et al. 2014).

Although standardised models provide a framework for improving clinical communication, they are fallible (Marshall & Robson 2005) if they become rules rather than guides, potentially causing clinicians to disengage from employing critical-thinking skills. As was shown in Chapter 7, poor communication can result in organisational inefficiencies (Randmaa et al. 2014); failing to achieve desired outcomes (Blair & Smith 2012); and even death and disaster (De Meester et al. 2013). It is therefore helpful to remember that models of communication are not used to reduce the need for clinicians to think; instead, they are designed as a guide or framework to focus thinking and doing by ensuring that only relevant information is communicated.

Standardised models for improving the safety of clinical communication exist for every context where information transfer occurs in healthcare. The following section explores some common models used in written and verbal communication, including strategies that bridge both contexts to enhance the quality of patient care.

Verbal communication

The use of verbal communication is pivotal to the quality of healthcare delivery. From conducting an initial patient interview, to building and maintaining patient rapport, the healthcare professional is required to be adept at verbal communication as part of their role. Furthermore, the need to communicate information about the patient's condition to a wide array of staff from different disciplines and with differing levels of expertise demands strong communication skills to avoid the potential for breakdowns in communication.

There are clinician-to-clinician communication frameworks or tools currently implemented across various healthcare settings, each designed to be flexible and adaptable to suit workforce, setting, organisational culture and purpose (Bakon et al. 2017; Mardis et al. 2017; Starmer et al. 2014). These include:

- SBAR (Situation, Background, Assessment, Recommendation)
- ISBAR (Identify, Situation, Background, Assessment, Recommendation)
- ISoBAR (Identity, Situation, Observations, Background, Agreed Plan, Read Back)
- SHARED (Situation, History, Assessment, Risk, Expectation, Documentation)
- I PASS the BATON (Introduction, Patient, Assessment, Situation, Safety concerns, Background, Actions, Timing, Ownership, Next).

Two common frameworks used to guide verbal communication and promote safety in the clinical environment are the AIDET, a tool for patient–clinician communication, and SBAR, a tool for clinician–clinician communication. These are discussed in more detail below. In addition, there are variations arising from the SBAR framework, such as ISBAR and ISoBAR.

The process of building rapport should transcend the adoption of a framework and result in the clinician having an awareness of how their communication style can impact on the less obvious issues in patient safety. In considering this, it is important to recognise that verbally communicating with patients is more than just the words being said. The tone, inflection and body language of the clinician can convey to a patient whether the person looking after them is attentive, professional and caring, or lacking these traits.

While clarity and efficiency of communication is vital in the clinical setting, the notion of warmth when communicating with patients can greatly impact upon whether the patient feels as though they are being safely cared for. For these reasons, using any communication framework must be undertaken in conjunction with an awareness of one's self. Empathy and compassion towards other human beings are often a strong motivator for people entering the healthcare professions. However, fatigue and burnout can result in clinicians becoming emotionally detached from patients, making it difficult to convey an empathetic and compassionate presence (Wright 2011). The frameworks discussed below should be employed with caution, as effective, efficient, safe and professional communication must be matched with the need to ensure that clinician–patient interactions are person-centred and marked by humanism.

AIDET

AIDET
A mnemonic outlining the framework that improves communication between clinicians and recipients of care:
A = Acknowledge;
I = Introduce;
D = Duration;
E = Explanation;
T = Thank.

The mnemonic **AIDET** was introduced in 2003 by the Studer Group as a template for improving communication between clinicians and patients (Studer 2003). AIDET was initiated in response to a perceived loss of interpersonal communication between the care provider and patient (Studer 2003). The AIDET framework guided the development of strong therapeutic rapport by providing a model for humanised conversations where the civilities of normal social communication colour what is otherwise a clinically orientated dialogue (see Figure 9.1).

Although the AIDET model is predominantly focused on providing a framework for improving interpersonal communication between clinicians and patients, its utility as a means of developing patient rapport is becoming more recognised. Since its introduction, it has been demonstrated to enhance safety in communication by establishing a framework for initiating interpersonal communication with patients (Katona et al. 2014) and improving patient compliance with care delivery (Zhang et al. 2013). Its simplistic structure, aimed at standardising how clinicians engage patients in communication, is a key tool in formalising what is designed to appear as an informal event. Many studies have addressed the critical window of opportunity available to those who rely on their initial conversations to make a positive impression on a person. In clinical contexts, the value of establishing an immediate rapport with the patient is widely recognised as fundamental to ensuring that the therapeutic relationship continues to be successful (Norfolk, Birdi & Walsh 2007). The AIDET model has distinct verbal and non-verbal communication elements; positive features associated with this communication model for patients include staff behaviours of smiling, knocking before entering and making eye contact (Allen, Rieck & Salsbury 2016).

FIGURE 9.1 The AIDET mnemonic

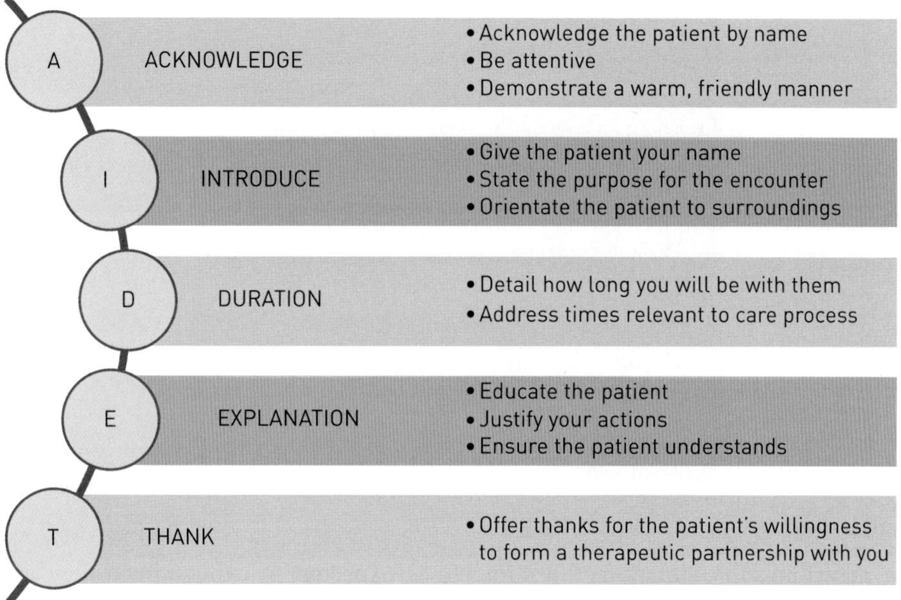

SBAR

SBAR is a mnemonic that stands for Situation, Background, Assessment, Recommendation. It is used globally in the healthcare environment to enhance communication, principally between clinicians, and is usually verbal (Hughes, Durham & Alden 2008).

SBAR was first developed by the US military as a means of promoting prompt and appropriate communication (Pope, Rodzen & Spross 2008). The model was subsequently adopted and implemented by staff at Kaiser Permanente (a leading US-based healthcare consortium) to improve communication between clinicians (Leonard et al. 2004). This model is particularly valuable for structured communication by telephone (Müller et al. 2018). The model focuses on communication necessary to the situation: background, assessment and recommendation articulated by the clinician, usually to another clinician.

SBAR
A mnemonic employed in healthcare communication between healthcare professionals:
S = Situation;
B = Background;
A = Assessment;
R = Recommendation.

FIGURE 9.2 The SBAR mnemonic

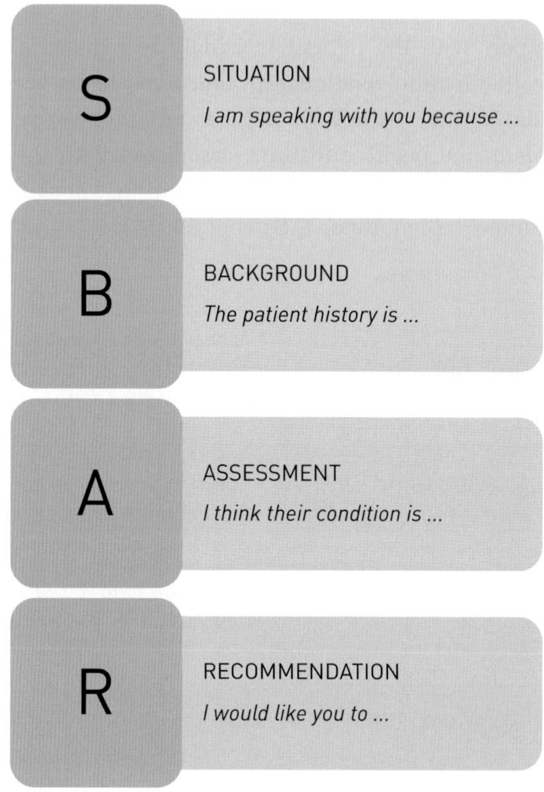

Situation

In describing the situation, the clinician is expected to explain *why* they are contacting another clinician to communicate with them. The clinician should explain the situation by:

- identifying themselves, their role and their work unit
- identifying the patient by name
- describing the current situation—for example, concerning change in health status.

An example of describing the situation: Hello Dr Jackson. My name is Nick and I am a registered nurse from Ward A. I am calling about patient Joan Grant. Joan seems to have deteriorated as she is confused and her breathing is increasingly laboured.

Background

Giving the patient's background is vital. The clinician should provide this by:

- giving the reason for admission
- detailing significant medical and social history
- addressing the patient's current treatment regime.

An example of providing the background: Joan was admitted three days ago for treatment of deep vein thrombosis and cellulitis of the left leg. She has a history of mild asthma and depression and is allergic to drugs. She has been treated until now with anticoagulants and antibiotics, to which she appears to have been responding well.

Assessment

One of the most vital aspects of the SBAR mnemonic is to give an accurate assessment of the patient. Communication using SBAR is usually between clinicians and the need to give an accurate picture of the patient is achieved by prioritising important information gleaned from the assessment of the patient. The clinician should provide:

- vital signs in terms of numbers *and* quality—for example, the heart rate and whether it is irregular or regular
- visual appearance and effect—for example, is the patient pale, sweating and confused?
- primary and secondary assessment information—for example, airway, breathing, circulation, etc.

An example of providing the assessment: I have just taken Joan's vital signs and her resting respiratory rate has increased significantly over the last 15 minutes from 12 breaths per minute to 24 breaths per minute. I have applied six litres of oxygen via a facemask. She is also becoming more agitated and confused and appears to be pale and diaphoretic.

Recommendation

The next step in the SBAR process is providing a recommendation. This step is not necessarily about validating the clinician's approach but stating their needs or expectations clearly. The clinician should:

- explain what they need clearly, including timeframes and care requirements
- suggest possible diagnoses or treatment options.

An example of giving a recommendation: I think Joan may have a pulmonary embolus and I would like you to urgently review her. Can you please let me know when you will be able to come? Can you also provide me with treatment options that I can undertake now?

The use of standardised communication tools is increasingly mandated for clinical handover in healthcare settings. Effective use of standardised models of communication such as SBAR in combination with other strategies can positively influence the safety and quality of care delivery. These strategies all aim to minimise the risks to patient safety that may arise from human error and miscommunication.

Reflect and apply

When you are next in the clinical environment, make a note of the models used for structuring verbal communication. Are they used consistently? Do they vary across healthcare professional groups?

Written communication

Written communication (documentation) occurs in a variety of ways throughout healthcare settings and can be electronic or paper-based, or a combination of both. Written communication is vital to the integrity of the healthcare system and occurs throughout the environment, whether it be documenting a patient's condition, detailing a hospital policy or describing aspects relevant to the administration of a hospital.

Poor documentation is a key safety and quality risk in healthcare settings, particularly during transitions of care where there is an even higher risk of information being miscommunicated or lost (ACSQHC 2019b). Healthcare professionals are required to maintain clear and accurate clinical records as part of their professional codes and responsibilities and in accordance with the National Safety and Quality Health Service (NSQHS) Standard Communicating for Safety 6.11 (ACSQHC 2012). Documentation of patient care information must:

- be objective, clear, legible, concise, contemporaneous, progressive, complete, relevant, consistent and accurate
- include information about assessments, action taken, and care provided, outcomes, reassessment, risks, complications and changes to the care plan
- meet all necessary medico-legal requirements for documentation.

Digital or electronic clinical information systems and technologies are increasingly used in healthcare settings and such systems must meet the same principles of best practice as patient care documentation. See the focus box 'Common forms of written communication in healthcare'.

BOX 9.1

COMMON FORMS OF WRITTEN COMMUNICATION IN HEALTHCARE

- Clinical records
- Patient monitoring—for example, vital signs equipment
- Electronic health records
- Discharge summaries
- Hospital policies
- Clinical guidelines
- Posters and signs—for example, handwashing, clinical waste sheets

- Dangerous drugs books—for example, scheduled medicines
- Surgical safety checklists
- Pathology or radiology results
- Specialist referral forms.

SOAP

A common standardised model of written communication is **SOAP**, which stands for Subjective, Objective, Assessment, Plan. SOAP is a way of guiding the structured documentation of clinical progress notes in the healthcare setting.

SOAP
A mnemonic used to help clinicians structure progress notes in a problem-specific clinical decision-making order:
S = Subjective;
O = Objective;
A = Assessment;
P = Plan.

The use of SOAP as a mnemonic is designed to assist clinicians in structuring clinical progress notes that encourage a holistic, systemically ordered and problem-specific approach to clinical decision making (Mowery et al. 2012; Pearce, Ferguson, George & Langford 2016). The SOAP structure is increasingly used in electronic health records to support clinician documentation, which also allows for the automated extraction and utilisation of data as a means of summarising the continuum of patient care (Mowery et al. 2012; Pearce et al. 2016). The purpose of SOAP is to eliminate uncertainty about how to structure the documentation of a patient's condition, as some clinicians experience hesitancy in knowing when, what, why, where and how to document important information. Figure 9.3 provides an example of SOAP documentation.

FIGURE 9.3 An example of SOAP documentation

S	SUBJECTIVE *A brief statement outlining the reason for presentation; patient status; and medical history*	Joan Grant is a 58-year-old patient presenting with diffuse pain in the left lower leg for the past three days. The patient has a history of mild asthma, depression and an allergy to sulphur drugs resulting in severe pruritus. She is not on any regular medication. She is a non-smoker and consumes approximately three glasses of wine per week.
O	OBJECTIVE *Information collected by measuring or observing the patient's health status*	Joan's vital signs are as follows at 1015: • BP: 128/84; HR: 94; Temp: 36^8; RR: 24; SPO_2: 97% on $6LO_2$ via Face Mask • Swelling evident left calf • Pain on palpation = 9/10; Resting 6/10 Absent pulses for *dorsalis pedis and posterior tibial* Breathing laboured and irregular
A	ASSESSMENT *Information collected to determine patient symptoms and diagnosis*	Patient currently receiving: • anticoagulant for DVT (left leg) • antibiotic therapy for cellulitis (left leg) Queried pulmonary embolus
P	PLAN *The plan for the patient – usually involving treatment and care delivery*	Contacted Medical Officer for urgent review at 1020 Medical Officer assessed patient at 1030 Patient sent for urgent radiology review at 1035

The merits of effective communication in the clinical setting have clear benefits for the clinician and the patient. It is vital that healthcare professionals are adept at employing written and verbal models of communication, thus enhancing the safety of the care environment.

Risks to communicating safely in the clinical setting

The delivery of healthcare is complex in nature; with these complexities come inherent risks that demand safety and quality in communication. These risks are compounded by the complex healthcare environment, where communication is affected by time and performance pressures, political and cultural divides, cross-disciplinary approaches to care, and scope-of-practice issues (Reader, Flin & Cuthbertson 2007). The clinician must navigate the process of care delivery in the healthcare environment context to ensure that risks to the patient are minimised (Kilpatrick 2013; Slade, Murray, Pun & Eggins 2018). Risks exist throughout the healthcare environment, but situations with a particularly heightened safety risk include clinical handover, transitions of care and medication management.

The process of medication administration serves as an excellent example of what can happen when communication breakdowns occur. First, the documented prescription may not be clear, concise, accurate and legible, which may cause the medication administrator to err. Second, this context might be further complicated by stressful emergency situations or patients with highly complex needs which, again, increase the likelihood of communication failures that translate to patient harm (Cheragi, Manoocheri, Mohammadnejad & Ehsani 2013; Keers, Williams, Cooke & Ashcroft 2013). Third, medication orders are sometimes provided verbally (e.g. at the bedside or over the phone) where immediate intervention is required. Contexts such as these have been strongly linked to medication errors, as orders can be misread or mistakes can occur during transcription of an order. Pharmacists also play a role in the communication process, and communication breakdown can occur during the dispensing phase of mediation management (Cheragi et al. 2013; Keers et al. 2013).

The patient plays a pivotal role in medication safety and must also be actively involved in the communication process (Wheeler, Scahill, Hopcroft & Stapleton 2018). Patients have the right to informed consent about prescribed medication. Lack of education and instruction on medication usage can lead to polypharmacy, medication omissions and overdose (Keers et al. 2013). The clinician plays a central role in reducing the likelihood of medication error, and can mitigate risk by using recognised communication tools, such as the strategy 'Six rights to medication safety' (see Figure 9.4):

- Right patient
- Right drug
- Right dose
- Right route
- Right time
- Right to refuse.

FIGURE 9.4 The six rights of medication administration

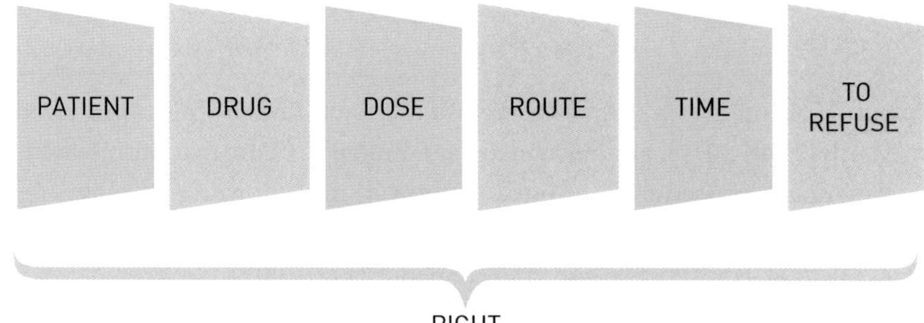

Depending on the clinical setting, the number of 'rights of medication administration' can be more expansive (e.g. right reason, right response).

Effective communication is critical in medication safety. Recognising this, there is a specific medication safety standard in the NSQHS Standards intended 'to ensure clinicians are competent to safely prescribe, dispense and administer appropriate medicines and to monitor medicine use…and to ensure that consumers are informed about medicines and understand their individual medicines and risks' (ACSQHC 2019a).

The World Health Organization (WHO) is also working to improve medication safety through its Global Patient Safety Challenge on Medication Safety program (Donaldson et al. 2017). A key strategy within this program is to improve the accuracy and communication of medication information using tools for medication reconciliation (MedRec) with the aim of obtaining the best possible medication history (Stark et al. 2019). Other strategies to improve communication for medication safety include electronic prescribing, personal electronic health records, and collaborative medicines reviews in the community (Wheeler et al. 2018). If these are coupled with good patient education, and demonstrated understanding from the patient, the risk of harm can be significantly lowered (Cheragi et al. 2013; Keers et al. 2013).

Reflect and apply

Consider the risks of communication at your university. What is the greatest risk that faces you—for example, failing, forgetting a deadline? What strategies do you have in place to overcome the risks you have identified?

Use the following table to identify risks you currently face and pose strategies that use various forms of communication (e.g. written or verbal) to minimise or eliminate them.

Identified risk	Minimising risk	Eliminating risk
1 Example: Not responding to assignment task appropriately.	• Review assessment task carefully • Highlight key words	• Communicate with the lecturer to ensure response is 'on topic'
2		
3		

Communication errors in healthcare are a known underlying cause of patient harm (Mardis et al. 2017), and have also been linked to coordination-of-care issues such as surgical procedures, clinical handover procedures, pathology results, mistimed procedures, examination errors and diagnostic errors (Collins, Newhouse, Porter & Talsma 2014; Mardis et al. 2017; Reader et al. 2007).

Failures in the pre-operative process safety checklist or failure to complete appropriate checklists have led to patient harm—for example, removal of the wrong body part during surgery or omissions of pre-medications for surgery. Failures to recognise early communication factors that provide signs of patient deterioration are very common in healthcare and often harm the patient because of the lateness of appropriate care intervention (Collins et al. 2014). The concept of 'failure to rescue' has strong links to communication competence and a clinician's ability to employ clinical reasoning (as in recognition of the deteriorating patient) in order to isolate important information through verbal and non-verbal cues and react in a timely and appropriate fashion (Johnston et al. 2015). Root cause analysis of many adverse patient situations has identified a lack of communication *and* clinical reasoning skills as a significant cause of failures in the healthcare process (Levett-Jones et al. 2010).

Barriers and enablers

The Swiss-cheese model of accident causation is a paradigm used in integrated risk management that has been widely used in healthcare for the past three decades. The Swiss-cheese model serves as an analogy of what can occur when holes in the system align and an issue 'falls through the gaps', creating harm or heightening the risk of harm. The model is also sometimes called the cumulative act effect. James Reason, the original author of the model, theorised that most accidents are traceable to four possible areas of failure. They are:

1. organisational influences
2. supervision
3. preconditions
4. specific acts (Reason 2000).

In healthcare professional practice, long working hours can result in fatigue that may lead to deficits in the safety of individual clinicians. Feeling tired or distracted can lead to poorer communication among staff (Collins et al. 2014; Reason 2000). Unsafe supervision or an inappropriate skill mix can be a common root cause of adverse situations (Haig et al. 2006). Organisations that have a positive workplace culture in nurturing and supporting inexperienced staff experience lower episodes of patient harm (Haig et al. 2006). Effectively communicating with staff on correct procedures and processes with repetitious communication and feedback is advantageous. Organisational influences that reduce expenditure on healthcare professional communication skills training have links to increased adverse patient situations. Once it is understood that communication is failing at certain points in the organisational process, solutions to prevent that failure can target the source of risk. In terms of the Swiss-cheese model, finding which slice—corporate, institutional, professional, team, individual, technical—provides the solution (Collins et al. 2014; Reason 2000).

As an example, root cause analysis may reveal that the communication breakdown is cultural in nature. Staff conflict can also hinder decision making or prevent effective communication; introducing sound conflict resolution should help to improve communication channels over time (Piening et al. 2012). Appropriately recognising the risks and correlating their presence with the implementation of a systematic risk management approach can address risk factors for effective communication. This process should begin with gathering background information, followed by the groundwork assembly of the intended message and its targeted dissemination and distribution, with a monitoring and review process.

Communication strategies in healthcare are really plans for transferring information related to a specific clinical issue, patient event or healthcare audience (Kilpatrick 2013; Parry & Land 2013; Reader et al. 2007). The strategies can act as blueprints for how staff should communicate and engage, making sure a consistent and accurate message is conveyed by more than one healthcare professional. For example, a patient may need information about the medications they will be taking home after discharge. The healthcare professionals providing this information (e.g. the nurses and pharmacist) must ensure they give the same accurate information to the patient; this is one way to reinforce the patient's knowledge. Conflicting messages will confuse the patient and lead to distrust (Parry & Land 2013) and such miscommunication is known to increase the risk of patient harm (Merten, van Galen & Wagner 2017; Starmer et al. 2014).

Communication strategies in healthcare should:

- outline key objectives and goals for the communication task
- ensure all key stakeholders are included in the communication—for example, patient, family
- define key messages
- explore and define common methods and tools for communicating information for a specific purpose
- specify the instruments that will be used to confirm the message has been received and understood.

Communication channels do not have to take the shape of formal written documents. Simply taking the time to deliberate about a communication problem and agreeing to implement a consistent approach to communicating a message or patient information is enough. Such an approach applies to simple issues healthcare professionals need to convey about low-risk patient issues that may escalate to a high-risk priority or require wider dissemination. However, issues with higher levels of risk for harm—or which are controversial—need a more formalised written plan to ensure that all key stakeholders are targeted and that all key messages are received and interpreted by a wider audience (Kilpatrick 2013; Parry & Land 2013; Reader et al. 2007).

Quality in communication

Quality in communication is often addressed in the literature, and principally focuses on strategies that elevate the transfer of information above the mere elimination of risk to approaches that offer improvements to the overarching quality of communication within systems. To elevate the quality of communication to *the next level*, utilising evidence to inform approaches is vital to achieving the goals of the system: high-quality communication processes that positively impact on care delivery.

Evidence-based measures of quality in communication

Lessons in risk mitigation have led to an array of evidence-based communication interventions designed to decrease the likelihood of human error. The introduction of the National Inpatient Medication Chart (NIMC) is a leading example of this action. Clearer documentation strategies are now apparent to ensure prescriptions are clearer to those healthcare professionals involved in the administration process, with a growing suite of national standard medication charts (ACSQHC 2019a). The NIMC signifies national consensus on standardised presentation and communication of medication information and the practices that underpin them. One significant constituent of the NIMC is the communication of medicine prescriptions to allow safe and precise dispensing, administration and reconciliation of medicines. As an example, the NIMC aids in the communication of known patient allergies to those staff who are about to administer a medication, as shown in Figure 9.5 (ACQSHC 2019a). Additional examples include an NIMC for paediatrics, day surgery, a national subcutaneous insulin chart, and a national residential medication chart (NRMC) specifically for residential aged care (ACQSHC 2019a).

FIGURE 9.5 Clear communication of known allergies and adverse drug reactions (ADR) in NIMC

ATTACH ADR STICKER		
ALLERGIES AND ADVERSE DRUG REACTIONS (ADR) ☐ Nil known ☐ Unknown (tick appropriate box or complete details below)		
Medicine (or other)	Reaction/Type/Date	Initials
Sign____________ Print_________________ Date______		

Shared effective communication strategies like the one shown in Figure 9.5 are necessary elements when aspiring to attain higher quality care and patient safety standards. The true source of breakdown in a communication chain is not always obvious, and patient incidents often require a thorough analysis to determine where failures have occurred. Retrospective analysis and concise mapping depicting how events unfolded is an effective way to discover factors that contribute to communication failure. Consequently, structured communication techniques and tools are increasingly mandated in many healthcare settings (Sharp et al. 2019; Slade et al. 2019).

As discussed in Chapter 7, silence can have negative consequences in the organisational setting. The ability to question or challenge colleagues' healthcare decisions can be instrumental in saving a patient's life. However, appropriately dealing with such situations requires employing the strategies of graded assertiveness effectively. Graded assertiveness is a learnt skill; it does not come easily to many novice clinicians, who can feel intimidated by their more senior, high-profile colleagues. When used well, graded assertiveness is a method of communicating, advocating and focusing with clarity in challenging or crisis scenarios (Lin et al. 2004). One form of graded assertiveness that has been embraced by healthcare professionals is represented by the acronym PACE: Probe, Alert, Challenge, Emergency. PACE consists of four stages or tiers of communication. Each stage is a measured intensification that meticulously—if the problem is not resolved—relocates power to an individual who has a right to refuse active participation in an activity that they believe will result in harm, such as the administration of a medication (Miller 2013).

Ensuring safe, high-quality communication in such circumstances relies on the presence or absence of the human factor. For instance, the presence of human dynamics between different healthcare professionals—such as junior and senior clinicians—can create a power differential and impose constraints on the flow of important information that could impact on the continuity or effectiveness of care. The context of care can also play a major role in *when* clinicians feel the need to speak up; an issue with a cancer patient, for instance, may resonate more deeply with some clinicians than others and lead them to communicate the importance they attach to certain issues. The absence of humanising influences on communication can also result in a rigid, robot-like manner of communicating, leaving patients believing that the person caring for them is simply 'going through the motions'.

PACE, along with other structured models of communication discussed in this chapter, assists healthcare organisations to ensure communication is clear, effective and timely. Collaborative communication strengthens both healthcare professional and patient satisfaction, as well as advancing positive patient safety outcomes by fostering teamwork and supporting working relationships (Beckett & Kipnis 2009). Patient satisfaction or opinion is fundamental to quality measures of effective communication in healthcare, so it is imperative that teamwork communication frameworks also incorporate the patient. Language must enable understanding, and patient understanding should help to alleviate risk (DeVoe, Wallace & Fryer 2009). Enabling patient understanding also includes support for people who need assistance with communication—for example, health literacy, language, speech, hearing or vision (ACSQHC 2019b).

Improving the quality of communication in the clinical setting is an ongoing priority in the healthcare sector. Understanding the root causes of good-quality (and poor-quality) communication is an essential step towards sound quality assurance. Evidence-based solutions must be piloted in order to measure a reduction in associated risk. PDCA, or the Plan-Do-Check-Act cycle, is a simple four-step model designed to help an organisation's quality team measure the longitudinal impact of a given solution (Tague 2005). Also known as the PDSA (Plan-Do-Study-Act) cycle, PDCA is considered a more pragmatic yet scientific method for testing changes in complex systems such as healthcare and minimises the risk of patient harm (Taylor et al. 2014). Figure 9.6 is an adaptation of the original PDCA cycle, and shows the organisational benefit gained through continuously monitoring and reporting communication risk. Through continuous quality improvement, a healthcare organisation can engender wide and positive growth in evidence-based communication processes and systems (Tague 2005).

FIGURE 9.6 The Plan-Do-Check-Act cycle

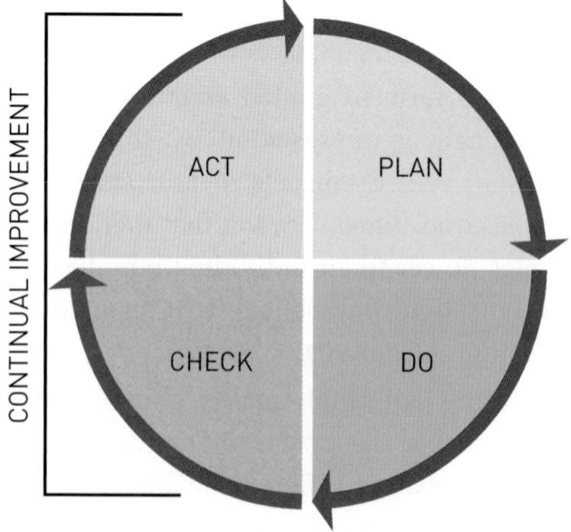

Research outcomes signify that there is positive correlation between clinicians' communication skills and patients' capacity to comply with medical recommendations, become effective self-managers of chronic conditions, and embrace preventive health behaviours. For these reasons, evidence-based strategies in communication can bring about a more inclusive, personalised patient experience through explaining, listening and empathising, as well as improving physiological, emotional, intellectual, spiritual and psychosocial health outcomes (Institute for Healthcare Communication 2011).

However, there are occasions when none of the strategies used to facilitate the delivery of care work. In these cases, it is worth noting that even the best studies reflect natural failures of communication attributed to 'human error'. Few studies reflect 100 per cent success in communication. The healthcare environment is an inherently unnatural context in which patients are unwell, away from home, constantly disturbed and feeling subordinate to the 'experts' in uniforms who often look after them. It is, for some, a very dehumanising experience that can result in an unwillingness to communicate. In these instances, the therapeutic relationship can be salvaged by asking other clinicians to communicate with the patient, or by communicating with the patient's family, where appropriate, to improve the transfer of information between people. Another approach clinicians can use to reconnect the lines of communication is speaking regularly with the patient and asking them to evaluate their experience and how it could be improved. Fundamentally, recognising that people wish to be cared for, listened to and advocated for is necessary, as is the process of acknowledging situations where communication has not been ideal.

CASE ACTIVITY 9.1

Plan-Do-Check-Act cycle

The hospital administration has informed ward staff that communication processes between them and the operating theatre have resulted in significant delays to the timely progression of surgical lists. These delays have affected the availability of after-hours surgical operating suites and compromised the implementation of the comprehensive model of service delivery the hospital is mandated to provide.

Key factors that have affected these delays are:

- inappropriate time estimates for surgical procedures
- inadequate ward staff during early morning shifts
- indistinct communication regarding the timely progression of operating theatre lists.

Using evidence, develop strategies for each part of the Plan-Do-Check-Act cycle that would address the issues raised across the ward, the operating theatre and hospital management.

Ward	Operating theatre	Hospital management
Plan		
Do		
Check		
Act		

Reflect and apply

How is clinical handover conducted at your healthcare service? Does the healthcare service use a structured communication tool to ensure patient safety? Are patients and their families involved in clinical communication activities (e.g. discharge, handover).

What other safety in communication strategies or measures are utilised at your healthcare service (e.g. surgical patient checklist, discharge checklist)?

Conclusion

In many respects, the goals of safety and quality in communication mirror the often-used dictum in healthcare: *primum non nocere*, meaning 'first, do no harm'. If safety is the avoidance of harm, then quality is concerned with establishing evidence-based mechanisms that create multiple layers of risk mitigation and positively affect patient outcomes and clinician performance. For clinicians, apprehending the notions of safety and quality in communication is of vital importance. The use of standardised models of communication is one approach to assuring safety and quality in healthcare. While communication can often be overlooked because it is so ubiquitous, individuals and healthcare systems should always prioritise identifying, investigating and articulating approaches that promote safety and quality of communication.

SUMMARY POINTS

- Communicating safely is defined by efforts to ensure a minimum standard of safety for patients in the context of healthcare delivery.
- Quality communication looks to enhance communication to achieve safety by improving efficiency, efficacy and proficiency in every facet of the healthcare environment.
- Several evidence-based approaches to safe, quality clinical communication (such as AIDET and SBAR) are useful tools for framing interpersonal communication between patients and healthcare providers, as well as between clinicians.
- Evidence-based communication models, such as the six rights of medication administration and the PDCA/PDSA cycle, have been proven effective in structuring

procedural or organisational communication, ensuring communication is clear and effective.
- While frameworks and guidelines are vital in guiding evidence-based approaches to communication, ensuring that communication is undertaken in a humanistic, empathetic, compassionate and professional tone is of equal importance to the safety and quality of communication.

CRITICAL THINKING QUESTIONS

1. The mnemonics used in this chapter highlight the differences between the various models of communication. Compare each model and identify situations when each would be acceptable.
2. Quality of communication is a necessary concept in healthcare and in other professional organisations. Examine communication quality measures in your university. Does your university pay attention to the quality of communication between staff, between students and staff, and between students and clinical colleagues? Make a list of the measures employed by your university to ensure that communication quality is maintained.

Group activity

Safety and quality in communication

In your study groups or via your subject discussion site, discuss your experiences of working in the clinical environment. What examples have you seen where examples of effective communication have enhanced quality and safety? Have any group members witnessed instances where quality and safety were compromised by poor communication? What could have been done differently in those instances?

WEBLINKS

Safety and Quality in Health Care

Australian Commission on Quality and Safety in Health Care:
www.safetyandquality.gov.au

Institute for Healthcare Improvement:
www.ihi.org

World Health Organization (WHO): Patient safety:
www.who.int/patientsafety/medication-safety/en

Clinical handover

Handover project:
http://handover.cmj.org.pl

I-Pass: Better handoffs. Safer Care:
www.ipasshandoffstudy.com/home

Documentation

Clinical Excellence Queensland (Queensland Health):
https://clinicalexcellence.qld.gov.au/resources/audit-tools-national-safety-and-quality-health-service-standards

NPS MedicineWise:
www.nps.org.au

REFERENCES

Allen, T., Rieck, T. & Salsbury, S.J. (2016). Patient perceptions of an AIDET and hourly rounding program in a community hospital: Results of a qualitative study. *Patient Experience Journal*, 3(1), 42–9.

Australian Commission on Safety and Quality in Health Care. (2012). *National Safety and Quality Health Service Standards*. Sydney: ACSQHC.

Australian Commission on Safety and Quality in Health Care. (2016). *Patient-Clinician Communication in Hospitals: Communicating for Safety at Transitions of Care*. Retrieved from www.safetyandquality.gov.au/sites/default/files/migrated/Information-sheet-for-executives-and-clinical-leaders-Improving-patient-clinician-communication.pdf.

Australian Commission on Safety and Quality in Health Care. (2019a). National standard medication charts. Sydney: ACSQHC. Retrieved from www.safetyandquality.gov.au/our-work/medication-safety/medication-charts/national-standard-medication-charts.

Australian Commission on Safety and Quality in Health Care. (2019b). *The State of Patient Safety and Quality in Australian Hospitals*. Sydney: ACSQHC. Retrieved from www.safetyandquality.gov.au/sites/default/files/2019-07/the-state-of-patient-safety-and-quality-in-australian-hospitals-2019.pdf.

Bakon, S., Wirihana, L., Christensen, M. & Craft, J. (2017). Nursing handovers: An integrative review of the different models and processes available. *International Journal of Nursing Practice*, 23(2), e12520. doi:10.1111/ijn.12520.

Beament, T., Ewens, B., Wilcox, S. & Reid, G. (2018). A collaborative approach to the implementation of a structured clinical handover tool (iSoBAR), within a hospital setting in metropolitan Western Australian: A mixed methods study. *Nurse Education in Practice*, 33, 107–13. doi:https://doi.org/10.1016/j.nepr.2018.08.019.

Beckett, C.D. & Kipnis, G. (2009). Collaborative communication: Integrating SBAR to improve quality/patient safety outcomes. *Journal for Healthcare Quality*, 31(5), 19–28. doi:10.1111/j.1945-1474.2009.00043.x.

Blair, W. & Smith, B. (2012). Nursing documentation: Frameworks and barriers. *Contemporary Nurse*, 41(2), 160–8.

Brewster, D. & Waxman, B.P. (2018). Adding kindness at handover to improve our collegiality: The K-ISBAR tool. *Medical Journal of Australia*, 209(11), 482–3, e481. doi:10.5694/mja18.00755.

Cheragi, M.A., Manoocheri, H., Mohammadnejad, E. & Ehsani, S.R. (2013). Types and causes of medication errors from nurse's viewpoint. *Iranian Journal of Nursing & Midwifery Research*, 18(3), 228–31.

Collins, S.J., Newhouse, R., Porter, J. & Talsma, A. (2014). Effectiveness of the surgical safety checklist in correcting errors: A literature review applying Reason's Swiss cheese model. *American Operating Room Nurses Journal*, 100(1), 65–79. doi:0.1016/j.aorn.2013.07.024.

De Meester, K., Verspuy, M., Monsieurs, K.G. & Van Bogaert, P. (2013). SBAR improves nurse–physician communication and reduces unexpected death: A pre and post intervention study. *Resuscitation*, 84(9), 1192–6.

DeVoe, J.E., Wallace, L.S. & Fryer Jnr, G.E. (2009). Measuring patients' perceptions of communication with healthcare providers: Do differences in demographic and socioeconomic characteristics matter? *Health Expectations*, 12(1), 70–80. doi:10.1111/j.1369-7625.2008.00516.x.

Donaldson, L.J., Kelley, E.T., Dhingra-Kumar, N., Kieny, M.-P. & Sheikh, A. (2017). Medication without harm: WHO's third global patient safety challenge. *The Lancet*, 389, 1680–1.

Fealy, G., Donnelly, S., Doyle, G., Brenner, M., Hughes, M., Mylotte, E., … Zaki, M. (2019). Clinical handover practices among healthcare practitioners in acute care services: A qualitative study. *Journal of Clinical Nursing*, 28(1–2), 80–8.

Forde, M.F., Coffey, A. & Hegarty, J. (2018). The factors to be considered when evaluating bedside handover. *Journal of Nursing Management*. 26(7), 757–68. doi:10.1111/jonm.12598.

Haig, K.M., Sutton, S. & Whittington, J. (2006). SBAR: A shared mental model for improving communication between clinicians. *Joint Commission Journal on Quality and Patient Safety*, 32(3), 167–75.

Halligan, M. & Zecevic, A. (2011). Safety culture in healthcare: A review of concepts, dimensions, measures and progress. *British Medical Journal: Quality & Safety*, 20(4), 338–43.

Hughes, R.G., Durham, C.F. & Alden, K.R. (2008). Enhancing patient safety in nursing education through patient simulation. In R. Hughes (ed.), *Patient Safety and Quality: An Evidence-Based Handbook for Nurses*. Rockville, MD: Agency for Healthcare Research and Quality.

Institute for Healthcare Communication. (2011). *Impact of Communication in Healthcare*. New Haven, CT: IHCC. Retrieved from http://healthcarecomm.org/about-us/impact-of-communication-in-healthcare.

Johnston, M.J., Arora, S., King, D., Bouras, G., Almoudaris, A.M., Davis, R. & Darzi, A. (2015). A systematic review to identify the factors that affect failure to rescue and escalation of care in surgery. *Surgery*, 157(4), 752–63.

Katona, A., Kunkel, E., Arfaa, J., Weinstein, S. & Skidmore, C. (2014). Methodology for delivering feedback to neurology house staff on communication skills using AIDET (Acknowledge, Introduce, Duration, Explanation, Thank You). *Neurology*, 82(10 supp.), P1.328–P321.328.

Keers, R., Williams, S., Cooke, J. & Ashcroft, D. (2013). Causes of medication administration errors in hospitals: A systematic review of quantitative and qualitative evidence. *Drug Safety*, 36(11), 1045–67. doi:10.1007/s40264-013-0090-2.

Kilpatrick, K. (2013). Understanding acute care nurse practitioner communication and decision-making in healthcare teams. *Journal of Clinical Nursing*, 22(1/2), 168–79. doi:10.1111/j.1365-2702.2012.04119.x.

Leonard, M., Graham, S. & Bonacum, D. (2004). The human factor: The critical importance of effective teamwork and communication in providing safe care. *Quality and Safety in Health Care*, 13(supp. 1), i85–i90.

Levett-Jones, T., Hoffman, K., Dempsey, J., Jeong, S., Noble, D., Norton, C., Roche, J. & Hickey, N. (2010). The 'five rights' of clinical reasoning: An educational model to enhance nursing students' ability to identify and manage clinically 'at risk' patients. *Nurse Education Today*, 30(6), 515–20. doi:http://dx.doi.org/10.1016/j.nedt.2009.10.020.

Lin, Y.-R., Shiah, I.S., Chang, Y.-C., Lai, T.-J., Wang,K.-Y. & Chou, K.-R. (2004). Evaluation of an assertiveness training program on nursing and medical students' assertiveness, self-esteem, and interpersonal communication satisfaction. *Nurse Education Today*, 24(8), 656–65. doi:http://dx.doi.org/10.1016/j.nedt.2004.09.004.

Mardis, M., Davis, J., Benningfield, B., Elliott, C., Youngstrom, M., Nelson, B., … Riesenberg, L.A. (2017). Shift-to-shift handoff effects on patient safety and outcomes: A systematic review. *American Journal of Medical Quality*, 32(1), 34–42. doi:10.1177/106286061561292.

Marshall, P. & Robson, R. (2005). Preventing and managing conflict: Vital pieces in the patient safety puzzle. *Healthcare Quarterly*, 8, 39–44.

Merten, H., van Galen, L.S. & Wagner, C. (2017). Safe handover. *BMJ*, 359, 5. doi:10.1136/bmj.j4328.

Miller, I. (2013). *Graded Assertiveness*. Retrieved from http://thenursepath.com/2013/11/24/graded-assertiveness.

Mowery, D., Wiebe, J., Visweswaran, S., Harkema, H. & Chapman, W.W. (2012). Building an automated SOAP classifier for emergency department reports. *Journal of Biomedical Informatics*, 45(1), 71–81. doi:http://dx.doi.org/10.1016/j.jbi.2011.08.020.

Müller, M., Jürgens, J., Redaèlli, M., Klingberg, K., Hautz, W.E. & Stock, S. (2018). Impact of the communication and patient hand-off tool SBAR on patient safety: A systematic review. *BMJ Open*, 8(8), e022202. doi:10.1136/bmjopen-2018-022202.

Norfolk, T., Birdi, K. & Walsh, D. (2007). The role of empathy in establishing rapport in the consultation: A new model. *Medical Education*, 41(7), 690–7.

Pape, T.M. (2003). Applying airline safety practices to medication administration. *Medsurg Nursing: Official Journal of the Academy of Medical-Surgical Nurses*, 12(2), 77–93;.

Parry, R.H. & Land, V. (2013). Systematically reviewing and synthesizing evidence from conversation analytic and related discursive research to inform healthcare communication practice and policy: An illustrated guide. *British Medical Council: Medical Research Methodology*, 13(1), 1–13. doi:10.1186/1471-2288-13-69.

Pearce, P.F., Ferguson, L.A., George, G.S. & Langford, C.A. (2016). The essential SOAP note in an EHR age. *The Nurse Practitioner*, 41(2), 29–36.

Piening, S., Haaijer-Ruskamp, F.M., de Graeff, P.A., Straus, S.M. & Mol, P.G. (2012). Healthcare professionals' self-reported experiences and preferences related to direct healthcare professional communications: A survey conducted in the Netherlands. *Drug Safety*, 35(11), 1061–72.

Pope, B.B., Rodzen, L. & Spross, G. (2008). Raising the SBAR: How better communication improves patient outcomes. *Nursing 2013*, 38(3), 41–3.

Randmaa, M., Mårtensson, G., Swenne, C.L. & Engström, M. (2014). SBAR improves communication and safety climate and decreases incident reports due to communication errors in an anaesthetic clinic: A prospective intervention study. *British Medical Journal Open*, 4(1), e004268.

Reader, R., Flin, R. & Cuthbertson, B. (2007). Communication skills and error in the intensive care unit. *Current Opinion in Critical Care*, 13, 732–6.

Reason, J. (2000). Human error models and management. *British Medical Journal*, 320(7237), 768–70.

Sharp, L., Dahlén, C. & Bergenmar, M. (2019). Observations of nursing staff compliance to a checklist for person-centred handovers—a quality improvement project. *Scandinavian Journal of Caring Sciences*, 3 March, 1–10. doi:10.1111/scs.12686.

Slade, D., Murray, K.A., Pun, J.K.H. & Eggins, S. (2019). Nurses' perceptions of mandatory bedside clinical handovers: An Australian hospital study. *Journal of Nursing Management*, 27(1), 161–71. doi:10.1111/jonm.12661.

Smeulers, M., Lucas, C. & Vermeulen, H. (2014). Effectiveness of different nursing handover styles for ensuring continuity of information in hospitalised patients. *Cochrane Database of Systematic Reviews*, 6. doi:10.1002/14651858.CD009979.pub2.

Stark, H.E., Graudins, L V., McGuire, T.M., Lee, C.Y.Y. & Duguid, M.J. (2019). Implementing a sustainable medication reconciliation process in Australian hospitals: The World Health Organization High 5s project. *Research in Social and Administrative Pharmacy*. doi.org/10.1016/j.sapharm.2019.05.011.

Starmer, A.J., Spector, N.D., Srivastava, R., West, D.C., Rosenbluth, G., Allen, A.D., … Landrigan, C.P. (2014). Changes in medical errors after implementation of a handoff program. *New England Journal of Medicine*, 371(19), 1803–12. doi:10.1056/NEJMsa1405556.

Studer, Q. (2003). *Hardwiring Excellence*. Pensacola, FL: Fire Starter Publishing.

Tague, N.R. (2005). *The Quality Toolbox* (2nd edn). Milwaukee, WI: ASQ Quality Press.

Taylor, M.J., McNicholas, C., Nicolay, C., Darzi, A., Bell, D. & Reed, J.E. (2014). Systematic review of the application of the plan-do-study-act method to improve quality in healthcare. *BMJ Quality and Safety*, 23(4), 290–8. doi:10.1136/bmjqs-2013-001862.

Tobiano, G., Bucknall, T., Sladdin, I., Whitty, J.A. & Chaboyer, W. (2018). Patient participation in nursing bedside handover: A systematic mixed-methods review. *International Journal of Nursing Studies*, 77, 243–58. doi.org/10.1016/j.ijnurstu.2017.10.014.

Wheeler, A.J., Scahill, S., Hopcroft, D. & Stapleton, H. (2018). Reducing medication errors at transitions of care is everyone's business. *Australian Prescriber*, 41(3), 73–7. doi.org/10.18773%2Faustprescr.2018.021

Wong, X., Tung, Y.J., Peck, S.Y., Goh, M.L. (2019). Clinical nursing handovers for continuity of safe patient care in adult surgical wards: A best practice implementation project. *JBI Database of Systematic Reviews and Implementation Reports*, 17(5), 1003–15.

Wright, K.B. (2011). A communication competence approach to healthcare worker conflict, job stress, job burnout, and job satisfaction. *Journal for Healthcare Quality*, 33(2), 7–14.

Zhang, L.-F., Tang, B., Zhu, Y.-M., Zhao, Y., Chen, L.-C. & Yan, M. (2013). The application of AIDET communication mode in the postoperative pain management. *Chinese Journal of Nursing*, 4, 4–15.

CHAPTER 10

CONFIDENTIALITY, PRIVACY AND COMMUNICATION

NARELLE BIEDERMANN AND JULIE SHEPHERD

CHAPTER FOCUS

After reading this chapter and completing the activities, you will be able to:

- define concepts relating to confidentiality, privacy and fidelity
- outline legislation that covers the issue of confidentiality for healthcare professionals relevant to your jurisdiction
- describe situations in which a healthcare provider may risk a breach of their duty of confidentiality
- discuss challenges to maintaining confidentiality, and identify measures for protecting information against such challenges.

KEY TERMS

Code of conduct
Code of ethics
Confidentiality
E-health record
Fidelity
Legislation
Privacy
Social media

Introduction

As we have learnt through the previous chapters, communication in healthcare is a uniquely complex but vital component of the relationship between the healthcare professional and the patient. It is essential for the provision of safe and quality care. In this chapter, we explore the concepts of privacy and confidentiality in relation to communication, and outline the legal, ethical and moral obligations that healthcare professionals must be aware of and abide by. The chapter provides guidance on common challenges encountered in maintaining confidentiality, and offers examples of contemporary considerations and provisions when the duty of confidentiality may be dismissed. It is by no means a complete rulebook; instead, it provides a foundational framework upon which the healthcare professional can explore confidentiality in communication within their own clinical world.

What is confidentiality?

Confidentiality refers to the explicit and tacit protection of personal information, which includes information held on paper; on a computer, videorecording or audio recording; or even held in human memory. Apart from the quintessential premise that a healthcare professional should do no harm (non-maleficence), there is likely no greater ethical principle that is more indoctrinated in the profession of healthcare than confidentiality. All healthcare professionals are duty-bound to maintain the confidentiality of information that becomes available to them in the course of their professional relationship with patients. This duty protects information created, disclosed, acquired and stored—directly or indirectly—in the context of the relationship between the patient and the healthcare provider. Without assurances of confidentiality, patients may be reluctant to seek medical attention, or fail to provide healthcare professionals with the information they need in order to provide good care.

Confidentiality
Implicit protection of personal information provided by individuals in the course of a professional healthcare interaction or relationship.

Historically, confidentiality was binding and absolute—a secret that went with the holder to the grave. The classic version of the Hippocratic Oath from 5 BCE puts confidentiality like this: 'What I may see or hear in the course of the treatment or even outside the treatment in regard to the life of men, which on no account one must spread abroad, I will keep to myself, holding such things shameful to be spoken about.' In the modern version, written in 1964, confidentiality is sworn as: 'I will respect the privacy of my patients, for their problems are not disclosed to me that the world may know.' The Florence Nightingale pledge, historically taken by nurses upon graduation from nursing training, espouses: 'I … will hold in confidence all personal matters committed to my knowledge in the practice of my calling.'

The Medical Board of Australia's (MBA) *Good Medical Practice: A Code of Conduct for Doctors in Australia* recognises that a doctor must protect their patients' 'privacy and right to confidentiality, unless release of information is required by law or by public-interest considerations' (MBA 2014, pp. 8–9). It further suggests that a doctor can share information about patients for the purpose of holistic healthcare, providing it is consistent with **privacy** laws and abides by professional guidelines about confidentiality.

Privacy
The right of an individual to keep information about themselves from being disclosed to others.

Code of conduct
Set of principles that govern how an individual, group or organisation should behave and practise.

Code of ethics
Set of guidelines prepared by an organisation or professional body to inform its members how they should conduct themselves to meet certain ethical and integrity standards.

Legislation
A collective body of laws or a single law (known as a statute).

Nursing **codes of conduct** identify a similar view. For example, the International Council of Nurses (ICN) provides a conduct statement that a nurse 'holds in confidence personal information and uses judgement in sharing this information' (ICN 2012, p. 2). Likewise, the International Confederation of Midwives (ICM) has also published a *Code of Ethics* for midwives that provides specific guidance about confidentiality and the ways in which it must be observed as 'holding in confidence client information in order to protect the right to privacy, and use judgment in sharing this information except when mandated by law (ICM 2008, p. 2).

Indeed, most healthcare professional bodies have their own **code of ethics** that outlines expectations on dealing with confidentiality. The Australian Psychological Society has a formalised Code of Ethics that requires psychologists to 'safeguard the confidentiality of information obtained during their provision of psychological services' (Australian Psychological Society 2007, p. 14). In the Australian Association of Social Workers' Code of Ethics, social workers are obliged to 'respect the rights of clients to a relationship of trust, to privacy and confidentiality of their information obtained in the course of professional service' (2010, p. 27). Pharmacists are bound by numerous principles of confidentiality, beginning with 'treating information about patients or clients as confidential and applying appropriate security to electronic and hard copy information' (Pharmacy Board of Australia 2014, p. 11). In addition to the various codes of conduct and ethics guiding healthcare professional practice, **legislation** (discussed later in this chapter) and organisational policies also determine how confidential information is managed.

Skills in practice

Breaching confidentiality

The following dialogue is between two hospital registrars and takes place in the hospital cafeteria while they are waiting in line to be served.

R1: 'How did the angioplasty go this morning?'

R2: 'Not much fun! It wasn't as straightforward as I would have liked. The patient was old and really obese, making access awkward, which wasn't a great start. Then he kept dropping his blood pressure and was unstable for the most part. It was hard to see the catheter tip and we needed a lot of contrast. I felt I was navigating blindly at times! I'm amazed he didn't crash during it!'

R1: 'That sounds like a nightmare! We should have weight limits on our patients!'

R2: 'Yeah, that would make *our* lives a heck of a lot easier!'

What's happening here?

Although the patient's name was never mentioned, the description of the patient provided to the colleague could easily be overheard by members of the public. A family member or friend of the patient may have been in the same queue in the cafeteria and would be very distressed to hear the treating doctor talking about their loved one in such a derogatory way. Discussions about patients should never occur in public places. This dialogue is an example of how patient confidentiality and the professional code of conduct is breached, even without disclosing the patient's name.

Students of the healthcare professions are not exempt from their profession's obligations of confidentiality. When in the clinical setting—even as an observer—students are given the same level of access to patient information as the healthcare professionals working around them. Healthcare professionals are generally afforded a privileged depth of access to private and personal information about health and illness not seen elsewhere in society. In the course of the therapeutic relationship, healthcare professionals will inquire about aspects of the lives and body functions of their patients that might reasonably be considered taboo in normal conversations. They will examine intimate parts of human anatomy typically kept private as part of a physical assessment. Patients place undeniable trust in the healthcare professional that these sensitive questions and examinations are relevant or important to the healthcare professional's ability to diagnose, care and treat their condition, and that their responses to such intimate questions will be equally guarded and used only for the purpose of diagnosis, care and treatment. In this way, patients are extremely vulnerable. As an acknowledgement of this vulnerability, healthcare professionals must hold in confidence knowledge and information gained during the therapeutic relationship without jeopardising health and safety, and have the utmost respect for privacy.

The terms privacy and confidentiality are often used interchangeably, but they are quite separate concepts. Unlike confidentiality, which concerns the actions of individual healthcare professionals, privacy concerns the practices of agencies, such as a hospital or community healthcare clinic. When we talk about privacy, we are referring to the right of individuals to keep certain information about themselves from being disclosed or shared with people who do not have a need to know. But it can also have a physical aspect related to protecting personal modesty or dignity. For example, a doctor who allows a patient to undress behind a curtain and cover herself with a sheet before performing a pelvic examination is demonstrating respect for the patient and their right to privacy.

The right to privacy is recognised in international treaties such as the United Nations' *Universal Declaration of Human Rights* (1948) and *International Covenant on Civil and Political Rights* (1966). It is based on the principle of autonomy or self-determination, because it relates to an individual being free to choose to be left alone and free from unwarranted interference or intrusion by others into their personal affairs, including the right to choose care based on personal beliefs, feelings and attitudes. This also implies that individuals have some control over their own personal, sensitive information, including control over how and for what purpose the information is to be gathered, kept, used and discarded (Prince 2018).

In a healthcare relationship between a patient and a healthcare professional, the patient must surrender some measure of privacy so that the professional can properly assess the situation and determine a course of action or treatment. The patient may need to share private or sensitive information, or allow the healthcare professional to examine or treat their body. This is why confidentiality is so incredibly important. While necessary for the healthcare relationship and the quality of care provided, sharing highly personal or intimate details is usually challenging for most people. Confidentiality provides the patient with a safety net for giving up their right to privacy in the context of the therapeutic relationship. The Australian Charter of Healthcare Rights was created by the Australian Commission on Safety and Quality in Health Care (ACSQHC) to ensure that patients know their rights, including the right to privacy and the right to expect that personal and health information will be kept securely and confidentially (ACSQHC 2019).

CASE ACTIVITY 10.1

Confidentiality and privacy

Amira is a nursing student on her first clinical placement. She introduces herself to her assigned patients and gets to know them all a little better throughout the shift. One of her patients, Pearl, consents to Amira performing a dressing change on a pressure area sore that has deteriorated into a deep wound. The wound is more complicated than anything Amira has seen before in labs, and provides an interesting learning opportunity to work with a more complex wound. Amira thanks Pearl for allowing her to perform this procedure on her, explaining that students don't often get to see these kinds of wounds; this seems to please Pearl, as though she is happy to have helped a student with her learning.

Later that shift, Amira excitedly tells the other students about Pearl's wound, and encourages them all to take the dressing down and look at the wound. As the room fills with students, eager to have a look at her wound, Pearl is surprised and a little overwhelmed. Despite the discomfort of removing the dressing, she reluctantly allows the students to have a look.

1. Was confidentiality breached here?
2. Amira shared the information with her fellow students so that they too could learn from the interesting wound. Is this a problem?
3. What are the legal and professional consequences for Amira and her colleagues?

One additional principle that must be considered in relation to ethical communication is **fidelity**. When we maintain confidentiality, we are making an implicit promise to keep the information provided during the course of the therapeutic relationship—or in the provision of the healthcare service—confidential. Fidelity refers to that promise. Under normal circumstances in the professional healthcare relationship, patients are fully informed and provide explicit consent; confidentiality ensues because healthcare professionals honour their promises.

Fidelity
To behave in a way that means the keeping the promises made as part of the professional role, whether that is to provide safe and competent patient care, to act ethically, or simply as part of the relationship with patients or clients.

The physical environment and other features of healthcare facilities present many challenges to maintaining confidentiality in healthcare interactions. Shared hospital wards offer very little to ensure confidentiality. A thin hospital curtain is certainly not a 'cone of silence', and discussions that occur between the patient and the healthcare professional at the bedside must be done with great awareness of this limitation. This challenge is described in the literature as a common source of breaches in confidentiality and privacy, especially in emergency departments (Hartigan, Cussen, Meaney & O'Donoghue 2018; Heskett, Preston & Maskell 2014) and operating theatre recovery rooms (Koivula-Tynnila, Axelin & Leino-Kilpi 2018) where healthcare providers may unconsciously neglect confidentiality for the sake of clinical urgency. Healthcare professionals must consider what they discuss with their patients at the bedside, and how/what they can do to support privacy and confidentiality. Clinical handovers can also present challenges for ensuring confidential communication, especially if the location does not allow for private conversations about clinical situations. Much research has been conducted on the practice of bedside handovers or, more correctly, handovers involving patients, and one detracting factor in this clinical process is its effect on confidentiality (Malfait et al. 2017; Tobiano, Whitty, Bucknall & Chaboyer 2017). The purpose of clinical handovers is for those involved in the healthcare of a patient to communicate care planning, patient progress and clinical findings, and responses to treatment, and thus is often detailed and clinically personal. The conduct of such exchanges of information within earshot of others—patients, visitors, family members, administrative and service staff—must be considered to ensure that breaches of confidentiality do not occur.

Awareness of confidentiality is paramount in relation to communication with all people for whom private information is often extremely sensitive, whether this concerns information concerning physical or mental health status, religion, gender or sexuality. For example, many lesbian, gay, bisexual, transgender, questioning, intersex, asexual + (signifying other possibilities on the gender and sexuality spectrum) (LGBTQIA+) people have added concerns about being 'outed' in contexts where being known to be LGBTQIA+ may carry a significant personal risk or risks to family and friends, whether due to the age of the patient or their cultural identification (Babst 2018). Closeted patients may be reluctant to disclose certain health information for fear of revealing their sexual orientation, or having it revealed to others. Older LGBTQIA+ people may also have had very different life experiences from younger LGBTQIA+ people, and are more likely to have experienced homophobia, and this may affect their willingness to disclose information about their sexuality and health concerns. The healthcare professional can eliminate much of this stress by providing a receptive, caring and non-judgmental environment for all patients, with an overt emphasis on confidentiality, respect and trust.

Communicating with people with cognitive impairments or mental health conditions also presents challenges. While it is often the families and carers who know the most about the people for whom they care, some people do not want their family members or carers involved in all aspects of their medical treatment. It is imperative that wherever possible the healthcare professional gains informed consent before discussing confidential matters with family members or carers. Healthcare professionals cannot assume to know the dynamics of patients' private family situations. However, it is not a breach of confidentiality to listen to family members and carers if they offer information that may help with the clinical picture of the patient.

Adolescents have unique needs when it comes to confidentiality. In early childhood, parents are responsible for their children's healthcare. As children mature through adolescence, they develop an increased capacity for decision making and for taking responsibility for their health. With this often comes the desire for greater privacy. Research informs us that one of the greatest barriers adolescents face in seeking medical treatment, particularly for sensitive issues like sexual healthcare, substance use and mental healthcare, is fear and mistrust surrounding issues of confidentiality and disclosure (Cuffe et al. 2016; Gilbert, Rickert & Aalsma 2014; McCann, Mugavin, Renzaho & Lubman 2016; Sasse, Aroni, Sawyer & Duncan 2013). The duty of confidentiality exists, but it is also a tenuous line that healthcare professionals must observe, especially when parents' expectations of their participation in the treatment of their adolescent child differs from current guidelines.

Legal obligations of healthcare professionals

The security of information gained in the course of therapeutic relationships is of vital importance. Australian law protects information obtained in therapeutic relationships, which is deemed confidential from disclosure. The *Privacy Act 1988* (Cth) is a federal law that standardises how personal information about individuals is collected, used, stored and disclosed (Federal Register of Legislation n.d.). The Act defines personal information as any information about an individual who is or could be identified by this information, regardless of the format of this information. Examples include name, date of birth, residential address, personal telephone number, bank account or superannuation account information, tax file number, medical or dental records, or even commentary or opinion about the individual.

The Act also outlines provisions as to who can access and correct that information in Commonwealth agencies, private sector organisations (including small businesses and non-profit organisations) and healthcare providers. This Act encompasses all information about Australians, but from a healthcare perspective, it establishes a legal obligation for employees in healthcare settings to keep health records confidential.

In Australia, each state and territory also has its own legislation that concerns confidentiality in healthcare. The multiple layers of federal, state and territory laws and regulations do, in some instances, confound privacy obligations. It is important to note that there are nine different legal jurisdictions that deal with the issue of confidentiality in healthcare: six states, two territories and the Commonwealth. In most cases, the privacy responsibilities required by federal and state or territory privacy laws are very similar, but each of the nine jurisdictions has a combination of legislation and case law that relates specifically to confidentiality. Table 10.1 provides examples of the Acts that are relevant to the disclosure of confidential information at state and territory level.

Like Australia, New Zealand has legislation that controls how personal information is collected, used, stored, disclosed and accessed; this is the *Privacy*

TABLE 10.1 Australian state and territory legislation relating to confidentiality

State or territory	Relevant Acts and sections within the Act
Australian Capital Territory	*Health Records (Privacy and Access) Act 1997*, parts 2–3
New South Wales	*Health Records and Information Privacy Act 2002*, health privacy principle 10 *Mental Health Act 2007*, s. 189
Northern Territory	*Health Services Act 2014*, s. 70 *Mental Health and Related Services Act 2005*, s. 91
Queensland	*Hospital and Health Boards Act 2011*, part 7 *Mental Health Act 2000*, s. 530
South Australia	*Public Health Act 2011*, s. 99 *Mental Health Act 2009*, s. 34
Tasmania	*Children, Young Persons and their Families Act 1997*, ss. 16 and 103 *Mental Health Act 2013*, s. 134
Victoria	*Health Records Act 2001*, part 3 *Mental Health Act 2014*, s. 120
Western Australia	*Health Services (Conciliation and Review) Act 1995*, s. 71 *Mental Health Act 1996*, s. 206

Act 1993 (Department of Prime Minister and Cabinet 2019). As part of this Act, codes of practice have been created to regulate practice in specific areas, including health information. Known as the Health Information Privacy Code, this code outlines 12 rules that are specific to healthcare.

Reflect and apply

Consider the types of information regularly collected by those working in your healthcare profession. Conduct an online search for the legislation relevant to your jurisdiction and review requirements for the collection, use and management of this information.

Exemptions to the general rule of confidentiality

While confidentiality is a fundamental principle in healthcare professionals' duty, it is also frequently the source of their most serious ethical dilemmas (Kadooka, Okita & Asai 2016; Knight & Papanikitas 2018; Resnik & Randall 2018). Confidentiality, as a principle, can never be absolute. There are a few exceptions to the general rule of confidentiality where healthcare professionals may be legally or ethically within their rights to breach confidentiality. Each has a legal basis for their exemption and they are generally applicable across the spectrum of healthcare professionals. Unless there exists a stronger conflicting duty or legal mandate, confidentiality and privacy are prima facie duties—that is, they are duties that must be honoured (Beauchamp & Childress 2012).

Exemptions to the general duty of confidentiality include those that are permitted by law, those where it is in the public interest, and those where consent is given for confidentiality to be breached. These are discussed in further detail below.

Exemptions mandated or permitted by law

These exemptions are:

- The patient is a child/elder and is being abused, or at risk of abuse.
- A patient has a 'notifiable disease'—for example, certain infectious diseases or sexually transmitted illnesses, bioterrorism agents such as anthrax or smallpox, epidemic diseases such as severe acute respiratory syndrome or the Ebola virus.
- Records must be made available to the police if they have a warrant to inspect documents.
- Records must be made available in the case of suspected or confirmed physical or sexual abuse.
- In response to a summons or subpoena.

Exemptions 'in the public interest'

These exemptions are:

- The healthcare professional is concerned that the patient is 'at risk', in that they are believed to be dangerous, and might harm themselves or an identifiable third party (also see the focus box).
- A patient discloses that they have committed a serious crime.

BOX 10.1

EXEMPTIONS IN THE PUBLIC INTEREST

Individuals can be considered at risk of harming themselves or others in many ways, such as by driving under the influence of drugs or alcohol, engaging in unsafe sexual practices, etc. For the purpose of disclosure 'in the public interest', it must be considered that the person is dangerous through the expression of a serious or imminent threat or intent to kill or seriously injure themselves or another identifiable person. Determining whether a threat is 'serious' is a matter of judgment. It requires consideration about how likely it is that the threat will occur and the seriousness of the consequences if it does eventuate. A threat is considered 'imminent' if it is about to occur or may escalate if action is not taken quickly. The threat posed might indicate that the harm is immediate, or within a few hours, or even within a few days, depending on the circumstances.

Consent given (implied or expressed)

If the patient does give consent to sharing of confidential information, the duty of confidentiality is overridden, but it must be noted that this is only to the extent that the patient has consented. For example, the patient may consent for confidential information to be shared with other members of the healthcare team but not with their family, and therefore there is still a duty of confidentiality in that context.

Miscellaneous

Exclusions also apply if the information is unspecific, trivial or common knowledge.

Grey areas do exist, and generally tend to compound the ethical dilemmas that present themselves to healthcare professionals, police, teachers and other professionals. For healthcare professionals, unique challenges to the rule of confidentiality are presented by dealing with adolescents and children; people who are mentally ill or developmentally disabled; and people who are considered to have impaired cognitive capacity. For example, do the same rules of confidentiality apply when an elderly patient discloses to her doctor that her carer hits her and deprives her of food? Or, what can a school-based counsellor do when her 12-year-old female patient tells her in a clinical interaction that she is participating in sex parties with older high school students and teachers on weekends?

TABLE 10.2 State and territory legislation relating to mandatory reporting relating to child protection in Australia

State or territory	Relevant legislation	Relevant section
Australian Capital Territory	*Children and Young People Act 2008* (ACT)	ss. 356, 357
New South Wales	*Children and Young Persons (Care and Protection) Act 1998* (NSW)	ss. 23, 27, 27A
Northern Territory	*Care and Protection of Children Act (NT)* 2007	ss. 15. 16, 2A
Queensland	*Public Health Act 2005* (Qld) *Education (General Provisions) Act* 2006 *Child Protection Act 1999* (Qld)	ss. 158 ss. 364, 365, 365A, 366, 366A ss. 13E, 186
South Australia	*Children's Protection Act 1993* (SA)	ss. 6, 8
Tasmania	*Children, Young Persons and Their Families Act 1997* (Tas.)	ss. 3, 4, 14
Victoria	*Children, Youth and Families Act 2005* (Vic.)	ss. 162, 182, 184
Western Australia	*Children and Community Services Act 2004* (WA)	ss. 124A-H

There is legislation in all Australian states and territories that mandates healthcare professionals to make a report (and, therefore, breach confidentiality) in cases where the professional holds a reasonable belief or suspicion that a child is at risk of harm, physical or sexual abuse, or neglect. Table 10.2 outlines the appropriate legislation concerning mandatory reporting in the case of child protection.

Mandatory reporting of crime also exists in some states and territories. For example, in New South Wales all citizens (including healthcare professionals) have a duty to inform the police or other authority if they know that another person has committed a serious indictable offence (*NSW Crimes Act 1900*, s. 316). In the absence of mandatory legal provisions, healthcare professionals may have a moral and a civil duty to disclose confidential information if it is perceived as the only means to stop an immediate and specifiable risk of harm to identifiable persons.

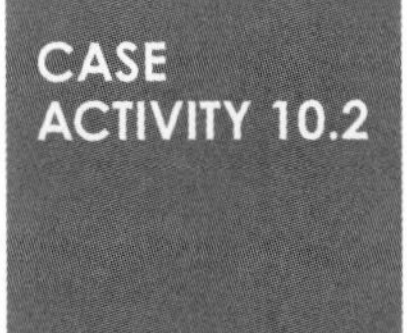

Mandatory reporting

Jacob is a 21-year-old male who has been brought in by ambulance to the emergency department with a stab wound to the abdomen. He was found under an overpass in an area known for gang-related crime. Jacob maintains that he accidentally stabbed himself and refuses to divulge any further information about the event. When the paramedic team arrived at the scene, they did not find a weapon on his person, nor was there a weapon around him.

There are three options for managing Jacob's case. What is the correct course of action?

1. Inform Jacob that you don't believe him, and will be informing the police of the incident, providing them with his name and details.
2. Inform the police that there is a patient with a knife wound in the emergency department, which may have been the result of an attack, but withhold the patient's name.
3. Inform Jacob that you respect his decision to not inform the police of the crime, and continue treatment regardless.

Reflect and apply

Dying patients are susceptible to revealing personal information. The secrets disclosed on a deathbed can be extremely confronting and intimate, and may pertain to matters that are illegal or immoral, as the dying person seeks absolution or attempts to lift the burden a secret has forced them to endure.

- Do the principles of confidentiality still exist in such circumstances? Do they exist even after their death?
- What if a patient confesses to an abhorrent crime, such as rape or child sexual abuse? Does it make a difference if the crime was for theft or burglary? What are the responsibilities of the healthcare professional in such cases?

Information technology and confidentiality

Globally, the healthcare system has undergone significant changes in the way information is handled, due to information technology (IT). We have answers to virtually any healthcare question at our fingertips, thanks to the growing sources of databases and websites on the internet that relate to health issues. There are online support groups and blogs relating to every imaginable illness or disease. The shift from paper records to electronic health **(e-health) records** has brought many benefits and challenges for healthcare providers and governments, as well as benefits and concerns for consumers of health services. However, medical data is generally considered more sensitive than other types of information because it goes beyond data such as height, weight and vital signs (McLeod & Dolezel 2018; Seckman 2018). Health records may contain sensitive personal information that most people would not want to be public knowledge, such as sexually transmitted illnesses, mental health issues, information about termination of pregnancies, genetic predispositions to illness and disease, and human immunodeficiency

E-health record
An electronic version of a person's healthcare record.

virus (HIV) status. The ways in which this information is handled, stored, accessed and used is of great concern. The ACSQHC developed the National Safety and Quality Health Service (NSQHS) Standards as one means to assist the healthcare industry in ensuring safety and quality standards, including standards for privacy and confidentiality of all patient data. For example, Standard 1, Clinical governance, sets out actions that healthcare providers and services should take to ensure documentation of information meets the safety and quality standards. Action 1.16 notes:

> Information about an individual's physical or mental health and wellbeing is both personal and sensitive, and there are many ethical, professional and legal restrictions on the way this information can be used. ... Consider the need to ... develop and implement specific policies and procedures addressing the use of clinical information for clinical, educational, quality assurance and research purposes, including authorising procedures for any uses of disclosures outside the usual provision of care. (ACSQHC 2017, Review privacy and confidentiality section, para. 1; point 4)

As Australia moves to a digital health records system, known as My Health Record, legislation has been passed to ensure that standards for privacy and security measures are mandated, making breaches prosecutable with harsher penalties. The My Health Records Amendment (Strengthening Privacy) Bill 2018 was passed by Australian Parliament in November 2018. The Bill ensures that those individuals who choose to have an e-health record can permanently delete their record at any time, with the assurance that no backup or archived copy will be kept. The Bill also directs who may have access and under what circumstances including access by insurers, researchers, employers, law enforcement and government agencies. Additionally, the legislation governs the age at which parents are removed as representatives on a child's e-health record, further ensuring privacy.

On the positive side, e-health records are less costly to produce, store and manage, and easier to share (although the cost of retrofitting current paper records to e-health records is enormous). Massive archives in the bowels of hospitals that once housed paper records are no longer required (with off-site records storage facilities taking over this task), and staff are no longer employed in the archives to retrieve, sort and manage paper records. Through the implementation of e-health networks and health information systems, patient information can be shared within organisations to ensure that continuity of care is provided. Healthcare professionals can gain access to previous medical records, medications, and even the results of previous tests that may be relevant to their current care. They also make it very timely for healthcare professionals to access patient information immediately, rather than waiting for the delivery of a paper-based chart to be located from patient records and delivered to the ward.

Skills in practice

IT and breaching confidentiality

The following dialogue between two midwives takes place in the maternity ward of a large city hospital, where a well-known celebrity has just been admitted.

M1: 'Sara! Did you hear? Rachel Musgrove has been admitted to our ward!'

M2: 'Rachel Musgrove! I love her movies! What is she admitted for? Who is assigned to her?'

M1: 'Tina is admitting her now, so we can ask her.'

M2: 'No, I can't wait, let's just look her up on the system.'

M1: 'OK, I will get her patient number from the ward clerk. Then we can read up on her together! Oh, I wonder how many weeks pregnant she is...'

M2: '...and who is the father! Come on, let's go, I can't wait to find out!'

What's happening here?

This communication exchange is a breach of the professional code of conduct, and if the midwives' plan is carried out, the patient's privacy is also breached. As health professionals, we are bound to our professional standards and the codes of ethics and conduct that are appropriate to our discipline. Breaches such as this planned reading of a patient's medical information by healthcare professionals who are not directly caring for her is a breach of all of these codes. It is imperative that healthcare professionals remain just that—professional and ethical in their duty of caring roles.

However, advances in technology are not without their drawbacks. There are strict guidelines about the storage and management of e-health records as they are vulnerable to hackers, malware, phishing and other fraudulent activities. No longer can we believe that personal information is sealed away in some locked room accessible only by a few very select key holders. The data within e-health records is easier to retrieve and, as a result, it might open the way for unethical access of information for research activities, despite new legislation designed to limit access to this data. The prevalence of unregulated health information and uncontrolled websites available on the web poses many concerns. Temptations abound for those who do have access to electronic patient data to access information for which they are not authorised, such as their own healthcare records or those of a friend or colleague. Despite the new legislation limiting access to My Health Records, paranoia about 'big brother' monitoring other forms of health information exists, particularly in relation to sensitive information that might be of interest to third parties such as employers, health insurance companies, the government or even other family members. While health information transmitted electronically is usually secure—because of the increasingly standardised use of encryption technologies—it is what might happen at the end point that is of most concern, as the sender has no control over what happens to the data once it has been sent (McLeod & Dolezel 2018; Shenoy & Appel 2017).

Of growing concern for healthcare consumers and the wider community is the control of the use of health data by secondary users, such as researchers and health companies. Electronic patient data is growing in volume, which means that opportunities exist to improve patient care and support public health decisions using data collated from multiple sources, including de-identified patient information. This information is exposed to additional threats, such as misuse, inappropriate access and privacy concerns. The National Health and Medical Research Council (NHMRC), in conjunction with the Australian Research Council, released a *National Statement on Ethical Conduct of Human Research* in 2007 (updated 2014), in which they made a point of noting they avoid using the phrase 'de-identified data', because it is not a clearly understood term (NHMRC 2007). The process of de-identifying information is not failsafe by any means, and this must be always be considered when attempting any form of 'de-identification'. Researchers and hackers have been able to 're-identify' people simply through knowledge of a combination of basic personal information including a person's date of birth, gender and postcode (Phillips, Dove & Knoppers 2017).

Although technological developments have changed the ways that health information is managed, the key issues about confidentiality and privacy remain. Who is authorised to access confidential information—and the purpose for which this information can be accessed—must be defined and understood within the organisation at all levels through clear guidelines and ongoing risk assessments and audits. Ultimately, information should and must be used for the purpose and intent for which the data was initially collected.

There are numerous issues that need to be resolved if we are to progress to a secure e-health environment. Even with legislation regarding privacy and confidentiality, no system is infallible. Data insecurity exists from the point of origin of patient records, and continues through into storage, access and dissemination of the same records and information. Organisations must accept the reality of risk. Security measures and dedicated processes must exist to provide ongoing assessment of the threat environment and prevent unauthorised access by those within the organisation, as well as those external to it. Seckman (2018) highlights that human error is the chief area of vulnerability when it comes to threats to electronic data in small business (including primary healthcare providers), followed by technology failure, so it is important that organisations factor these vulnerabilities into their development and staff training. At a government level, legislation must keep abreast with the changes and developments in electronic health information, as well as the management, access, storage and archiving of such data.

Confidentiality and social media

As an avenue for communication that is becoming universal in contemporary consciousness, **social media** has been largely neglected when discussing patient confidentiality. There is no doubt that social media is now a significant and normal part of everyday life for many people and, for the most part, use of social media is an unregulated form of publishing. Social media describes the online and mobile tools that are used to share opinions, information, evidence, experiences, images and video or audio clips. It also is an umbrella term that includes websites and applications used for social networking and interaction. The most common networking sites used today are highlighted in the focus box 'Social networking sites', along with some astounding statistics relating to their use.

Social media
A collective term given to online websites and applications (such as Facebook, Twitter, Instagram, etc.) that enable people to communicate, create and share information and ideas.

BOX 10.2

SOCIAL NETWORKING SITES

Facebook	829 million daily users 1.49 billion daily active users on Facebook on average for September 2018
Twitter	500 million tweets per day
LinkedIn	Over 313 million members worldwide 562 million users
Instagram	75 million daily users 500 million daily users.
Snapchat	161 million daily

Sources: Facebook Newsroom 2019; Instagram 2019; LinkedIn 2019; Twitter 2019.

Social media tools that connect healthcare providers with patients and caregivers offer an ideal landscape for providing opportunities to allow people to access health advice, receive and provide social support, manage chronic conditions and make informed day-to-day health decisions. Many healthcare organisations use social media routinely as part of their health promotion, health education, distribution of research, news and events, and even marketing. As will be discussed in Chapter 15, social media affords healthcare professionals a range of benefits: the opportunity to contribute to discussions and debate, to comment on trending issues of the day, the opportunity for conversation, the opportunity to collaborate with anyone, anywhere, and the opportunity to establish a community. Health consumers can 'follow' healthcare providers and organisations, and be kept abreast of developments in technologies and advances in treatments. However, despite the benefits for health communication, it is not without its dangers.

Social media can create a perception of anonymity and detachment from social cues and consequences for online actions, meaning that a healthcare professional may say or do things online that they would not do or say in person. Social media takes any breaches in confidence beyond tearoom storytelling or recounting an interesting clinical event at a party onto an international stage, where it is not possible to control or contain any breaches in confidentiality. In other words, a slip in confidentiality made online can have a far greater impact than one made over lunch with a colleague. When we join social networking sites, we surrender control of the information we share. We lose the right to choose which of the images we upload to our personal pages of ourselves and our family will become public, even with the tightest of privacy settings. We cannot control the images that other people upload of us. We also lose our personal privacy, often forgetting that millions of people have the potential to 'eavesdrop' on any of our conversations and pry through photographs that we have uploaded. Additionally, those professional boundaries that exist in the 'real world' can become blurred in the online social networking space, where consumers of healthcare and healthcare providers can interact so readily. The line between professional and personal lives in the online world can be difficult to distinguish when we use our social media accounts so readily.

CASE ACTIVITY 10.3

Social media and breaching confidentiality

Frank is a fourth-year physiotherapy student on clinical placement at a small rural healthcare facility. He makes a comment on his Facebook page about an adverse event that occurred to one of his patients that day. He was careful not to name the person or the hospital in his post. However, in a post the previous week on his Facebook page, he mentioned that he was on placement at this particular facility, so his friends knew where he was. Friends offered him supportive comments, and Frank described a little more about what had happened to the patient, saying he felt so sad and helpless because he was so young and was all alone with no family nearby.

Later that week, the aunt of the patient conducts a search on Facebook in order to find the hospital's Facebook page so she can make contact with her nephew. When the search results are displayed, Frank's Facebook post about him doing placement at the hospital is shown. With some further reading, the aunt sees Frank's more recent post about the adverse event involving a patient, along with his descriptions of the patient and the family situation, and the aunt knows that Frank is talking about her nephew.

1. Outline all the ways in which confidentiality was breached in this scenario.
2. The post was not derogatory or defamatory about the patient. Could Frank argue he was simply venting to his friends on his private page about an anonymous situation that left him feeling sad and helpless?
3. Frank has the tightest possible security settings for his Facebook profile. Is that enough to assume that what he posts on his private page is private? Why, or why not?

Writing about specific patient cases while protecting their identity may be more difficult than many healthcare professionals believe. It is not simply a matter of changing or omitting key patient details, such as name and date of birth. Even avoiding a description of particular medical conditions or locations might not be enough to de-identify the patient, living or dead. A study of 271 medical blogs authored by healthcare professionals found that 42 per cent of them described individual patients. Of those, 17 per cent included sufficient information for patients to be able to identify themselves or their healthcare providers, and a further three blogs included photos in which patients were clearly recognisable (Lagu, Kaufman, Asch & Armstrong 2008). Although revealing an isolated piece of information about a patient may not in itself represent a breach of confidentiality, it might do so when combined with other items of information. In some cases, the fear held by healthcare professionals that they may accidentally or inadvertently breach patient privacy or confidentiality actually drives them away from engaging in certain social media platforms (Baird et al. 2018; Panahi, Watson & Partridge 2016).

Importantly, healthcare professionals are subject to their profession's code of conduct, both when they are on and off duty. Social media sites are not exempt from this code of conduct. The Australian Health Practitioner Regulation Authority's (AHPRA) social media policy (2014) clearly reminds health professionals who use social media that the national law and their National Board's code of ethics and professional conduct apply. The argument that there needs to be a line between a private life and a professional life is not relevant in the sphere of social media. Several research studies have explored the potential and actual public disclosure of confidential information as a result of cases of breaching of confidentiality in social media (Chretien, Greysen, Chretien & Kind 2009; Garner & O'Sullivan 2010; Lagu et al. 2008; Levati 2014; Neville 2017). The studies found that despite university or healthcare agency guidelines about acceptable online behaviour and standards, users were generally unaware of the implications their breaches could have. Often this was because the individuals perceived that there was a large, impermeable gap between their online personal life and professional obligations.

Conclusion

Healthcare professionals work within a complex framework of legislation, policy directives, protocols and professional codes of conduct, ethics and practice. Confidentiality is a principle that crosses the moral, ethical and legal boundaries for all healthcare professionals. The duty and obligation to maintain confidentiality are reinforced by legal and professional standards. This duty creates an expectation within the community that personal health information will be treated with the utmost attention to avoid breaches. However, confidentiality and privacy are not absolute. Communication of information shared among healthcare professionals is vital to high-quality care. Information shared among healthcare professionals must be pertinent to the patient encounter and provided on a need-to-know basis. Furthermore, rights to privacy and confidentiality may be superseded when society deems that collective needs are more important than those of the individual's right to privacy and confidentiality. The duty of confidentiality is one of the most important principles by which healthcare professionals must abide; it is also a major cause of significant dilemma for the healthcare professional and distress for the patient when it is breached. It is because of this complexity and the consequences that it must be taken extremely seriously.

SUMMARY POINTS

- Confidentiality is the implicit protection of information gained in the course of a therapeutic relationship between a healthcare professional and an individual seeking the services of the healthcare professional or healthcare service.
- Healthcare students are not exempt from the provision of confidentiality, being bound by the same standards of practice as registered health professionals.
- Even in a healthcare relationship, patients and clients have the right to privacy. Sensitive information will only be shared by those who have trust that their information will only be used in the course of treatment and only by those who need to know.
- Healthcare professionals are legally obliged to protect the information—how it is used, stored and disclosed—provided to them. However, legal exemptions do exist that allow a healthcare professional to disclose certain information under specific conditions.
- Health-registering bodies have developed policies regarding the use of social media, particularly in relation to assuring confidentiality.

CRITICAL THINKING QUESTIONS

1. A fellow student has expressed interest in starting a blog about the trials and tribulations of being a health student. What advice and cautions would you give them?
2. A patient was admitted to the emergency department with a severe reaction to alcohol. He had driven himself to the hospital, and you learn that he is taking Naltrexone for the treatment of alcohol dependence. Upon discharge, he is still intoxicated but you learn that he is planning to drive himself home. Can you contact the police about the patient? Are you breaching patient confidentiality in informing the police of this person's actions?
3. Is it permissible to access an e-health record to get a date of birth or other generic piece of information from a patient's file? Why, or why not?

Group activity

Maintaining confidentiality

In your study groups or via your subject discussion site, discuss how you might handle the following scenarios:

- An internationally renowned actor is filming a sequel to their latest blockbuster movie on location in your area and has been admitted to your unit following an injury on set. Your friends and family known the actor has been admitted to your hospital and is keen to hear everything you know about their case.
- A local football player has overdosed on illicit drugs following celebrations after a big win on the field. He is admitted to your facility and you are assigned to his care. As you are leaving work at the end of your shift, you are approached by local media for a statement.

WEBLINKS

Legislation and statutes

Commonwealth Legislation (Australian Government):
www.australia.gov.au/about-government/publications/commonwealth-legislation

Federal Register of Legislation (Australian Government):
www.legislation.gov.au

New Zealand Legislation:
www.legislation.govt.nz

Privacy laws, policies and codes

ASHM: Guide to Australian HIV Laws and Policies for Healthcare Professionals:
www.hivlegal.ashm.org.au

Privacy Commissioner (New Zealand):
www.privacy.org.nz/the-privacy-act-and-codes/privacy-act-and-codes-introduction

The Privacy Act (Australian Government):
www.oaic.gov.au/privacy/the-privacy-act

REFERENCES

Australian Association of Social Workers. (2010). *Code of Ethics*. Canberra: AASW. Retrieved from www.aasw.asn.au/practitioner-resources/code-of-ethics.

Australian Commission on Safety and Quality in Health Care. (2017). *NSQHS Standards*. Retrieved from www.nationalstandards.safetyandquality.gov.au/1.-clinical-governance/patient-safety-and-quality-systems/healthcare-records.

Australian Commission on Safety and Quality in Health Care. (2019). *Australian Charter of Healthcare Rights*. Retrieved from www.safetyandquality.gov.au/national-priorities/charter-of-healthcare-rights.

Australian Health Practitioners Regulation Agency. (2014). *National Board Policy for Registered Health Practitioners: Social Media Policy*. Retrieved from www.nursingmidwiferyboard.gov.au/Codes-Guidelines-Statements/Codes-Guidelines/Social-media-policy.aspx.

Australian Psychological Society. (2007). *Code of Ethics*. Melbourne: APS.

Babst, B.A. (2018). Privacy and outing. In A. Cudd & M. Navin (eds), *Core Concepts and Contemporary Issues in Privacy* (pp. 219–233). Cham: Springer International.

Baird, S.M., Marsh, P.A., Lawrentshuk, N., Smart, P. & Chow, Z. (2018). Analysis of social media use among Australian and New Zealand otolaryngologists. *ANZ Journal of Surgery*. Advance online publication.

Beauchamp, T.L. & Childress, J.F. (2012). *Principles of Biomedical Ethics* (7th edn). New York: Oxford University Press.

Chretien, K.C., Greysen, R.S., Chretien, J.P. & Kind, T. (2009). Online posting of unprofessional conduct by medical students. *Journal of the American Medical Association*, 302(12), 1309–15.

Cuffe, K.M., Newton-Levinson, A., Gift, T.L., McFarlane, M. & Leichliter, J.S. (2016). Sexually transmitted infection testing among adolescents and young adults in the United States. *Journal of Adolescent Health*, 58(6), 512–19.

Department of Prime Minister and Cabinet. (2019). *Privacy Act 1933*. New Zealand Government. Retrieved from https://dpmc.govt.nz/our-business-units/cabinet-office/supporting-work-cabinet/cabinet-manual/8-official-information-3.

Facebook Newsroom. (2019). Our mission. Retrieved from http://newsroom.fb.com/company-info.

Federal Register of Legislation. (n.d.). *Privacy Act 1988*. Australian Government. Retrieved from www.legislation.gov.au/Details/C2014C00076.

Garner, J. & O'Sullivan, H. (2010). Facebook and the professional behaviors of undergraduate medical students. *The Clinical Teacher*, 7(2), 112–15.

Gilbert, A.L., Rickert, V.I. & Aalsma, M.C. (2014). Clinical conversations about health: The impact of confidentiality in preventative adolescent care. *Journal of Adolescent Health*, 55(5), 672–7.

Hartigan, L., Cussen, L., Meaney, S. & O'Donoghue, K. (2018). Patients' perception of privacy and confidentiality in the emergency department of a busy obstetric unit. *BMC Health Services Research*, 18(978), 1–6. doi:10/1186/s12913-018-3782-6.

Heskett, A., Preston, J.C. & Maskell, P.M. (2014). 'A curtain around a bed, not very private is it?': Thematic analysis of survey responses of medical patients in shared compared with single accommodation. *Age & Ageing*, 43(suppl. 1), i31.

Instagram. (2019). InfoCenter. Retrieved from http://instagram.com/press.

International Confederation of Midwives. (2008). *International Code of Ethics for Midwives*. The Hague: ICM.

International Council for Nurses. (2012). *The ICN Code of Ethics for Nurses*. Geneva: ICN.

Kadooka, Y., Okita, T. & Asai, A. (2016). Ethical obligations in the face of dilemmas concerning patient privacy and public interests: The Sasebo schoolgirl murder case. *Bioethics*, 30(7), 520–7.

Knight, S. & Papanikitas, A. (2018). Confidentiality. *InnovAiT: Education and Inspiration for General Practice*, 11(11), 639–45.

Koivula-Tynnila, H., Axelin, A. & Leino-Kilpi, H. (2018). Informational privacy in the recovery room: Patients' perspective. *Journal of PeriAnesthesia Nursing*, 33(4), 479–89.

Lagu, T., Kaufman, E.J., Asch, D.A. & Armstrong, K. (2008). Content of weblogs written by health professionals. *Journal of General Internal Medicine*, 23, 1642–6.

Levati, S. (2014). Professional conduct among registered nurses in the use of online social networking sites. *Journal of Advanced Nursing*, 70(10), 2284–92.

LinkedIn. (2019). About LinkedIn. Retrieved from http://press.linkedin.com/about.

Malfait. S., Eecklook, K., Lust, E., van Biesen, W. & van Hecke, A. (2017). Feasibility, appropriateness, meaningfulness and effectiveness of patient participation at bedside shift reporting: Mixed-method research protocol. *Journal of Advanced Nursing*, 73(2), 482–94.

McCann, T.V., Mugavin, J., Renzaho, A. & Lubman, D.I. (2016). Sub-Saharan African migrant youths' help-seeking barriers and facilitators for mental health and substance use problems: A qualitative study. *BMC Psychiatry*, 16(275), 1–10.

McLeod, A. & Dolezel, D. (2018). Cyber-analytics: Modeling factors associated with healthcare data breaches. *Decision Support Systems*, 108, 57–68.

Medical Board of Australia. (2014). *Good Medical Practice: A Code of Conduct for Doctors in Australia*. Retrieved from www.medicalboard.gov.au/Codes-Guidelines-Policies/Code-of-conduct.aspx.

National Health and Medical Research Council. (2007). *National Statement of Ethical Conduct in Human Research (updated March 2014)*. Canberra: Australian Government.

Neville, P. (2017). Social media and professionalism: A retrospective content analysis of fitness to practice cases heard by the GDC concerning social media complaints. *British Dental Journal*, 223(5), 353–7.

Panahi, S., Watson, J. & Partridge, H. (2016). Social media and physicians: Exploring the benefits and challenges. *Health Informatics Journal*, 22(2), 99–112.

Pharmacy Board of Australia. (2014). *Code of Conduct*. Melbourne: Pharmacy Board of Australia. Retrieved from www.pharmacyboard.gov.au/codes-guidelines/code-of-conduct.aspx.

Phillips, M., Dove, E.S. & Knoppers, B.M. (2017). Criminal prohibition of wrongful re-identification: Legal solution or minefield for big data? *Biomedical Inquiry*, 14, 527–39.

Prince, C. (2018). Do consumers want to control their personal data? Empirical evidence. *International Journal of Human-Computer Studies*, 110, 21–32.

Resnik, D.B. & Randall, D.C. (2018). Reporting suspected abuse or neglect in research involving children. *Journal of Medical Ethics*, 44, 555–9.

Sasse, R.A., Aroni, R.A., Sawyer, S.M. & Duncan, R.E. (2013). Confidential consultations with adolescents: An exploration of Australian parents' perspectives. *Journal of Adolescent Health*, 52, 786–91.

Seckman, C.A. (2018). Electronic health records and applications for managing patient care. In R. Nelson & N. Staggers (eds), *Health Informatics: An Interdisciplinary Approach* (2nd edn) (pp. 90–110). St Louis, MO: Elsevier.

Shenoy, A. & Appel, J.M. (2017). Safeguarding confidentiality in electronic health records. *Cambridge Quarterly of Healthcare Ethics*, 26(2), 337–41.

Tobiano, G., Whitty, J.A., Bucknall, T. & Chaboyer, W. (2017). Nurses' perceived barriers to bedside handover and their implication for clinical practice. *Worldviews on Evidence-Based Nursing*, 14(5), 343–9.

Twitter. (2019). Our company. Retrieved from https://about.twitter.com/company.

United Nations. (1948). *Universal Declaration of Human Rights*. Paris: UN.

United Nations. (1966). *International Covenant on Civil and Political Rights*. New York: UN.

CHAPTER 11

ADVOCACY AND THE HEALTHCARE PROFESSIONAL ROLE

SOPHIA COUZOS

CHAPTER FOCUS

After reading this chapter and completing the activities, you will be able to:

- define advocacy, and describe commonly recognised forms of advocacy related to healthcare provision
- describe policy advocacy and give examples of policy levers used to develop health policy
- outline the features of professional disciplines and the social contract and relate these to advocacy
- describe how advocacy by health professionals can be used to empower and disempower communities
- compare and contrast the health professional role in facilitational advocacy, representational advocacy and individual advocacy and in reference to community participation, public trust and healthcare outcomes
- analyse the debates that surround public health activism and individual liberties as a caution to consider in public health advocacy.

KEY TERMS

Advocacy
Facilitational advocacy
Health policy
Individual advocacy
Patient-centred care
Personal autonomy
Policy advocacy
Representational advocacy
Social contract

Introduction

Advocacy in healthcare can form an integral part of the care healthcare professionals provide to patients and the community. For most healthcare providers, regulations and societal laws bind the scope of practice concerning advocacy. In this chapter, advocacy is defined and applied to individuals and community situations. The role of the healthcare professional as an advocate is delineated and challenges to this role are highlighted and discussed. The concept of social justice and ethical decision making in **health policy** development are also debated. Real-life scenarios allow the reader to examine the various ways in which effective advocacy can be achieved. Finally, the chapter poses questions, encouraging the reader to pause and think about how they would manage various challenges related to healthcare advocacy.

Advocacy
The 'combination of individual and social actions designed to gain political commitment, policy support, social acceptance and systems support for a particular health goal or program' (WHO 1998).

Health policy
'Includes actions or intended actions by public, private and voluntary organizations that have an impact on health...policy may refer either to a set of actions and decisions, or to statements of intent' (Palmer & Short 2010).

An overview of advocacy

Healthcare professionals will inevitably be advocates for some issue or for someone at some time. Anyone who negotiates for the needs of another, or supports another person's cause, is acting as an advocate. Politicians who are democratically elected act as advocates on behalf of their constituents, constantly aiming to persuade others of a needed and preferred course of action. Healthcare professionals, in particular, have a core obligation to be advocates for their patients and for the public good. Advocacy has a political dimension. The World Health Organization (WHO 1998) defines advocacy as the 'combination of individual and social actions designed to gain political commitment, policy support, social acceptance and systems support for a particular health goal or program'.

Advocacy has also been defined by experts as 'taking a position on an issue, and initiating actions in a deliberate attempt to influence private and public policy choices' (Labonte 1994, p. 263). Similarly, health advocacy occurs when 'individuals or groups endeavour to change some of the factors that shape people's environments and health behaviours by restructuring a range of elements such as institutions, policies and laws' (Gould 2012).

The French chemist Jean-Baptiste Boussingault acted as a public health advocate in 1833 when he urged his government to add iodine to salt to prevent goitre (Kamien 2006). In 2007, healthcare professionals advocated for the mandatory fortification of bread with iodised salt because of the high prevalence of iodine deficiency in Tasmania (Seal et al. 2007). Iodine fortification of bread was subsequently mandated throughout Australia, reversing the trend towards iodine deficiency (DePaoli, Seal, Burgess & Taylor 2013).

Most public health advocacy aims to influence population health outcomes, as in the example of bread fortification with iodine. The goal of advocacy is thus not merely to raise public awareness about an issue, but to *influence outcomes*.

Public health advocacy thus involves contesting differing ideas, ideologies, traditions, research findings, personal and social values, political interests and ambitions in order to influence an outcome; these have been called 'competing rationalities' (Lin 2003). Interest groups have differing views about the importance of the outcomes being sought or what policy levers might best work to bring about these outcomes. Public health advocacy thus invites debates and challenges over a range of issues. A competing rationality, for example, might be how the loss of **personal autonomy** is valued if public health advocates seek to impose government regulation on people's behaviour in order to achieve a 'greater good': a public health outcome. Other competing rationalities are debates over the use of limited resources. This creates what are called 'opportunity costs', as there are consequences when a choice is made that forgoes the alternative. In addition, the broader consequences of the proposal being put forward need to be considered (sometimes this is phrased as the 'slippery slope' argument). The public expects governments to pay attention to competing rationalities, as poor decisions could mean that 'the policy outcomes of today become the policy problems of tomorrow' (Biggs & Helms 2006, p. 407). The issues that matter to policymakers, such as competing rationalities, should also matter to public health advocates because these understandings can lead to more effective advocacy.

Personal autonomy
An ethical principle that people should be allowed to be self-governing and make decisions for themselves.

Advocacy often only involves awareness raising, or framing issues in a certain way to maximise public exposure to the issue and create a context for policymaking. Such advocacy strategies aim to change or modify the beliefs or values of the public and political leaders. Most public health advocacy toolkits focus on ways to frame issues, especially through social marketing techniques (International Council of Nurses 2008; Public Health Advocacy Institute of Western Australia 2013). This focus has been criticised, especially when the success of advocacy has been judged not by the achievement of outcomes, but by the advocacy effort itself: 'we advocated, therefore we were successful' (McCubbin, Labonte & Dallaire 2001).

Research findings are often used to advocate for an issue. However, research evidence alone often plays a small role in gaining the attention of policymakers and effecting change. Research is highly contestable as it may be small-scale and context-specific, raising doubts over its generalisability, and it may provide merely a small fraction of the information needed to make policy decisions. On the other hand, even small-scale research can support advocacy efforts if it is framed in a way that is consistent with the values and ideologies of policymakers (Gibson 2003, p. 19). This is discussed in more detail later in the chapter.

Forms of advocacy

Health advocacy takes many forms. Individual advocacy describes efforts towards partnerships with individuals to advocate on their behalf as 'patient advocates' or to foster self-advocacy so that people can speak for themselves and assert their own needs when they face specific difficulties. Advocacy efforts on a broader population scale, which may be community, national or international, and which serve to influence health policy, are known as systems or systemic advocacy, or **policy advocacy**. Some authors have described these differences as advocacy for 'cases' as compared with advocacy for 'causes' (Carlisle 2000). Other forms of advocacy include citizens and legal advocacy (note these are not discussed in this chapter as being of less relevance to healthcare professionals).

Policy advocacy
Efforts on a broader population scale (community, national or international) to influence policy and enhance health outcomes.

Individual (or 'case') advocacy

Each healthcare professional discipline has different approaches to patient advocacy, depending on the patient's needs and their circumstances. Generally, patient advocates work to empower others. This role may take the form of supporting patients to access services, facilities, and entitlements or opportunities. The type of support depends on the patient's physical and mental capacity, their contextual situation, and their desires and aspirations towards independence. The type of advocacy healthcare providers offer is placed somewhere in the 'empowerment continuum' within which patients are situated (see Figure 11.1).

FIGURE 11.1 The empowerment continuum

EMPOWERMENT CONTINUUM	
	Description of individual advocacy
Disempowered	Doing 'for'
↕	Doing 'with'
	Coaching
	Mentoring
Empowered	Doing 'for oneself'

Source: Adapted from New Zealand Government 2016.

Another way to conceptualise the different forms of patient advocacy is when advocates adapt their relationship to the specific situations of clients or patients. Advocates who support clients to self-advocate (i.e. represent themselves and their needs) demonstrate a form of advocacy that is highly empowering for the client. Other situations may require advocates to assume greater professional control in order to protect those who are most vulnerable (Freddolino, Moxley & Hyduk 2004). Essentially, **individual advocacy** needs to be matched to the functional needs of the person.

Individual advocacy
Partnering with individuals to advocate on their behalf or to foster self-advocacy so that people can speak for themselves, asserting their own needs when they face specific difficulties.

Governments often fund such advocacy efforts. For example, the Australian Government provides funding to advocacy agencies across Australia through the

National Disability Advocacy Program (NDAP) run by the Department of Social Services (DSS). This funding enables people with disability to access advocacy services to overcome barriers that impact on their ability to participate in the community. Disability advocacy agencies receive funding under the *Disability Services Act 1986* (Cth). Most of the program funds support people either through:

- *individual advocacy*: paid advocates employed by an advocacy agency
- *systemic advocacy*: when peak bodies receive funds to employ policy officers to advocate for the rights of those with disabilities (DSS 2018).

Policy or 'cause' advocacy

Policy advocacy draws from skills gained through experience and a thorough knowledge of the health policy environment (McCubbin et al. 2001). This type of advocacy is usually associated with health promotion, or efforts to improve the health of individuals and populations through upstream strategies using a range of policy levers, such as regulation and legislation. The goal of policy advocacy is to effect policy change or bring about changes to programs to enhance health outcomes. Some examples of policy advocacy are shown in the activities throughout this chapter.

Health promotion is the process of enabling people to increase control over their health and its determinants, and thereby improve their health (WHO 1986, 2005). The participation of people and communities is integral to efforts towards health promotion. Policy advocacy thus not only requires knowledge of structural or social barriers to health—it requires knowledge of the policy process to influence these determinants, as well as meaningful engagement with community. Community participation is an ideal aspiration in policy advocacy, and just like individual advocacy, such efforts can be understood within an empowerment continuum that defines several levels of community participation, as shown in Table 11.1 on page 229.

Policy advocacy without community participation risks both failure and irrelevancy. Healthcare professionals can play a role in supporting community efforts and priorities through **facilitational advocacy** (advocating 'with') or representational advocacy (advocating 'for'). Representational advocacy is discussed later in this chapter in relation to policy advocacy. Communicating with communities is discussed in detail in Chapter 8.

Facilitational advocacy
Advocacy that empowers disadvantaged groups to lobby for change by providing individuals and communities with the skills to tackle health issues.

Healthcare professions and advocacy

All healthcare professionals commit to a code of conduct to promote the best interests of their patients, to protect their autonomy, promote health and prevent disease, reduce health inequalities and promote the public good. Such codes of conduct have originated from human rights declarations. Patient-centred care, for example, typifies the partnership between healthcare professionals and patients whereby patients' needs and preferences are identified and met (ACSQHC 2011). Advocacy has thus emerged as a core obligation of the healthcare professional committed to serving patients and the community.

Increasingly, healthcare providers are broadening their attention to address the social determinants of health. For example, clinicians have an obligation to explore a range of upstream (social) health determinants with their patients such as employment, housing and transport; as well as midstream factors such as access to healthcare services; and psychosocial risk factors such as social exclusion, job stress and social networks. Strategies to address inequities and social disparities can then be prepared in an individual care plan and may involve individual advocacy or policy advocacy efforts. Healthcare providers also act as advocates for health equity when they accept a lesser fee from those who find it difficult to afford the cost of the service. General practitioners will fervently act as advocates for their patients to have earlier specialist appointments or elective surgery within the public sector (Porter, Blashki & Grills 2014).

Being an effective advocate for patients is a core competency for medical students and other healthcare professionals. Learning how to advocate for the health needs of a community is a core part of physician and general practice training in Australia (ACRRM 2013; RACGP 2016; RACP 2014). In particular, rural and remote general practitioners are expected to be aware of the social and economic impacts on health, the political context in which they are working, and to have the ability to engage with governments, community leaders and a range of agencies in order to effect positive health outcomes (ACRRM 2013). High-profile health advocates are also often public healthcare professionals.

Healthcare professionals, non-professionals, government and non-government organisations (NGOs), community groups and politicians practise advocacy every day. Governments may also fully or partly sponsor NGOs and consumer groups to advocate on health issues for their constituencies (Health Consumers Queensland 2017). Examples include Australian Government funding of national bodies such as the Heart Foundation, Consumers Health Forum of Australia, Federation of Ethnic Communities' Councils of Australia, and the National Aboriginal Community Controlled Health Organisation (NACCHO).

The professional role

Does it matter if an advocate is a healthcare professional? And what is meant by the professional role anyway? Isn't expert knowledge more important than that of lay advocates?

Belonging to a profession gives certain rights and privileges as well as public responsibilities, and those responsibilities are tied up into what is known as the **social contract**. The healthcare professional's relationship with, and accountability to, society can be traced back to the Hippocratic Oath.

Social contract
The bargain struck between a profession and society to provide specialised skills and a guaranteed commitment to professional attributes (integrity, altruism, etc.), in return for autonomy in practice and the privilege of self-regulation. The 'profession' is then trusted to provide specific services to society.

BOX 11.1

THE SOCIAL CONTRACT

The social contract describes societal expectations of healthcare professionals in return for health professionals' autonomy, self-regulation and other rewards. Society expects health professionals to commit to a code of ethics and profess a commitment to competence, integrity and morality, altruism, and the promotion of the public good within their domain. Professionals are accountable to those served, to the profession and to society.

Source: Cruess, Johnston & Cruess 2002.

The Hippocratic Oath was a covenant for ethical practice developed around the fourth century BCE and is attributed to Hippocrates who was a Greek physician. This formed the foundation for what we now call 'professional attributes'. The Oath has enduring appeal because it emphasises the primacy of the patient's interests over the interests of physicians, the responsibility towards beneficence and non-maleficence when treating patients, the vital importance of maintaining patient confidentiality, the need to be just, and a physician's responsibility to be held accountable to society (Hulkower 2010). The body of published works that make up the Hippocratic Corpus discuss the influence of the natural world over the supernatural world, and individual, diet and lifestyle factors as determinants of disease. Scholars have reflected that these Hippocratic writings and traditions laid the foundations for what are now recognised as preventive medicine and the biopsychosocial model of health (Merikas 1992; Tsiompanou & Marketos 2013). All this means that healthcare professionals have been advocates for healthy living for over 2000 years!

However, being an advocate for patients is not enough. A healthcare professional also has duties to society (for the public good), and must be accountable to those served, the profession and society.

Current definitions of professionalism are contained in the international Charter on Medical Professionalism, which first appeared in 2002. The Charter refers to three common facets of professionalism from which principles of practice and professional responsibilities arise. Professionalism demands 'placing the interests of patients above those of the physician; setting and maintaining standards of competence and integrity; and providing expert advice to society on matters of health' (Medical Professionalism Project 2002). Personal attributes considered essential in professional practice are:

- altruism: placing the interests of individual patients and society above their own
- integrity: being honest, moral, virtuous and consistent
- devotion towards the public good: responding to, and addressing the concerns of society, using resources responsibly, and advocacy for public health (Cruess et al. 2002; Sinha 2011).

The profession is then trusted to provide specific services to society, as citizens know that their interests and those of the public as a whole will be paramount.

Healthcare providers commit to professionalism through an unwritten social contract. The profession provides these specialised skills and guarantees commitment to these attributes, in return for professional autonomy in practice, the privilege of self-regulation and a more prominent role in society than the average citizen. Self-regulation confers prestige and public trust, and minimises the government's role without completely eliminating it. This shared accountability supports a good relationship with government that allows the profession to express its own view and, in particular, to gain privileged access to government with respect to policy and advocacy (Balthazard 2010).

Professional self-regulation in turn benefits the government because the costs of regulation are met by the profession, as well as insulating it from the actions of the profession. If the profession cannot be trusted to serve the public interest while self-regulating, society may need to impose external regulation on professions to constrain inappropriate practice.

The social contract means that healthcare professionals are in a unique and privileged position to advocate for programs and policies that may benefit individual clients, subpopulations, and society as a whole. Some would say that this privilege means healthcare professionals have a civic duty to tackle health inequity both at the individual and systems levels. This privilege also entails the responsibility to be professional, to align efforts with the priorities of the community, minimise conflicts of interest, and be mindful of the use of public resources and the consequences of such use.

Advocacy through primary healthcare

The individual advocacy efforts of healthcare professionals and other professionals such as social workers to assist patients and to empower them to access resources and to address social disparities (Freddolino et al. 2004) intersects with the role of general practitioners within primary healthcare systems. The general practitioner is often the first point of contact within the primary healthcare system and serves as a pivotal advocate for all patients, 'acting as the coordinator and interpreter of care for the patient over time and across services' (AMA 2010). Primary healthcare aims to provide holistic, comprehensive care that is not just biomedical, but involves a collaborative team that is both interprofessional and multisectoral.

Aboriginal Community Controlled Health Services (ACCHSs) are specific primary healthcare services that have a central advocacy role for Aboriginal and Torres Strait Islander people (Hunter et al. 2004). They employ general practitioners and allied health professionals such as nurses, Aboriginal Health Workers, and others.

There are over 140 of these services situated across Australia (NACCHO 2018) with activity mostly consistent with the Alma Ata Declaration on Primary Health Care (WHO 1978), including programs that address all the five action areas of the Ottawa Charter for Health Promotion (WHO 1986). Importantly, they empower individuals and the community by acknowledging the social determinants of health. They are community-controlled, operating a governance structure comprising elected members of the community. A range of community development efforts result in the employment of Indigenous Australians, support for their career pathways, community cohesion, the expression of leadership (e.g. Board appointments), as well as policy advocacy (Grant, Wronski, Murray & Couzos 2008).

Individual advocacy in the primary healthcare context

An example of individual advocacy to address social determinants of health within a general practice or an ACCHS setting is shown through the process of developing a chronic disease care plan. This example demonstrates processes to improve the health circumstances of individual patients and to find solutions to problems that patients identify as a priority, and doing so collaboratively. The development of chronic disease care plans is a particularly valuable way of enhancing patients' self-management of their health, identifying the issues that are most important to them and outlining the agreed pathway towards improved health (Dennis et al. 2008).

The care plan in the 'Skills in practice' feature below can be expanded if the setting is an ACCHS. Trust is enhanced in culturally appropriate environments; home visits may be more readily negotiated; transport support may be provided by the service; allied health services may be delivered on-site; communication may occur in 'language'; some services can assist with short-term financial support if needed; and remote-area Aboriginal health services can provide medicines on-site without the patient needing to visit a community pharmacy (*National Health Act 1953*, s. 100—Federal Register of Legislation n.d.).

Skills in practice

Example of a care plan

Care plans are an example of a mechanism of advocacy for social circumstances in a common general practice. An example of a care plan for Kathy is provided below. Some abbreviations have been used to make the table easier to read:

- My Aged Care: This Australian Government program provides aged care support and can refer Kathy to the National Aboriginal and Torres Strait Islander Flexible Aged Care Program. Eligibility starts from age 50 years.
- PBS: Pharmaceutical Benefits Scheme.

Patient problems, needs or concerns	Goals	Required treatments and services	Arrangements for treatments and services
Overcrowded housing	Alleviate stress	Seek support for larger, more suitable housing.	Letter of support to the local Aboriginal Housing Corporation. Referral to social worker.
Build trust in the doctor–patient relationship	Support Kathy to return for regular care	Address Kathy's clinical and social priorities incrementally. Offer home visits from the practice nurse or Aboriginal Health Worker (AHW).	Frequent contact to assess priorities; involve practice nurse/AHW; maximise home support for disability and aged care—consider referral to My Aged Care.
Financial struggles	Manage finances independently	Maximise access to available welfare support. Develop personal skills to manage home budgets.	Letter to the social worker.
Needs transport support to attend clinic	Source transport support for Kathy to attend the clinic	Provide transport support.	Register with the local government transport subsidy scheme for pensioners. Source My Aged Care for transport support.
Unable to meet medication costs	Enhance adherence by reducing the burden of the cost of medicines	Enhance access to medicines.	Optimise the medications list. Assess for adherence. Register for co-payment relief for Indigenous Australians (medicines will be free of the co-payment). Assess eligibility for the PBS safety net. Liaise with pharmacist to monitor the PBS safety net.

Tips: Care plans are generally developed as part of a general practice consultation. These usually include the management of a person's primary condition, along with any existing comorbidity, risk factors and preventive interventions. The plan should be written in a way that is understandable to the patient and others who will refer to it in providing care to the patient.

CASE ACTIVITY 11.1

Care plan in action

The above care plan was developed for Kathy, a 50-year-old Aboriginal woman with type 2 diabetes mellitus. She is seeing a general practitioner (GP) at a rural private general practice for a repeat prescription. The GP invited Kathy to talk about what concerned her the most about her health and if she would like the GP to assist her. The GP specifically enquired about her social situation. Kathy lives in overcrowded rental accommodation. She has custody of three children aged between 8–12 years of age living in the same house as Kathy and her mother. This is causing Kathy to be stressed because the house only has three bedrooms. Because of illness, Kathy has not been employed since she was in her mid-20s. She is on a disability support pension, and her mother receives the aged care pension, but she is struggling financially with the family's living expenses and caring for the children. At times, she does not fill her prescription because she cannot meet the co-payment for each of her medicines. She finds it difficult to attend the clinic, as it is too costly by bus or taxi. Kathy grew up at a time when there was a much greater wariness of doctors. The GP is a new doctor whom she has never met before.

1. What other issues and strategies would you include in a care plan to tailor management of Kathy's healthcare needs to her social circumstances, and to change some of the social factors that affect her life?
2. How might these or other mutually agreed strategies empower Kathy towards better self-management of her chronic disease and its social determinants?
3. If this service was an Aboriginal Community Controlled Health Service, what additional supports could be offered to Kathy?

Policy advocacy in the primary healthcare context

Classic examples of public health advocacy relevant to primary healthcare include efforts promoting breastfeeding, decreased tobacco smoking, vaccination efforts, needle and syringe exchange programs and stroke prevention (Gruszin, Hetzel & Glover 2012).

Reflect and apply

In 2004, the NACCHO undertook research to explore health services access to a federal government program encouraging the self-management of asthma. (The advocacy efforts were undertaken by a health professional employed by NACCHO, with oversight and direction from the Aboriginal leadership.) Data revealed that 80 per cent of ACCHSs—24 from 28 services—reported their clients had difficulty accessing asthma spacer devices due to their cost. Some staff reported using 390 mL plastic Coke bottles as makeshift spacer devices for clients, as conventional spacers were unaffordable. A makeshift device was photographed and published in the research paper (see Figure 11.2) (Couzos & Davis 2005).

Advocacy efforts included the conduct of research, the publication of findings, meetings with policymakers from the Department of Health, and the briefing of a senator. At the time, the Department of Health was heavily invested in evaluating asthma initiatives and had discretionary access to funds for asthma initiatives through a Federal Budget allocation.

The publication of the research with the Coke-bottle image led a senator to pose questions to the Department of Health in the upper House of Parliament regarding Aboriginal people's lack of access to these devices. In response, the Department supported a scheme to provide asthma spacers to ACCHSs at a subsidised rate (Asthma Spacers Ordering System [ASOS]) developed with NACCHO and Asthma Australia. This was accompanied by an education campaign to enhance Aboriginal peoples' awareness of asthma. Over 1000 spacers were purchased by ACCHSs for their needy clients within 12 months of the scheme operating. The scheme is still in operation and is now supported independently through Asthma Australia (Asthma Australia n.d.).

FIGURE 11.2 Plastic Coke bottle used as an asthma spacer device, with instructions for use

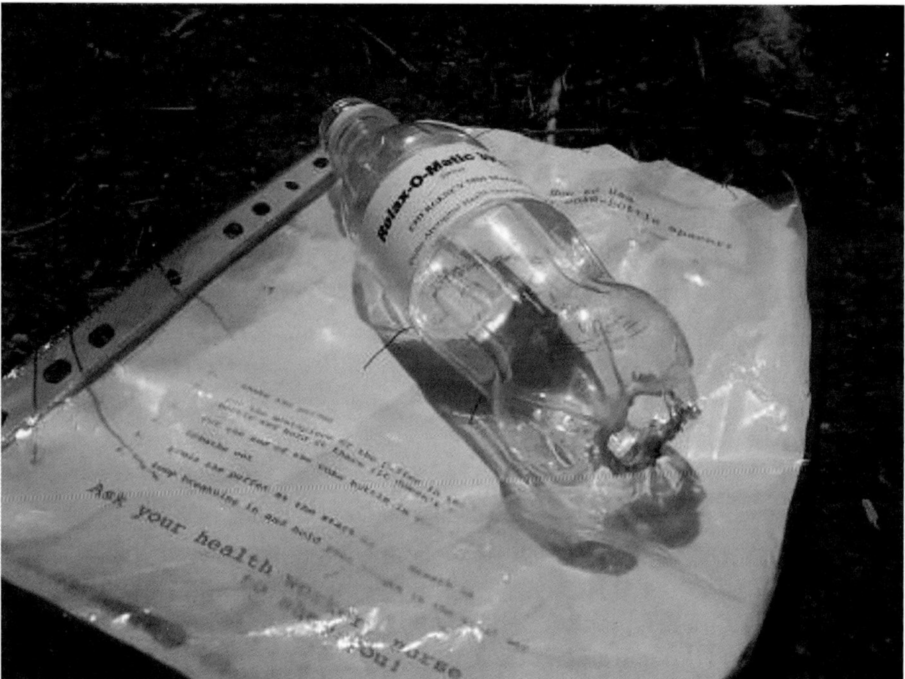

Source: Sophia Couzos.

- What type of policy lever is being used for the provision of asthma spacers through Asthma Australia in this example?
- What other policy measures might have enhanced access to asthma spacer devices for those who could not afford them?
- Are the efforts of the healthcare professional described in this example facilitational advocacy or representational advocacy?

Challenges to the professional role as an advocate

We have seen how being an advocate for patients is an inherent part of being a healthcare provider in a professional capacity (Schwartz 2002). We have also seen how healthcare professionals are in a privileged position to advocate for programs and policies that may benefit clients and society as a whole. The social contract obliges professionals to act and advocate for the good of society, but the form this takes can sometimes be contentious.

Healthcare providers can face potential conflicts of loyalty when acting as patient advocates. Specifically, acting in the patient's best interest can often conflict with the healthcare professional's own ethical responsibility for non-maleficence and codes of conduct to promote the public good. Policy advocacy by experts may promote expert interests while disempowering community views. We will explore these issues by asking: when does advocacy become paternalism?

Being a patient advocate in a professional capacity means:

- empowering the patient, protecting patient autonomy and ensuring informed consent
- protecting a patient's rights and interests when they cannot protect their own
- ensuring the patient has fair access to available resources (Schwartz 2002).

But when health professionals advocate for their patients, does this also mean supporting any decision the patient makes without regard for their needs or potential costs and consequences? Consider the following examples.

- *Example 1:* A euthanasia specialist chose not to intervene to prevent the suicide of a former patient in the belief that the patient's decision was clear and rational even in the absence of a terminal illness, and because such action would be contrary to that person's wishes (Medew 2014; Worsley 2014).
- *Example 2:* Many doctors refused to support parents who conscientiously objected to vaccinating their children. Vaccination of children in Australia was linked to the receipt of family tax benefit supplements—an annual sum of just under $750 and families who objected to vaccination could receive an exemption from their doctor so they could still receive the payment. However, many doctors (up to 18%) refused to acknowledge a parent's conscientious objection to vaccination (Leask et al. 2008) and facilitated the application of financial penalties to these families by denying their access to the financial supplement (Hansen 2014). Conscientious objection is no longer acceptable to the Australian Government, so this decision no longer resides with the doctor.

These two examples illustrate opposing positions. Example 1 refers to an advocate who places high moral value on a former patient's wishes by providing unconditional support, even in the face of overwhelming condemnation for failing to prevent suicide as a duty of professional care. Example 2 advocates for the public good (collectivism) when doctors place their own personal moral values and an assessment of the public good above the values of the individual patient. The latter can also be described as paternalism, because the doctor's interference was (in their view) for the good of the family (i.e. 'doctor knows best').

The professional role always requires a balance between the commitment to a patient's autonomy and their best interests. The patient's autonomy also needs to be balanced against the responsibility the healthcare professional has towards the broader public good. Being a professional and being the best advocate means that paternalism is sometimes a consequence (i.e. making a decision to override a patient's preferences), although there are many ways this and the potential for harm can be avoided.

Reflect and apply

Many Aboriginal patients in non-remote Australia have been unable to afford co-payments for their medicines. In response, ACCHSs reported paying for some clients' prescriptions out of their core operating budget, knowing that these patients would otherwise forgo their medicines. National health expenditure data for PBS medicines confirmed that for every dollar spent by a non-Indigenous Australian, an Indigenous Australian spent only 32 cents. This figure was worse for Indigenous peoples in non-remote Australia, at 26 cents per person (2001–02) (AIHW 2005).

NACCHO embarked on an advocacy strategy to address this inequity by raising the issue with government departments in several submissions that proposed waiving the co-payment for medicines. These approaches on their own were unsuccessful due to government concerns about setting a precedent for co-payment relief. NACCHO subsequently formed a coalition with the Pharmacy Guild of Australia that offered a timely opportunity to fund a trial program. In 2006, through this partnership with other healthcare professionals, a strategy to improve quality use of medicines and enable equitable access to pharmaceuticals for Aboriginal peoples in non-remote areas was born: the Quality Use of Medicines Maximised for Aboriginal and Torres Strait Islander People (QUMAX) program.

The Australian Government approved the QUMAX program as part of the Fourth Community Pharmacy Agreement (Commonwealth of Australia 2005, 2007). This $11 million program began in early 2008 and enabled access for Aboriginal and Torres Strait Islander clients who were not accessing medicines under existing arrangements. The program provided medicines support to over 70 ACCHSs in non-remote areas through partnerships with community pharmacists. A customised package of interventions was developed with each ACCHS under agreed work plans. The packages included QUM training to ACCHSs and cultural training to community pharmacies; transport support to ACCHSs for medicines access from a community pharmacy; Dose Administration Aids to high-risk clients; after-hours pharmacy support; and a waiving of the co-payment for eligible and needy clients facing financial barriers who were at risk of not complying with their prescribed medicines (Couzos, Sheedy & Thiele 2011).

The program was independently evaluated and found to have substantially increased access to medicines (Urbis Pty Ltd 2011). It was subsequently extended to general practices across Australia in the 2007–08 Federal Budget and commenced in 2010 as the PBS Co-payment Measure, also known as Closing the Gap scripts (CTG) (Australian Government 2018b; Couzos et al. 2011). Between 2010 and 2016, over 407 000 Aboriginal peoples and Torres Strait Islander people have benefited from the CTG script measure.

- Did the advocacy efforts change policy in the desired direction?
- What was the outcome: the advocacy effort itself, altered health policy or health outcome?
- Were health outcomes improved? Can you attribute potential health outcomes to the advocacy effort, or would these outcomes have occurred anyway?
- How important was the combination of Aboriginal community involvement and support from healthcare professionals in this example of policy advocacy? Why did that matter?

CASE ACTIVITY 11.2

Professionals as advocates

Caleb is a fifth-year medical student sitting in with a general practitioner to observe their interaction with patients. Caleb notices that the doctor is very friendly and readily agrees to patients' requests for medical certificates, investigations and prescriptions for drugs of dependence. One patient requests total body MRI 'because I am sure something is wrong with me, and I know my own body', but the doctor is only prevented from ordering this because the hospital requires a referral from a specialist.

1. Is this doctor behaving professionally? What aspects of professionalism are being undermined in this example?
2. Is the doctor acting as a patient advocate and respecting this patient's autonomy to make independent decisions?
3. What should Caleb do in this situation?

Many patients expect healthcare professionals to be paternalistic, as this suggests they are advocating for the patient's best interests (Taylor 2009). A healthcare professional's expert knowledge and their commitment to the social contract can engender public trust, which is a powerful tool for advocacy in itself. For example, a factor that significantly influences a mother's decision to vaccinate her child when exposed to messages from anti-vaccination lobby groups is the mother's strong trust in healthcare professionals. In the face of increased consumer willingness to question medical interventions, and anti-vaccination messages that are framed to foster greater parental autonomy and freedom over powerful vested interests such as government or pharmaceutical bodies, the professionalism of the doctor can outweigh those influences.

However, mothers also value healthcare professionals who trust them and regard them as competent decision makers (Leask, Chapman, Hawe & Burgess 2006). Only a very small proportion of parents who question vaccination are strongly against vaccination. Rather, they may express hesitancy due to safety concerns that have been unsatisfactorily answered by clinicians, or experienced a transitory but frightening adverse experience following vaccination of their child, or they may be seeking a health professional to trust (Leask 2015). Adversarial advocacy that shames people, restricts or eliminates consumer choice to question (such as banning vaccine-related searches on global social media) (McMillan & Hernandez 2019) or forcefully vaccinates under threat of imprisonment (Khan & Chiau 2015) may paradoxically amplify exposure to radical anti-vaccination messages and do considerably more harm to vaccination uptake (Leask 2015).

The vital healthcare paradigm of **patient-centred care** means that paternalism in healthcare delivery is no longer seen as acceptable (see Institute of Medicine Committee on Quality of Health Care in America 2001). Treating the patient as a person, respecting their values, identifying and managing healthcare issues through a biopsychosocial lens, sharing power and responsibility, and developing an enduring and meaningful therapeutic alliance are core concepts defining patient-centredness (Mead & Bower 2000). For many public health issues, healthcare professionals will grapple between competing rationalities such as upholding the rights of the individual versus the need to protect society as a whole (the collective) and, if necessary, using the power of government to achieve that (Calman 2009). This issue is discussed further later in the chapter.

Patient-centred care Healthcare that respects and responds to individual people's preferences, needs and values, and ensures that the patients' values and involvement guide all decision making.

Advocacy and the community

Policy advocacy by experts is often constructed in paternalistic ways, even though it may be well intentioned. One of the most well-known scholars on community empowerment, Ronald Labonte, has written: 'Professionals…remain the controlling actor, defining the terms of the interaction [with communities]. Relatively disempowered individuals or groups remain the objects, the recipients of professional actions' (Labonte 1994, p. 255). Professionals who advocate as experts may inadvertently be reinforcing the view that 'non-professional groups are incapable of their own powerful actions.' He refers to professionals as exercising 'power over' others, to educate clients to a particular way of viewing the world in contrast to 'power with' others, which finds common ground by respecting what communities and people think and know about the issues (Labonte 1994).

Advocacy should ideally involve community engagement and capacity building as communities and people 'provide the stories, lived problems and issues', while professionals have privileged access to mechanisms and language of advocacy

(Labonte 1994). This is the notion of advocacy that is authentic, 'starting where people are', where the priorities and lived realities are, where the professional role is facilitational, collaborative and supportive, which to some extent entails giving up some professional autonomy.

Just as there is an empowerment continuum with regard to individual advocacy, collaborations for policy advocacy can also be expressed as a community empowerment continuum. This has been termed the 'ladder of participation' (see Table 11.1) (Arnstein 1969). It has been applied in various forms to describe levels of community participation in strategies, programs, policies and services. The ladder has eight levels of participation from the highest, where the community exercises control over the issue, to the lowest, which occurs when communities are neither consulted nor informed, or may even be re-educated or diverted away from an issue by authorities or professionals. This has also been used to describe 'grassroots' or 'bottom-up' advocacy (community led) or 'top-down' advocacy (by experts outside the community) (Loue 2006). The eight levels are illustrative and do not represent discrete stages or steps, as different contexts will define different roles for stakeholders.

TABLE 11.1 Ladder of community participation

Degree of participation	Participant's role	Definition
High	Control	Community groups have control over the identification of issues, including resourcing, and exercise managerial power over strategies and actions.
	Delegated power	The community identifies the needs, determines and implements programs, and is accountable to the community, while the external organisation provides resources (finances and other assistance)—e.g. through subcontracting.
	Partnership	There is partnership between community/representative bodies and external organisations. The relationships are formalised, roles and responsibilities are clear, there is interdependence, commitment, integrity, sharing of information, sufficient resources and balanced power relationships. This enables community groups to negotiate with external organisations.
	Plan jointly	External organisations permit and enable community direction on predefined issues and scope, provided the outcome is acceptable to the external organisation.
	Influence	Community representatives are invited to influence predefined issues or programs and their implementation, as developed by external organisations. Channels of influence might occur through committees, and representatives may be in a minority. This level has been viewed as 'placation'.

Degree of participation	Participant's role	Definition
Low	Consulted	Community representatives are invited to make comment on predefined issues and scope—e.g. through submissions. There is no guarantee of any community influence over the issue.
	Receive information	External organisations develop programs or plans and announce them. Community may be ad hoc recipients of information or forums are convened for informational purposes only. There are no channels for feedback or negotiation.
	None	Community not involved in any program plan or issue, or may be distracted from playing any role in the issue.

Source: Adapted from Arnstein 1969.

This ladder may also be considered as a way of viewing the levels of community participation related to the 'ends' of advocacy as well as the 'means' of advocacy. For example, the degree of control over what advocacy seeks to achieve has been termed the 'ends' and degree of control over the capacity to advocate and the form it takes has been termed the 'means' (Freddolino et al. 2004). Community groups that have the means to advocate by having an organised powerbase, structures that make their leaders directly accountable to the community, and sufficient resources, can exercise a high degree of control over advocacy efforts. This means that community leaders can be active participants in the policymaking and political arena—making advocacy happen—while healthcare professionals play a largely facilitational role.

Reflect and apply

How much control does the community have over what advocacy seeks to achieve? Consider levels of control over: what groups are going to advocate for (the 'ends'), and how groups are going to get there (the 'means').

Applying a lens to policy advocacy efforts is instructive. It is possible to ascertain how inclusive they are and at what level the target community has been involved in those efforts. Community participation and control over the means and ends of advocacy can generate some unease among health professionals and advocates (Robertson & Minkler 1994). For example, a remote Aboriginal community negotiated trading their rights to land in exchange for much needed satellite kidney dialysis services, a contentious arrangement with government that disappointed many. A community spokesperson said: 'some may be critical of land being exchanged for community services, but the old people said there are no sacred sites here; there are no ceremony places; it is not a hunting area. We worry about countrymen with kidney disease…' (Loff & Cordner 1998, p. 1451). The trade arrangement was eventually withdrawn and a satellite unit has since been established (Couzos et al. 2008).

Healthcare professionals advocating at the forefront of political forums and structures may deprive community groups of the opportunity to speak for themselves and to influence forums directly. It promotes learned helplessness and undermines the advocacy effort, as it is the 'authentic voice which needs to be heard for advocacy efforts to be both successful and on target' (McCubbin et al. 2001, p. 25). For example, the majority of health policy targeting Aboriginal people over the past few decades has been formulated at a level least inclusive of this community, purportedly for their benefit. Of this, the late Dr Puggy Hunter, Aboriginal leader and human rights champion, said in 2001: 'We were driving the car; all they had to do was put fuel in it' (Hunter 2001).

The ideal role of the healthcare professional is to facilitate community's advocacy efforts by supporting democratic participation, utilising the professional's expertise to provide quality information, and empowering people and communities to define problems, pose solutions and express those needs themselves. This particularly aligns with the ideals of the Ottawa Charter, because communities are seen as the agents of change towards health promotion (Robertson & Minkler 1994).

Facilitational and representational advocacy by healthcare professionals

As discussed earlier, advocacy that empowers disadvantaged groups to lobby for change is egalitarian and is called facilitational advocacy. Facilitational advocacy can take any of the following forms:

- Professionals lend their skills to community organisations as employees who undertake research, analyses, and prepare submissions for use by these organisations.
- Community groups commission independent professionals or organisations to undertake analyses for them.
- Professionals or organisations undertake their own policy analyses, which independently support the advocacy efforts of community groups.
- Professionals or organisations provide statements of support for community groups.
- Professionals or organisations form coalitions with community groups in formalised relationships.

Representational advocacy
A type of advocacy that speaks for or represents the needs of vulnerable groups.

In contrast, advocacy that speaks for or represents the needs of vulnerable groups is **representational advocacy**. Representational advocacy may be necessary when communities are unable to participate in processes for health, even if the opportunity is available (Carlisle 2000).

Advocacy and the policy process

Given that the goal of advocacy is to influence outcomes, policy advocacy can utilise the same methods as political advocacy, but with the goal of bringing about health improvements.

Any deliberate attempt to influence private and public policy choices requires knowledge of the policy process and an ability to influence policymakers and public opinion through certain means. The organisational factors in the focus box below summarise much of what has already been discussed in this chapter, including the importance of community participation, especially at the highest level with unified positions on the issue, a large constituency, coalitions of support (such as from professional bodies), adequate resources to advocate, and access to expert knowledge on the issue, including the environment within which efforts to change policy occur—all supported by political intelligence.

BOX 11.1

ORGANISATIONAL FACTORS THAT BEST INFLUENCE THE POLICY PROCESS

- Credible information on available policy options and their likely impacts.
- Recurrent interactions with policymakers, especially using policy entrepreneurs who are able to shape ideas and make them palatable to governments.
- Large and geographically dispersed membership.
- Group cohesion and unified positions on priority issues.
- Coalitions of support from other agencies and relationships with professionals or bodies.
- Organisational resources, such as staff size and expertise.
- Campaign funds and political intelligence.
- Strategic position in a policy niche and recognition as a coalition leader.
- Timing and opportunism through continuous environment scanning and networking.

Sources: McCubbin et al. 2001; Oliver 2006.

The policy process in Australia is a fluid and complex system that has been described by some scholars as a 'policy cycle' (Althaus, Bridgman & Davis 2017). Advocacy efforts that are mindful of the policy process are generally more convincing and less risky for policymakers, and can galvanise political will by minimising operational challenges and reframe competing rationalities. Having said this, many advocacy proposals may be so straightforward that adoption and implementation by policymakers is rapid (as was the case in some of the earlier examples in this chapter).

Policy analysis will lead advocates and policymakers to define what might be the most appropriate policy instrument or policy lever to implement the policy objective. A simple way to view the main types of policy instruments available to government to influence people's behaviour or health outcomes is shown in the focus box 'Traditional policy levers'. Some policy levers are more suited to achieving a policy outcome than others. Effective advocacy requires careful analysis and negotiation of the policy instruments that could both achieve the objective and avoid unintended consequences.

Policy levers are also evolving to adapt to increasingly networked societies and shift away from government-centred structures, steering advocacy towards new and innovative directions. Examples include crowdfunding of programs and projects, prizes to change behaviour, open access to data, redefined boundaries of authority and delegation to other parties, better use of the private sector, and enhanced opportunities for collaborations between community bodies and the business sector (which might be used to leverage matched funding from government or philanthropic bodies) (Policy Horizons Canada 2012).

BOX 11.2

TRADITIONAL POLICY LEVERS

Regulation and legislation

Direct regulation

Direct regulation is often called 'command and control' intervention, such as when the government enforces behaviour of individuals or organisations. It is often used when the risks to the community of non-compliance are high— for example, age restrictions on cigarette purchases; immunisation requirements for school-entry; mandatory food fortification.

Self-regulation

Self-regulation is when government supports industry to adhere to codes of conduct, with industry responsible for enforcement—for example, accreditation schemes for healthcare professionals; professional limits to the scope of practice.

Taxes, subsidies and incentives

Taxes, subsidies and incentives are economic instruments to influence behaviour and equitable access to healthcare services through price signals or market systems, without direct interference into the lives of individuals or organisations—for example, tobacco taxes; financial incentives to healthcare providers, such as the Practice Incentive Program; Medicare rebates; subsidies for pharmaceuticals and vaccines (PBS); subsidies for health devices, such as the National Diabetes Supply Scheme.

Education

Education strategies can be used to enhance individual and organisational decision making—for example, public health campaigns such as healthy nutrition, anti-smoking, safe sex, vaccination.

Direct expenditure

Direct expenditure for health services and infrastructure can enable the delivery of programs—for example, grants to ACCHSs in return for service provision and quality care; community sport and recreational facilities.

Source: Modified from Couzos & Murray 2008.

Policy advocacy: distilling the issues

In light of policy advocacy, we might consider whether government intervention is really necessary. Do advocates merely want to capture the attention of policymakers or do they want to effect an outcome? The following questions (linked to stages of the policy cycle identified in brackets) provide some guidance when undertaking policy advocacy and assist with identifying competing rationalities (Oliver 2006):

- Is the issue of public health significance? How much of a risk does it pose for the community in terms of health impact and issues of justice and equity? (Identifying the issues)
- Who is held responsible for this issue? Is this issue a government responsibility? Can it be managed as a civil matter or by fostering greater personal responsibility? (Policy analysis)
- Is the policy proposal financially affordable? (Policy analysis)
- Can this proposal be a pilot for a subsequent much larger and comprehensive policy reform? (Policy analysis)
- Is this issue aligned with political priorities? Is there a 'window of opportunity' that makes this policy proposal particularly timely? (Policy analysis)
- Is the issue amenable to an incremental policy change? (Policy analysis)
- In providing benefits to subpopulations, is the imposition on taxpayers diffuse or does it have a traceable impact on them? (Policy analysis)
- Can the policy objective be met by simple forms of leverage, such as through education? Or does it require complex and comprehensive policy levers such as new legislation, taxation and regulation? (Policy instruments)
- Does the issue have the support of stakeholders? (Consultation)
- What impact does the proposed policy objective and instrument have on existing policies and broader financing across the health portfolio? Does the policy reform take away existing benefits? (Coordination)
- Is there a clear mechanism for the implementation of the proposed policy? (Implementation)
- Is there a plan for evaluating the proposed initiative? (Evaluation)

Healthcare professionals should consider whether they are playing a facilitational or representational advocacy role, or whether there is any community engagement at all. They should consider to what degree dialogue is occurring only between healthcare professionals and policymakers in the absence of the target group or community representatives. Moreover, the issue may not warrant engaging in the policy process at all and may merely warrant greater community engagement and public discourse. Finally, the degree to which top-down policy influences operate—especially 'command and control' measures—versus other policy levers that may better support local action needs to be considered. In other words, is government intervention really the best response to the problem (Gibson 2003)?

Public health activism and ethics

There is the perception that the values and preferences of public health advocates (who are usually healthcare professionals) dominate the agenda for public health reform. It has been said that this needs to be challenged and that 'promoting the community's capacity for autonomy instead of taking it away from them is the key' (Mooney 2000). It is often said 'that a public health advocate will identify solutions that focus on political, legislative and social action rather than on individual behaviour change' (Wise 2001, p. 70), even though behaviour change can be achieved with little or no government coercion—for example, the population-wide acceptance and use of sunscreen to prevent skin cancer.

Healthcare professionals can be disillusioned by conservative community views and the distraction of having to consult on an issue. Some public health advocates have referred to experts being besieged by the views and values of the 'ennobled community'. The act of consulting may require advocates to 'slavishly engage with communities about every effort [which would] surely paralyse our modest efforts in a delirium of permission seeking' (Chapman 2001, p. 338). Advocates with this view have argued that citizens need to be protected from the unhealthy manipulations of the marketplace, and that unhealthy behaviours are irrational or a product of the social gradient. In other words, those with the least autonomy over their lives experience the worst health, and therefore only a flawed argument supposes that people can change their circumstances without some coercion. This has been termed the 'cruel illusion' of individual control over health (Davison & Davey-Smith 1995, p. 99). Many public health advocates take a utilitarian view: a policy lever that restricts individual autonomy is justified if it provides the greatest gain for the greatest number. This end justifies the paternalism of health advocates because ordinary peoples' decision making is seen as largely defective. All citizens are subject to restraint in some form or another, but paternalism assumes that others are 'less than moral equals' and that it is therefore necessary to supplant their decisions (Buchanan 2008, p. 16).

A counterargument calls for strategies that expand people's autonomy, as the ability to be autonomous is itself a promoter of human wellbeing. Health professionals dismissive of competing rationalities or the 'authentic voice' of community can be accused of abusing their privileged position in society, and significantly risk damaging public trust and the social contract. The libertarian view encourages less attention focused on ways to limit or control unhealthy behaviours through state regulation, and more attention placed on levers that enhance personal responsibility. Healthcare professionals can best use their skills to empower communities and to recall the libertarian principles of John Stuart Mill (1869) commonly known as the 'harm principle', which affirms the:

> only purpose for which power can be rightfully exercised over any member of a civilized community, against his will, is to prevent harm to others. His own good, either physical or moral, is not sufficient warrant. He cannot rightfully be compelled to do or forbear because it will be better for him to do so ... [or] because in the opinions of others, to do so would be wise, or even right. Over himself, over his own body and mind, the individual is sovereign.

Where can the line be drawn between paternalism and respect for individual liberty in public health advocacy? Some argue this is increasingly difficult to do. Controversy was generated in the United States when public health advocates pointed out the potential of underutilised government tax powers to penalise (or incentivise against) unhealthy behaviour. Proposals included taxing those who don't declare that they are tobacco-free, or giving tax credits (rebates) to those who declare their body mass index is in the normal range or decreasing, or their glycated haemoglobin is controlled if diabetic, or a health check was performed in the previous year (Mello & Cohen 2012). Such taxes, however, are unlikely to influence disease patterns in the community and may worsen health inequalities, given the significant role that social determinants play on tobacco consumption, obesity and diabetes health outcomes.

Public opinions change over time. When experts first suggested that people stop smoking, or that car seat belts become mandatory, these were considered affronts to people's liberty, yet few would argue against the coercive structures now in place. Applying an ethical framework to inform policy advocacy may assist in defining the degree to which well-intentioned public health efforts for behaviour change eliminate or restrict people's choices over how they wish to live their lives that may be inadvertently harmful (Calman 2009). Analysing these issues will complement the policy advocacy process outlined earlier in this chapter.

A widely cited ethical framework by the UK Nuffield Council on Bioethics (2007) recommended that policies to improve public health that eliminate or restrict individual choice (such as removing 'unhealthy' ingredients from food), or coerce through the application of penalties and disincentives (such as loss of payments or increased taxes), need a much higher level of justification than policies that are more respectful of liberties (such as enabling choice, use of incentives, providing information, or doing nothing and monitoring the situation) (Calman 2009). This ethics framework explores beneficence, non-maleficence, protecting autonomy, and ensuring justice and fairness in public health policies by balancing the cost to liberty against the benefits to public health. These principles aim to minimise the selection of unnecessarily intrusive interventions to effect a public health outcome.

But still, the question remains—how much justification is enough justification to warrant that state powers be used to eliminate or restrict personal choice to benefit the collective? Vaccination policy in Australia shifted in 2016 from a voluntary system to a more coercive system under the 'no jab no pay' policy that withdrew welfare support to families who did not comply. This policy was considered controversial by some public health experts, who argued it was unwarranted as existing national vaccination rates were already high, and strategies targeting subpopulations with lower vaccination coverage needed attention, particularly where vaccine access barriers persisted. In addition, there was limited evidence that monetary sanctions were effective; monitoring rates of conscientious objections to vaccination would cease (an important source of data to target interventions); those families facing barriers to vaccine access would be unfairly financially penalised; and the policy risked worsening social inequalities in children of vaccine-refusing families, and public distrust especially from those parents who were initially merely vaccine-hesitant (Beard, Leask & McIntyre 2017). The 'no jab no pay' policy has not yet been evaluated.

Whatever argument is used by public health advocates, the right balance between paternalism and respect for individual liberty is not easily achieved, and only debate and consensus can help resolve this (Jochelson 2005). Such a debate hinges on community voices that are empowered and a growing public trust in the health advocate whose identity is informed by the values of professionalism.

Conclusion

This chapter presented the concept of advocacy in all its usages related to healthcare of individuals and community. Both individual and policy advocacy efforts by healthcare professionals ideally aim to empower individuals and communities to increase control over their health and its determinants, and the degree to which such control can be exercised has been represented as a continuum. As advocacy is central to the role of healthcare professionals, it is vital they are skilled in the various communication patterns associated with this function.

Professionalism means there is a responsibility that the best interests of the patient or the public will always come first when acting as an advocate. But this sometimes means that healthcare professionals will advocate for strategies to coerce the public towards certain behaviour in order to achieve a public good. Such activities can undermine the autonomy an individual has to make their own decision about their own behaviour. Ethical frameworks, debate and consensus can help healthcare professionals walk the fine line between paternalism and respect for individual liberty in public health advocacy. The ideal role of the professional is to facilitate the community's advocacy efforts by supporting democratic participation, utilising the professional's expertise to provide quality information, and empowering people and communities to define problems, pose solutions and express those needs themselves.

SUMMARY POINTS

- Advocates aim to shape people's environments and health behaviours in order to achieve a particular outcome, and do so using a variety of tools and political and policy levers.
- Individual or 'case' advocacy refers to efforts to support and empower individuals. Policy or 'cause' advocacy refers to efforts directed at the population level using a range of policy levers, such as regulation and legislation. Policy advocacy is usually associated with health promotion strategies.
- Communities may have a high or low level of control over what they seek to achieve or how they aim to achieve it. This continuum extends from the highest level where the community exercises control over the issue, to the lowest, which occurs when communities are neither consulted nor informed, or may even be re-educated about or diverted from an issue by authorities or healthcare professionals. This has also been described as 'bottom-up' advocacy (community-led) or 'top-down' advocacy (by experts outside the community).
- Effective advocacy requires community participation, especially at the highest level, with unified positions on the issue, a large constituency, coalitions of support (such as from professional bodies), adequate resources to advocate and access to expert knowledge on the issue, including the environment within which efforts to change policy occur, all supported by political intelligence.
- Advocacy efforts that are mindful of the policy process are generally more convincing and less risky for policymakers, and can galvanise political will by minimising operational challenges.

CRITICAL THINKING QUESTIONS

In 2008, then British Conservative Party leader David Cameron delivered a speech titled 'Fixing our Broken Society' and referred to increasing personal responsibility for our health.

> I think the time has come for me to speak out about something that has been troubling me for a long time. I have not found the words to say it sensitively. And then I realised, that is the whole point ...In order to avoid injury to people's feelings, in order to avoid appearing judgmental, we have failed to say what needs to be said...Instead we prefer moral neutrality, a refusal to make judgments about what is good and bad behaviour, right and wrong behaviour. [...] Refusing to use these words...means a denial of personal responsibility and the concept of a moral choice. We talk about people being 'at risk of obesity'

instead of talking about people who eat too much and take too little exercise. We talk about people being at risk of poverty, or social exclusion: it's as if these things—obesity, alcohol abuse, drug addiction—are purely external events like a plague or bad weather.

Of course, circumstances where you are born, your neighbourhood, your school and the choices your parents make—have a huge impact. But social problems are often the consequence of the choices people make...*in the end, the state cannot do it all. In the end, the best regulation is self-regulation, not state regulation.*

Source: Cameron 2008.

1. If you were to advocate addressing obesity in the community, what type of strategies or policy levers would you be recommending? Why?
2. Consider whether your approach supports self-regulation or state regulation and taxes, as referred to in David Cameron's speech.
3. Discuss how state regulation and taxes may be used to manage obesity. For example, a 'fat tax', such as a consumption tax on foods with a high fat content, or a tax on sugar sweetened beverages, or giving tax credits or rebates for those who declare their body mass index is in the normal range or has decreased.
4. Discuss whether this form of state regulation/taxes is paternalistic or supports people to make individual choices. What are the potential ethical harms in reducing individual choice? Discuss how a policy lever that eliminates or restricts individual choice is able to be sufficiently justified.
5. How could you advocate in a way that empowers the community to take action that enhances the personal responsibility of citizens?

Group activity

Public health advocacy

In your study groups or via your subject discussion site, brainstorm to produce a list of terms that have been used over the years to describe public health advocacy. Think in particular about controversial programs such as those referred to in this chapter. Challenge each other to come up with the most 'colourful' examples, such as nanny-state, moral vanity, new morality, adversarial advocacy, big government, over-regulation, sin taxes, safety-police, etc. Discuss in your groups the effect such terms have had, and continue to have, on the effectiveness of public health advocacy programs.

WEBLINKS

Advocacy and healthcare

Health Consumers Queensland: Consumer and Community Engagement Framework 2017:
www.hcq.org.au/our-work/framework

Nationwide Health and Disability Service (New Zealand):
www.advocacy.org.nz

Policy advocacy

Royal Australian College of Physicians:
www.racp.edu.au/advocacy

WHO: The Ottawa Charter for Health Promotion:
www.who.int/healthpromotion/conferences/previous/ottawa/en

REFERENCES

Althaus, C., Bridgman, P. & Davis, G. (2017). *The Australian Policy Handbook* (6th edn). Sydney: Allen & Unwin.

Arnstein, S.R. (1969). A ladder of citizen participation. *Journal of the American Institute of Planners*, 35(4), 216–24.

Asthma Australia. (n.d). *Asthma Spacers Ordering System*. Brisbane: Asthma Australia. Retrieved from www.asthmaaustralia.org.au/national/about-asthma/manage-your-asthma/spacers.

Australian College of Rural and Remote Medicine. (2013). *Primary Curriculum: Fellowship* (4th edn). Brisbane: ACRRM.

Australian Commission on Safety and Quality in Health Care. (2011). *Patient-centred Care: Improving Quality and Safety through Partnerships with Patients and Consumers.* Sydney: ACSQHC.

Australian Government. (2018a). *Aboriginal and Torres Strait Islander Health Performance Framework (HPF) Report*. Canberra: Australian Institute of Health and Welfare.

Australian Government. (2018b). *Closing the Gap: PBS Co-payment Measure*. Canberra: Department of Health. Retrieved from www.pbs.gov.au/info/publication/factsheets/closing-the-gap-pbs-co-payment-measure.

Australian Government (2019). *My Aged Care: Aboriginal and Torres Strait Islander People*. Canberra: Department of Health. Retrieved from www.myagedcare.gov.au/eligibility-diverse-needs/aboriginal-andor-torres-strait-islander-people.

Australian Institute of Health and Welfare. (2005). *Expenditures on Health for Aboriginal and Torres Strait Islander Peoples 2001–02*. Health and Welfare Expenditure Series no. 23. cat. no. HWE 30. Canberra: AIHW.

Australian Medical Association. (2010). *Advocacy (Section 7). AMA Position Statement—Primary Health Care*. Retrieved from https://ama.com.au/position-statement/primary-health-care-2010.

Balthazard, C. (2010). *What Does It Mean to Be Regulated?* Human Resource Professionals Association, Canada. Retrieved from http://s3.amazonaws.com/pchem/files/208/professional_self_regulation_article.pdf?1397506082.

Beard, F.H., Leask, J. & McIntyre, P.B. (2017). No Jab, No Pay and vaccine refusal in Australia: The jury is out. *Medical Journal of Australia*, 206(9), 381–3.

Biggs, S. & Helms, L.B. (2006). *The Practice of American Public Policymaking*. New York: ME Sharpe Inc.

Buchanan, D.R. (2008). Autonomy, paternalism, and justice: Ethical priorities in public health. *American Journal of Public Health*, 98(1), 15.

Calman, K. (2009). Beyond the 'nanny state': Stewardship and public health. *Public Health*, 123(1):e6–e10. doi:10.1016/j.puhe.2008.10.025.

Cameron. D. (2008). Fixing our broken society. Speech, Glasgow. Retrieved from www.britishpoliticalspeech.org/speech-archive.htm?speech=348.

Carlisle, S. (2000). Health promotion, advocacy and health inequalities: A conceptual framework. *Health Promotion International*, 15(4), 369–76.

Chapman, S. (2000). Public health should not be a popularity contest: A reply to Gavin Mooney. *Australian and New Zealand Journal of Public Health*, 24(3), 337–9.

Chapman, S. (2001). Advocacy in public health: Roles and challenges. *International Journal of Epidemiology*, 30(6), 1226–32.

Commonwealth of Australia. (2005, 2007). *Compilation of the Fourth Community Pharmacy Agreement between the Commonwealth of Australia and the Pharmacy Guild of Australia*. Retrieved from www.guild.org.au/__data/assets/pdf_file/0013/6034/fourth-community-pharmacy-agreement-2005-2010.pdf.

Couzos, S. & Davis, S. (2005). Inequities in Aboriginal health: Access to the Asthma 3+ Visit Plan. *Australian Family Physician*, 34(10), 837–40.

Couzos, S. & Murray, R.B. (2008). *Aboriginal Primary Health Care: An Evidence-Based Approach* (3rd edn). South Melbourne: Oxford University Press.

Couzos, S., Sheedy V. & Thiele D. (2011). Improving Aboriginal peoples' access to medicines: The QUMAX Program. *Medical Journal of Australia*, 195(2), 62–3.

Couzos, S., Thomas, M. & Cass, A. (2008) Chronic kidney disease. In S. Couzos & R. Murray (eds), *Aboriginal Primary Healthcare. An Evidence Based Approach* (3rd edn, Chapter 15). South Melbourne: Oxford University Press.

Cruess, S.R., Johnston, S. & Cruess, R.L. (2002). Professionalism for medicine: Opportunities and obligations. *Medical Journal of Australia*, 177(4), 208–11.

Davison, C. & Davey-Smith, D. (1995). The baby and the bath water: Examining socio-cultural and free-market critiques of health promotion. *The Sociology of Health Promotion*, 91–103.

Dennis, S.M., Zwar, N., Griffiths, R., Roland, M., Hasan, I., Davies, G.P. & Harris, M. (2008). Chronic disease management in primary care: From evidence to policy. *Medical Journal of Australia*, 188(8), S53.

DePaoli, K.M., Seal, J.A., Burgess, J.R. & Taylor, R. (2013). Improved iodine status in Tasmanian schoolchildren after fortification of bread: A recipe for national success. *Medical Journal of Australia*, 198(9), 492–4.

Department of Social Services. (2018). *National Disability Advocacy Program*. Retrieved from www.dss.gov.au/our-responsibilities/disability-and-carers/program-services/for-people-with-disability/national-disability-advocacy-program-ndap.

Federal Register of Legislation. (n.d.). *National Health Act 1953*. Australian Government. Retrieved from www.legislation.gov.au/Series/C1953A00095.

Freddolino, P.P., Moxley, D.P. & Hyduk, C.A. (2004). A differential model of advocacy in social work practice. *Families in Society: The Journal Of Contemporary Social Services*, 85(1), 119–28.

Gibson, B. (2003). Beyond 'two communities'. In V. Lin & B. Gibson (eds), *Evidence-Based Health Policy: Problems and Possibilities*. Melbourne: Oxford University Press.

Gould, T. (2012). Ethics and public health. In M.L. Fleming & E. Parker (eds), *Introduction to Public Health*. Livingstone, NSW: Churchill.

Grant, M., Wronski, I., Murray, R.B. & Couzos, S. (2008). Aboriginal health and history. In S. Couzos & R. Murray (eds), *Aboriginal Primary Healthcare: An Evidence-Based Approach* (3rd edn, Chapter 1). South Melbourne: Oxford University Press.

Gruszin, S., Hetzel, D. & Glover, J. (2012). *Advocacy and Action in Public Health: Lessons from Australia over the 20th Century.* Canberra: Australian National Preventive Health Agency.

Hansen, J. (2014). Scientists call for end of handouts to parents who don't vaccinate children. *The Daily Telegraph*, 6 April. Retrieved from www.dailytelegraph.com.au/news/nsw/scientists-call-for-end-of-handouts-to-parents-who-dont-vaccinate-children/story-fni0cx12-1226874673399?nk=86e37acb6509af79f86f09741b2aeabf.

Health Consumers Queensland. (2017). *Consumer and Community Engagement Framework 2017.* Brisbane: Health Consumers Queensland.

Hulkower, R. (2010). The history of the Hippocratic oath: Outdated, inauthentic, and yet still relevant. *Einstein Journal of Biology and Medicine*, 25, 2009–10.

Hunter, P. (2001). *Aboriginal Health: Achievements Through Partnership.* Keynote presentation. 6th National Rural Health Conference, Canberra, March.

Hunter, P., Mayers, N., Couzos, S., Daniels, J., Murray, R., Bell, K., … Tynan, M. (2004). Aboriginal community controlled health services. *General Practice in Australia, 2004*, 337–56.

Institute of Medicine Committee on Quality of Health Care in America. (2001). *Crossing the Quality Chasm: A New Health System for the 21st Century.* Washington, DC: National Academies Press.

International Council of Nurses. (2008). *Promoting Health: Advocacy Guide for Health Professionals.* Geneva: ICN.

Jochelson, K. (2005). *Nanny or Steward? The Role of Government in Public Health.* London: King's Fund.

Kamien, M. (2006). The repeating history of objections to the fortification of bread and alcohol: From iron filings to folic acid. *Medical Journal of Australia*, 184(12), 638–40.

Khan, T.M. & Chiau, L.M. (2015). Polio vaccination in Pakistan: By force or by volition? *Lancet*, 386(10005), 1733. doi:10.1016/S0140-6736(15)00689-3.

Labonte, R. (1994). Health promotion and empowerment: Reflections on professional practice. *Health Education & Behavior*, 21(2), 253–68.

Leask, J. (2015). Should we do battle with antivaccination activists? *Public Health Research and Practice*, 25(2), e2521515. doi:10.17061/phrp2521515.

Leask, J., Chapman, S., Hawe, P. & Burgess, M. (2006). What maintains parental support for vaccination when challenged by anti-vaccination messages? A qualitative study. *Vaccine*, 24(49), 7238–45.

Leask, J., Quinn, H.E., Macartney, K., Trent, M., Massey, P., Carr, C. & Turahui, J. (2008). Immunisation attitudes, knowledge and practices of health professionals in regional NSW. *Australian and New Zealand Journal of Public Health*, 32(3), 224–9. doi:10.1111/j.1753-6405.2008.00220.x.

Lin, V. (2003). Competing rationalities: Evidence-based health policy? In V. Lin & B. Gibson (eds), *Evidence-Based Health Policy: Problems and Possibilities.* Melbourne: Oxford University Press.

Loff, B. & Cordner, S. (1998). Aboriginal people trade land claim for dialysis. *The Lancet*, 352(9138), 1451.

Loue, S. (2006). Community health advocacy. *Journal of Epidemiology and Community Health*, 60(6), 458–63.

Mayers, N. & Couzos, S. (2004). Towards health equity through an adult health check for Aboriginal and Torres Strait Islander people. *Medical Journal of Australia*, 181(10), 531–2.

McCubbin, M., Labonte, R. & Dallaire, B. (2001). *Advocacy for Healthy Public Policy as a Health Promotion Technology*. Toronto: Centre for Health Promotion.

McMillan, R. & Hernandez, D. (2019). Pinterest takes on anti-vaxxers by blocking vaccine-related searches. *The Australian*, 22 February. Retrieved from www.theaustralian.com.au/business/wall-street-journal/pinterest-takes-on-antivaxxers-by-blocking-vaccinerelated-searches/newsstory/105620eeb51b34bf21bbcf90562028dd.

Mead, N. & Bower, P. (2000). Patient-centredness: A conceptual framework and review of the empirical literature. *Social Science and Medicine*, 51, 1087–110.

Medew, J. (2014). Peter Singer questions ethics of suspending Dr Philip Nitschke. *The Age*, 17 August. Retrieved from www.theage.com.au/victoria/peter-singer-questions-ethics-of-suspending-dr-philip-nitschke-20140817-1052jw.html#ixzz3DRaVUcFh.

Medical Professionalism Project. (2002). Medical professionalism in the new millennium: A physicians' charter. *Medical Journal of Australia*, 177(5), 263–5.

Mello, M.M. & Cohen, I.G. (2012). The taxing power and the public's health. *New England Journal of Medicine*, 367(19), 1777–9.

Merikas, G. (1992). Hippocrates: Still a contemporary. *Humane Medicine*, 8(3), 212–18.

Mill, J.S. (1869). *On Liberty* (4th edn). London: Longman, Roberts, & Green Co. Retrieved from www.econlib.org/library/Mill/mlLbty.html.

Mooney, G. (2000). The need to build community autonomy in public health. *Australian and New Zealand Journal of Public Health*, 24(2), 111.

National Aboriginal Community Controlled Health Organisation. (2018). *Aboriginal Community Controlled Health Services Are More than Just Another Health Service—They Put Aboriginal Health in Aboriginal Hands*. Canberra: NACCHO. Retrieved from www.naccho.org.au.

New Zealand Government. (2016). *Models of Patient Advocacy: Evidence Brief*. NZ Government, Health Research Board. Retrieved from https://health.gov.ie/wp-content/uploads/2016/12/Final-Version-Patient-Advocacy-Services.pdf.

Nuffield Council on Bioethics. (2007). *Public Health: Ethical Issues*. London: Nuffield Council on Bioethics. Retrieved from http://nuffieldbioethics.org/project/public-health.

Oliver, T.R. (2006). The politics of public health policy. *Annual Review of Public Health*, 27, 195–233.

Palmer, G.R. & Short, S.D. (2010). *Health Care and Public Policy: An Australian Analysis* (4th edn). South Yarra: Palgrave Macmillan.

Policy Horizons Canada. (2012). *Driving Policy on a Shifting Terrain. Understanding the Changing Policy Environment Amid 21st Century Complexity*. Retrieved from http://publications.gc.ca/site/eng/432053/publication.html.

Porter, G., Blashki, G. & Grills, N. (2014). General practice and public health: Who is my patient? *Australian Family Physician*, 43(7), 483–6.

Public Health Advocacy Institute of Western Australia. (2013) *Advocacy in Action: A Toolkit for Public Health Professionals* (3rd edn). Perth: Curtin University.

Robertson, A. & Minkler, M. (1994). New health promotion movement: A critical examination. *Health Education & Behavior*, 21(3), 295–312.

Royal Australian College of General Practice. (n.d). *Becoming a GP in Australia*. Retrieved from www.racgp.org.au/becomingagp/what-is-a-gp/what-is-general-practice.

Royal Australian College of General Practice. (2016). *Population and Public Health: The RACGP Curriculum for Australian General Practice*. Melbourne: RACGP.

Royal Australasian College of Physicians. (2014). *Advanced Training Curriculum—Australasian Faculty of Public Health Medicine*. Sydney: RACP.

Schwartz, L. (2002). Is there an advocate in the house? The role of healthcare professionals in patient advocacy. *Journal of Medical Ethics*, 28(1), 37–40.

Seal, J.A., Doyle, Z., Burgess, J.R., Taylor, R. & Cameron, A.R. (2007). Iodine status of Tasmanians following voluntary fortification of bread with iodine. *Medical Journal of Australia*, 186(2), 69.

Sinha, M.S. (2011). Rousseau at the roundtable—The social contract and the physician's responsibility to society. *Virtual Mentor*, 13(10), 703.

Taylor, K. (2009). Paternalism, participation and partnership—The evolution of patient centeredness in the consultation. *Patient Education and Counseling*, 74(2), 150–5.

Tsiompanou, E. & Marketos, S.G. (2013). Hippocrates: Timeless still. *Journal of the Royal Society of Medicine*, 106(7), 288–92.

Urbis Pty Ltd. (2011). *Evaluation of the Quality Use of Medicines Maximised for Aboriginal And Torres Strait Islander Peoples (QUMAX) Program*. Prepared for the Australian Government Department of Health and Ageing. Sydney: Urbis.

Wise, M. (2001). The role of advocacy in promoting health. *Promotion & Education*, 8(2), 69–74.

World Health Organization. (1978). *Alma Ata Declaration on Primary Health Care*. Geneva: WHO. Retrieved from www.who.int/social_determinants/tools/multimedia/alma_ata/en.

World Health Organization. (1986). *The Ottawa Charter for Health Promotion*. Geneva: WHO. Retrieved from www.who.int/healthpromotion/conferences/previous/ottawa/en.

World Health Organization. (1998). *Health Promotion Glossary*. Division of Health Promotion, Education and Communications (HPR), Health Education and Health Promotion Unit (HEP). Geneva: WHO. WHO/HPR/HEP/98.1

World Health Organization. (2005). *The Bangkok Charter for Health Promotion in a Globalized World*. Geneva: WHO. Retrieved from www.who.int/healthpromotion/conferences/6gchp/bangkok_charter/en.

Worsley R. (2014). A duty of care or a duty to care? *6 Minutes*, 1 August. Retrieved from www.6minutes.com.au/blogs/6minutes-insight/a-duty-of-care-or-a-duty-to-care.

CHAPTER 12
MANAGING CONFLICT

MICHELLE FRANCIS AND LEE STEWART

CHAPTER FOCUS

After reading this chapter and completing the activities, you will be able to:

- discuss conflict as an inevitable component of human interaction
- recognise helpful and unhelpful responses to conflict
- identify sources and types of conflict
- apply a variety of approaches to managing conflict in personal and professional situations
- identify responses to conflict in personal and professional settings.

KEY TERMS

Conflict
Conflict management
Cooperation
Mediation
Negotiation

Conflict
An inevitable aspect of human interaction when two or more individuals or groups pursue mutually incompatible goals; if managed well, conflict can be beneficial.

Introduction

Conflict has been defined as:

> ...a form of relating or interacting where we find ourselves (either as individuals or groups) under some sort of perceived threat to our personal or collective goals. These goals are usually to do with our interpersonal wants. These perceived threats may be either real or imagined. (Vallence & McWilliam 1987, cited in Condliffe 2012, p. 3)

Conflict among people is as inevitable as the sun rising every day. Because we have needs, interests and values that differ, human beings are given to fighting over those differences. For healthcare professionals, the phenomenon of workplace conflict can be particularly fraught. Not only can poorly managed conflict cause distress for nurses, midwives, doctors, physiotherapists and others, it can also result in poorer outcomes for clients of the healthcare service. This chapter examines the concept of conflict and explores strategies for its effective management.

Understanding conflict

There are various types of conflict that can occur within healthcare settings, and these are described below.

- *Circumstantial conflicts:* Circumstances can create conflict. Where there is not enough information, or differing information, conflict can arise. For example, a staff member at a hospital is parking, and their car is hit by another car. Both drivers have provided the same account of the accident and how it happened, yet disagree about who is at fault. The circumstance and the different interpretation of liability have been the source of the conflict. By clarifying the facts of legal responsibility and road rules, the conflict can be resolved (Proksch 2016).
- *Conflicts of interest:* Conflicts of interest arise not from facts but from differing interests (Proksch 2016)—for example, in a respiratory unit where a nurse wants a patient to have a shower before a respiratory therapy session and a busy physiotherapist wants to attend to the patient so she can move on to the next patient. The nurse has put the patient's interests first and the physiotherapist has put their workload interests first. In this type of conflict, the central cause is competing interests.
- *Relationship conflicts:* The heart of relationship conflicts is emotional. They result from feelings such as fear and frustration (Proksch 2016). For example, a psychologist arrives at a case conference five minutes early to make sure they are on time as punctuality is important to them. They notice that the community nurse is constantly late to case conferences—for the community nurse, punctuality is less important. The psychologist may see the lack of punctuality as passive aggressive behaviour or contempt towards them. This may result in feelings of frustration and disappointment.
- *Value conflicts:* Value conflicts arise when there is not a shared understanding around values (Proksch 2016). In the healthcare setting, value conflicts can arise between differing values of disciplines—for example, in a case where a patient's mental health may be impacted by a physical procedure. Medical staff may prioritise the physical health of the person, whereas mental health staff may prioritise their mental health. For example, Jean needs to have a colonoscopy, without which medical staff will not be able to diagnose what is causing her

symptoms and how to treat them. Jean has also recently lost her job and left her husband, she is very anxious about her circumstances and is overwhelmed at the thought of having a colonoscopy. Conflict may arise between these healthcare professionals about what is most important in Jean's care at that moment. The medical staff may prioritise the colonoscopy, while the mental health nurse may see attending to Jean's anxiety and unemployment as more immediately important.

- *Structural conflicts:* Structural conflicts, as the name suggests, are not differences between people but arise from differences in structures (Proksch 2016)—for example, lawyers in a trial have deliberate structural conflict—one is representing one party and the other is representing another party (Proksch 2016). In the healthcare system structural conflict that may arise around patient movement. For example, a busy psychiatric ward has goals to discharge patients to clear beds for incoming patients and a busy community mental healthcare clinic may be at capacity and unable to take more patients. The conflict that arises is because of structural, not personal, reasons.
- *Inner conflict:* Inner conflicts are not about interaction, but are about the internal world of a person. They arise when goals, values and requirements are not aligned (Proksch 2016)—for example, a busy social worker values her work with vulnerable patients, yet it is also her daughter's birthday today and she values being a mother. Her work involves a lot of overtime, and she knows it's best for her patient if she stays back a little tonight, but it's also best for her daughter and family if she gets home on time to be part of the birthday celebrations. Here, her professional and personal goals, values and requirements come into conflict.

Reflect and apply

Consider the type of conflict that is occurring in each of the following scenarios:

- A new facility has been built and the multipurpose room has not yet been used. Nurses want it for group activities, the social workers want it for counselling, and the physiotherapists want it for using the exercise balls.
- Your colleague is engaging in a potentially unsafe work practice. You value your friendship with her yet you also value maintaining professional standards.
- It seems that Dave from IT takes forever to respond to your repeated telephone calls. You are feeling frustrated and perceive Dave to be disinterested in helping you resolve your IT issue so you can return to your clinical work.

The inevitability of conflict

It is vital to recognise that conflict is a basic social process; some conflict will always be present within healthcare organisations, whether they are hospitals, community healthcare services or clinics. The key is to understand that if conflict is managed well, performance tends to improve. Poorly managed conflict usually results in both personal and organisational damage (Katz & Flynn 2013). '**Conflict management**' is a more useful term, than 'conflict resolution'. This is 'for the simple reason that some conflicts cannot be resolved, but most conflicts can be managed' (Condliffe 2012, p. 2).

Conflict management Minimising the negative aspects of conflict while increasing the positive aspects.

Unhelpful responses to conflict

Unhelpful responses to conflict arise from a poor understanding of conflict management and the positive opportunities conflicts present. They can also be automatic responses when we don't take a step back and try to understand the source of the conflict, our own thoughts and feelings about the conflict, and possible solutions to conflict. Some common unhelpful responses to conflict are:

- *Opposition and rejection:* This response can be conscious or unconscious. A person facing conflict may see another's point of view as threatening and feel fearful about change or a perceived lack of power (Proksch 2016). A person responding in this way sees the other as a threat and seeks to hinder them by not passing on information and doing the bare minimum, thus making the other person's job difficult. For example, a new nurse unit manager starts on the medical ward and has ideas about changes that could be made to the documentation system. Some of the staff have had negative experiences with new managers in the past, largely because of lack of consultation about change. They are immediately opposed to any changes and the new manager. They avoid meetings that she calls and do not participate in consultation processes.
- *Withdrawal and indifference:* Poorly managed and understood conflict can result in a loss of motivation and an emotional withdrawal from work. People in this situation do not see the importance of being honest about emotions and issues and remain silent about them (Proksch 2016). For example, a senior clinician regularly asks staff how they are feeling and if they have the resources to do their job. One of the occupational therapists is angry, feels let down and does not have enough time to complete her case notes; however, she does not believe anything will ever change so she always responds that she is 'fine'.
- *Hostility, irritability and aggression:* Issues that have not been dealt with in the past may have resulted in feelings of anger that have been pushed to the side, but which sometimes surface unexpectedly and abruptly (Proksch 2016). In the occupational therapist example, above, after several weeks of her withdrawal behaviour and the feelings of anger building, she loudly verbalises her displeasure in an unprofessional manner.
- *Intrigue and rumours:* These have a purpose to undermine the perceived threat from another person and win people over to a particular point of view. The result is often division and suspicion among working teams (Proksch 2016).

continuing the example of people in a team rejecting a new nursing unit manager, staff members start a rumour that she has poor motives for the team. The team is divided between those in support and those not in support of the new unit manager.

- *Formality and conformity:* Excessive conformity and submission to the leader of a group can result in emotions, ideas and innovations that are not communicated, and valuable opportunities and feedback are missed, as in the example described above where the occupational therapist has become withdrawn and indifferent (Proksch 2016).
- *Physical symptoms:* Poorly managed conflict can have serious effects not just on patient care and organisational functioning, but can have a huge impact on healthcare professionals, leading to a myriad of physical symptoms such as headaches, stomach problems and lack of sleep. The organisational result is a high absenteeism and staff turnover (Proksch 2016).

There is a significant body of literature indicating that if people can understand how and why they habitually respond to certain situations, they can develop more effective solutions to conflict management, instead of trying to solve the same old problems using responses that do not work. The notion here is that we do not have to persist with only those habitual behaviours. Instead, we can discover a broader repertoire of skills and styles. People in conflict will usually choose their first 'solution' (e.g. 'I'll fight for my weekend off' or 'Management are always unhelpful', 'Things will never get better', 'There's no point speaking up'), rather than thinking strategically about the long-term outcomes of such conflict in terms of damaged relationships.

Effective approaches to conflict

The Conflict Resolution Network in Australia (see the Weblinks at the end of the chapter) has been educating people for decades about how to manage conflict to achieve good outcomes. They describe several conflict resolution skills that can be readily applied by healthcare professionals. Understanding conflict and having strategies to manage it can result in a better perception of conflict situations, reducing people's perception of threat when confronted with conflict and meaning there is less likelihood of engaging in unhelpful responses.

Emotional intelligence and conflict management

The Conflict Resolution Network identifies 'empathy', 'appropriate assertiveness' and 'managing emotions' as essential skills for effective conflict resolution (Conflict Resolution Network 2019). These can be readily linked to Salovey and Mayer's seminal work (1990) around emotional intelligence, which continues to be refined (Salovey, Mayer & Caruso 2008). Other contemporary writers have further developed the impact of emotional intelligence within organisational culture (e.g. see Cherniss 2010; O'Boyle et al. 2011; Ybarra, Kross & Sanchez-Burks 2014). While emotional intelligence is discussed in more detail in Chapter 3, the following activity deals will emotional intelligence in respect of conflict.

CASE ACTIVITY 12.1

Emotional intelligence and conflict

Emotional intelligence describes traits such as comprehending one's own mental models, having empathy for other people's outlooks and feelings, and being able to control one's emotions in ways that enhance the community. The physiological explanation underpinning emotional intelligence emanates from the work of neuroscientists such as Joseph LeDoux, who describes the role of the brain's hippocampus in recognising fact and the amygdala in storing emotional responses to those facts. The brain is therefore described as having essentially two memory systems—one storing ordinary facts and one storing emotionally charged ones. The significance of the discoveries by LeDoux and his colleagues is that they explain how the brain can be short-circuited, allowing emotions to dictate behaviour rather than intelligence (Johnson et al. 2009).

What this means is that our feelings, emotions and beliefs are interpreted by our brain and can influence how we behave or make decisions. This can be of benefit in critical situations, such as when feeling afraid, they may help us to run away quickly from a life-threatening situation; but fear can also make us unnecessarily uncertain and avoidant in other situations. For example, John and Sandy are both asked to do a presentation on their research project. John is feeling happy and motivated about it and gets to work straight away. Sandy on the other hand is feeling fearful; she believes she will look stupid and embarrass herself in front of everyone, even though her content is really impressive. She puts off preparing for it.

Another example involves anger. Jess is feeling angry as a result of a tough morning before work. When Leah asks her if she has had a chance to respond to an email that she to her, Jess becomes irritable with Leah, even though the question is reasonable. Sometimes when we feel angry, we may be impatient and make impulsive decisions. Excitement may make us rush decisions without thinking of their consequences.

1. Have you ever delayed making a decision or taking action because you felt fearful? What was the outcome?
2. Have you ever made an impulsive decision as the result of your emotions at the time? What were the consequences?

The case activity show how emotions play a large part in our decision making, yet they may not always lead good decisions. There is a risk that without awareness of our emotions, we may have unconscious biases, and display poor judgment or impulsivity. The good news is with self-awareness and effective communication, we have huge potential to manage ourselves and conflict in the workplace. The rest of the chapter is concerned with constructive approaches to managing conflict.

Win-win approach

The first of these constructive approaches to conflict, the 'win-win approach', means moving away from seeing conflict as being about taking fixed positions and fighting with each other, and instead learning to apply a joint problem-solving approach to a situation. A great way to understand 'win-win' is to compare this with the commonplace 'I win, you lose' approach, which many people learn from the time they are children.

From the Harvard Negotiation project in the United States (see the Weblinks), the seminal text by Fisher, Ury and Patton (1997) provides a major insight into moving away from a 'win/lose' approach by allowing people to see themselves as working side by side, tackling problems rather than each other. The authors outline two principles that can be used in conflict management:

1. Separating the people from the problem.
2. Focusing on interests.

Using Fisher, Ury and Patton's principles, we will analyse conflict situations.

Separating the people from the problem

The first principle can be seen often within work environments. For example, Bill keeps borrowing John's stapler and it drives John mad! He thinks that Bill is irritating and disrespectful. He feels annoyed. By separating Bill from the issue, John has a better chance of managing the conflict. Putting John's feelings aside and analysing the conflict, we can see that this situation is both a structural and circumstantial, which is easily rectified by supplying a stapler to Bill.

Focusing on interests

The second principle involves moving away from a rigid opinion about an issue by putting that opinion or 'position' to one side for a time, and focusing on interests rather than on positions. When we focus on our opinion or position, we tend to be very stubborn about our view of the world and either use our 'rights' (e.g. 'I deserve the weekend off because I've worked three weekends in a row and you haven't') or our 'power' (e.g. 'I've been a nurse here longer than you so I get the weekend off'). When people focus on interests, they start to ask good questions, such as: 'What is the reason you need this weekend off?' or 'What are the consequences for you if you have to work this weekend?' Focusing on interests and asking good questions invariably leads to better outcomes and greater satisfaction for everyone rather than focusing on rights or power, which is more about 'win/lose'. Interests are the things we care about, things we are frightened of or things we desire.

BOX 12.1

FOCUSING ON INTERESTS

Where interests cannot be reconciled, the use of Fisher, Ury and Patton's (1997) principle is vital: Insist on using objective criteria. In this situation, you can ask questions such as 'What is fair here?', 'What would an independent outsider think was fair here?' or 'What are the rules applied to rosters and numbers of weekends off in this unit or organisation?'

Alternative dispute resolution

Negotiation

So far the discussion about conflict has generally referred to personal qualities and behaviours that can lead to successful conflict management. Importantly, during the past decades, the alternative dispute resolution (ADR) movement has emerged. Significantly, the ADR movement came about because of the high cost and lengthy delays in resolving serious conflicts via litigation and court systems. The most common ADR method is **negotiation**. Negotiation is a process for resolving conflict between two or more parties whereby both (or all) have conversations with a view to achieving an agreement. With negotiation, when conflict occurs, people will talk through the issues and arrive at some sort of resolution that everyone thinks is reasonable. This is particularly so in healthcare agencies, where healthcare professionals are most concerned about the outcomes for their clients and patients. There are no formal rules governing how negotiations are to be conducted, although there are culturally accepted styles and approaches for doing so. A healthcare organisation is essentially a massive negotiating table. With everything healthcare professionals do at work, they are negotiating. Representatives of healthcare agencies negotiate with governments about funding and policy decisions. Executive members of the agency or health area negotiate about targets, money and other resources. All healthcare professionals negotiate with their supervisors, their colleagues, their subordinates and their clients and patients—all day, every day.

Negotiation
The process of communication and bargaining between people seeking to arrive at a mutually acceptable outcome on issues of shared concern.

Any negotiation has three components that are equally important in any interaction. These are:

1. the substance or issue: what people are negotiating about
2. the procedure: how people negotiate
3. the psychology or relationship: how people feel treated in the negotiation, and how their future relationship will be after the negotiation is concluded.

Everyone needs to pay equal attention to all three components in any interaction or negotiation. Unfortunately, people often focus only on the 'substance'—the thing they are negotiating about—and forget how important the future relationship is.

As Deresky and Christopher (2008) point out, negotiation can be difficult to achieve, even when it occurs among people from the same background. Negotiating when people are from different cultural backgrounds brings with it another set of challenges. Differences in 'perception, attitudes, social organisation, thought patterns, roles, language, non-verbal language and time' (p. 150) must be considered when communicating with people from different cultures.

CASE ACTIVITY 12.2

Negotiating with people from different backgrounds

Xavier was scheduled to spend two weeks of clinical placement in a small rural hospital. On his first morning at work he was instructed to undertake a physical assessment on a young man who had recently emigrated from Iran. He went to the young man's bedside and said: 'Hi, mate, I'll get you to take your shirt off so I can listen to your heart sounds.' The young man looked distressed and said, 'No, I will not do that.' Xavier became frustrated, replying, 'Come on, mate, I'm really busy, can you just do it please.' The young man shook his head and folded his arms. Xavier called on his clinical facilitator to assist him, and mediate between the young man and himself. This did not go well, and the young man continued to refuse to cooperate.

1. What might you have done in this situation?
2. In what way does Xavier's response to the young man create conflict?

Cooperation

In Case activity 12.2, there may have been multiple reasons for the client's refusal, but what Xavier did not understand as the communication progressed is that the notion of 'compromising' is not generally part of Iranian cultural norms (Deresky & Christopher 2008). By capitulating, the young man may have felt he was surrendering his principles. Bringing the clinical facilitator into the communication may also have been problematic, as 'mediators' can be seen as meddlers in Iranian culture (Deresky & Christopher 2008). Xavier will need to learn that there are not only personal and emotional factors influencing conflict management, but also social, cultural and environmental considerations to take into account. While it is important to avoid stereotyping people based on their culture, the healthcare professional should also develop an understanding of general patterns of belief and behaviour held by people from cultures that differ from their own.

This case is also an example of feelings influencing behaviours and decisions. Xavier was in a rush and became frustrated at the young man's refusal. Realising that the situation was not going well, he called in his clinical facilitator, which was not well received. A cue that Xavier missed was that the young man looked distressed by the request to take his shirt off. If Xavier had been more self-aware regarding his own stress (because of his busy day), he may have been able to acknowledge the distress and taken a more courteous approach. He could have acknowledged the young man's discomfort and sought to understand it, explained the physical examination and its importance, and worked with the young man on a way to complete the physical examination that was comfortable for him.

However, all is not lost for Xavier and the young man. As healthcare professionals sometimes we miss the mark or we do not realise important information until we look back on the situation. Xavier felt terrible when he reflected on the situation and realised his mistake. He returned to the young man the next day and apologised for his shortness and not noticing his discomfort. Xavier explained the importance of the physical examination and asked the young man if he would like to participate. The young man agreed that it was important and they negotiated he would keep his singlet on for the next examination. Even though there was initial conflict and misunderstanding, Xavier and the young man were able to return to the conflict and resolve it through **cooperation**.

Cooperation
The process of working together to achieve an outcome satisfactory to all parties.

Mediation

Mediation has been a popular form of dispute resolution processes for the past four decades. It essentially involves a way of thinking about the world, a philosophy, and is also a process to follow that optimises the chance of a conflict being resolved. Mediation can be defined as 'a form of intervening in conflicts where a neutral independent expert guides the communication and negotiations between parties in order to reach agreements about desired behaviours and a mutually beneficial optimal solution, both based on parties' actual interests' (Brenninkmeijer 2009, in Iles, Ellemers & Harinck 2014, p. 332).

Mediation
A method of negotiation where a mutually acceptable third party helps people find a solution to a conflict that they cannot find by themselves.

Formal mediation

In a formal setting, mediation processes generally follow a similar pattern and usually include the following.

- A mediator instruction, where the process is explained and ground rules for reasonable behaviour are outlined.
- Statement taking, where each person tells their story about the conflict, without interruption from the other person.
- Agenda setting is established for negotiation; the agenda is derived from the list of issues and the participants' stories.
- Participants then explore each of the issues in turn, talking about what has happened in the past and the problems they have experienced with each other. During this stage, the mediator uses good communication skills to help participants keep talking with each other. Participants then negotiate about the issues, moving on from what has happened previously and starting to talk about what might happen in the future about each issue on the agenda. The mediator's

role is to remain neutral, while displaying empathy for the participants and helping them continue with their discussion.

- Often, the mediator will meet with each participant privately to clarify 'how things are going' for each individual.
- Following the private meetings, participants move on to discussing and establishing some form of agreement for what will happen in the future. Sometimes this agreement is written down for the participants to take away with them, but not always (Condliffe 2012).

Mediation is not always such a formal process. Often in a healthcare environment, practitioners are mediating without recognising that this is happening—that someone is taking on the role of a 'neutral third party' to help resolve a conflict between two or more people, whether they be other healthcare professionals or patients. Iles et al. (2014, p. 331) refer to the 'variety of tactics that may be employed when intervening in different types of conflicts'.

Reflect and apply

- What are some of your automatic responses to conflict in social and professional settings? Do they differ?
- Can you identify any times where you have used unhelpful responses to conflict?
- Can you identify times when you have used constructive responses to conflict?
- Have you ever been in a conflict situation where you have been a neutral third party?
  - What was the source/type of the conflict?
  - What were the unhelpful responses you witnessed?
  - What were the constructive responses you witnessed?
  - What did you navigate being a neutral party?
  - Did you take sides?
  - Did you agree with one party more than the other?
  - What was the outcome?

As mentioned earlier in the chapter, we use the term conflict management rather than conflict resolution because some conflicts cannot be resolved, despite using conflict management skills. This can be for a variety of reasons, both structural and personal. What is important to know is where to get help if you are affected by unresolved conflict. In the workplace there are mechanisms for support. Informal mechanisms can include speaking with a trusted colleague for perspective and advice or with your supervisor or line manager. Formal mechanisms can include the complaints procedure, formal mediation and accessing the organisation's employee assistance program (EAP), which is a confidential service made available to all employees. EAP offers free confidential counselling with trained professionals to provide support to employees for personal and professional concerns.

CASE STUDY 12.3

Formal processes in managing conflict

Ben has noticed that Stephanie talks to everyone in the office except him. She makes negative comments about his work in front of his peers while making positive comments about everyone else. Ben uses two informal processes to address this. He first talks to a trusted colleague and explains he feels uncomfortable about Stephanie's behaviour and gets some advice on how to raise the issue with her. The second informal process Ben uses is having a conversation with Stephanie. He lets her know he feels uncomfortable about her negative comments and that she does not speak to him. Unfortunately, Ben's efforts to resolve this issue are not effective because Stephanie is dismissive of his concerns and the conversation results in her increasing her negative comments and gossiping about Ben in the office.

Ben starts to feel more and more uncomfortable at work. He speaks with his supervisor, who validates his concerns and encourages him to make a formal complaint. Ben is also encouraged to access the EAP for external support. Ben sees a counsellor through the EAP, who also validates his concerns, helps him clarify the issues, and supports Ben to make the formal complaint. His supervisor investigates the complaint and finds that Stephanie's behaviour is inappropriate, and she was unreasonable when Ben tried to raise his concerns with her.

Stephanie is formally disciplined and asked to apologise to Ben. She ceases excluding Ben and making negative comments. She is provided with extra supervision to develop her awareness of how her behaviour impacts on others.

This is an example of using formal processes to address conflict.

1. Have you ever used a formal complaint mechanism to resolve a conflict?
2. Was your outcome as positive as the one in the case study?
3. How did the outcome affect the ongoing working relationship you had with the other person?

Yet another avenue for hearing issues of conflict is the professional agency. Most healthcare professionals have an affiliated organisation that offers advice, mentorship and, in some cases, professional legal assistance for issues in the workplace.

The Australian Medical Association (AMA) is the peak body representing doctors and medical students (see https://ama.com.au). Likewise, the Australian Nursing and Midwifery Federation is the union for registered nurses, enrolled nurses, midwives and assistants in nursing in each state and territory (see http://anmf.org.au). The Australian Physiotherapy Association is a not-for-profit organisation that supports professional members. It was initially set up in 1906 (as the Australasian Massage Association) to protect the general public from sham or untrained practitioners.

These organisations are available to registered healthcare professionals and many have a student enrolment so that qualified and would-be practitioners can avail themselves of assistance.

Conclusion

This chapter has shown how valuable the skills of conflict management are, both personally and professionally. In this chapter, we defined conflict and identified the inevitability of conflict in human interaction. Rather than identifying conflict as a 'bad' thing, the idea of well-managed conflict as a constructive process was highlighted. The skills of conflict management were touched upon, as were the processes for moving towards a 'win-win' approach to conflict management. The role of emotional intelligence and reflection was touched upon to highlight the importance of moving away from habitual behaviours. Developing emotional intelligence to enable adjusting behaviours for good outcomes was discussed, as was the vital role of the ADR movement. Skills of negotiation and mediation were explored and applied to clinical situations. This knowledge, and the accompanying skill set, can enable healthcare professionals to be technically competent and learn the communication skills needed to optimally care for clients and contribute as valued members of the healthcare team.

SUMMARY POINTS

- Conflict is a basic social process in life.
- Conflict can occur when there is disagreement about information or the reasons for decisions; differences in ideas or principles; different understandings of the same words; or misunderstanding other people's principles, ideas or expectations.
- Organisational conflict has common elements:
  - there are recognised opposing interests
  - each side believes that the other is willing to act against them
  - the belief can be justified by actions
  - conflict is a process learnt from past interactions of the two parties.
- Unhelpful responses to conflict can occur when people fail to understand the source of the conflict, their own thoughts and feelings and possible solutions to conflict.
- Effective responses to conflict include alternative dispute resolution mechanisms such as negotiation, cooperation and mediation, and cooperation.

CRITICAL THINKING QUESTIONS

1. Conflict occurs every day. Examine your own daily life—how many conflicts have you experienced today and were they resolved? Are you harbouring negative feelings about any unresolved conflict, and how might you change this?
2. Often we witness organisational conflict. Conflict arises between two of your closest work colleagues. What strategies do you use to remain neutral in such situations? Are they effective?

3. The win-win negotiation is said to be the panacea of negotiation. However, can a win-lose or a lose-lose outcome be successful? Examine these possibilities for your workplace.

Group activity

Causes of conflict

In your study groups or via your subject discussion site, brainstorm to produce a list of the most common causes of conflict. Identify which of these causes are preventable. What strategies can you implement in your own life to manage preventable causes of conflict?

WEBLINKS

Conflict resolution

Australian Disputes Centre:
www.disputescentre.com.au/knowledge-resources

Conflict Management (Education and Training, Victorian Government):
www.education.vic.gov.au/hrweb/safetyhw/Pages/conflictmgt.aspx

Conflict Resolution Network:
www.crnhq.org

Harvard Negotiation Project:
www.pon.harvard.edu/category/projects/harvard-negotiation-project

Online DIY Managing Conflict Workshop:
https://crana.org.au/education/courses/programs/online-diy-managing-conflict-workshop

Workplace conflict

Better Health Channel: Workplace conflict (Victorian Government):
www.betterhealth.vic.gov.au/health/healthyliving/workplace-conflict

REFERENCES

Cherniss, C. (2010). Emotional intelligence: Toward clarification of a concept. *Industrial and Organizational Psychology*, 3(2), 110–26.

Condliffe, P. (2012). *Conflict Management: A Practical Guide* (4th edn). Chatswood: LexisNexis Butterworths.

Conflict Resolution Network. (2019). 12 skills summary. Retrieved from www.crnhq.org/12-skill-summary.

Deresky, H. & Christopher, E. (2008). *International Management: Managing Across Borders and Cultures*. Frenchs Forest: Pearson Education Australia.

Fisher, R., Ury, W. & Patton, B. (1997). *Getting to Yes: Negotiating an Agreement Without Giving In* (2nd edn). London: Arrow Books Limited.

Iles, R., Ellemers, N. & Harinck, F. (2014). Mediating value conflicts. *Conflict Resolution Quarterly*, 31(3), 331–53.

Johnson, L.R., LeDoux, J.E. & Doyere, V. (2009). Hebbian reverberations in emotional memory micro circuits. *Frontiers in Neuroscience*, 3(2), 198–205.

Katz, N.H. & Flynn, L.T. (2013). Understanding conflict management systems and strategies in the workplace: A pilot study. *Conflict Resolution Quarterly*, 30(4), 393–409.

O'Boyle, E.H. Jr, Humphrey, R.H., Pollak, J.M., Hawver, T.H. & Story, P.A. (2011). The relation between emotional intelligence and job performance: A meta-analysis. *Journal of Organizational Behavior*, 32, 788–818.

Proksch, S. (2016). *Conflict Management*. Vienna: Springer.

Salovey, P. & Mayer, J.D. (1990). Emotional intelligence. *Imagination, Cognition and Personality*, 9, 185–211.

Salovey, P., Mayer, J.D. & Caruso, D.R. (2008). Emotional intelligence: New ability or eclectic traits? *American Psychologist*, 63(6), 503–17.

Ybarra, O., Kross, E. & Sanchez-Burks, J. (2014). The 'big idea' that is yet to be: Toward a more motivated, contextual, and dynamic model of emotional intelligence. *Academy of Management Perspectives*, 28(2), 93–107.

PART 4
COMMUNICATION LITERACY

OXFORD UNIVERSITY PRESS

CHAPTER 13
COMMUNICATION AND HEALTH LITERACY

LOUISE YOUNG

LEARNING OBJECTIVES

After reading this chapter and completing the activities, you will be able to:

- describe the features and characteristics of functional literacy, health literacy and technology literacy
- evaluate the health implications of low literacy for individuals and healthcare professionals
- evaluate readability and literacy measures for healthcare settings using formal and informal techniques
- analyse the literacy levels of written and electronic texts and resources
- create plain English health resources for a range of literacy levels
- identify strategies to support low literacy healthcare communication.

KEY TERMS

E-health literacy
Functional literacy
Health literacy
Information processing skills
IT literacy
Literacy
Numeracy
Plain English
Readability

Introduction

The concept of literacy has changed over the years. In previous centuries, people were considered literate if they could write or sign their name, while more recent definitions include whether they can read and write (Boudard & Jones 2003). As education became more widespread during the twentieth century, UNESCO defined literacy as having completed four or five years of schooling (UNESCO 2004). However, this last criterion is an imprecise measure as natural talent, motivation, work ethic and variations in education quality affect education level in many ways. Health literacy has been mentioned in the literature for over 40 years (Nutbeam 2000). This chapter explores concepts of literacy and their relevance to communication in healthcare professional practice.

Literacy

Literacy
Ability to read and write and to use language proficiently.

Literacy involves the ability to understand, evaluate, use and engage with written texts to participate in society, to achieve one's goals and to develop one's knowledge and potential. Skills involved include decoding written words and sentences, comprehension, and interpretation and evaluation of written, numerical and digital text.

Literacy skills are required for people to be proficient in:

- obtaining and using information in job applications, payroll forms, transport timetables, maps, tables and charts
- managing text or prose, such as editorials, news stories, brochures and instruction manuals
- problem-solving involving goal-directed thinking where no routine solution is available; **numeracy**
- understanding knowledge related to health matters such as drugs, alcohol, disease prevention and treatment, safety and accident prevention, first aid, emergencies and staying healthy.

Numeracy
Ability to work with numbers and apply basic principles of mathematics.

Functional literacy

Functional literacy
The ability to understand short and familiar texts, and to obtain information from everyday sources.

Functional literacy refers to the ability to use literacy to participate in society. It involves the ability to understand straightforward texts on familiar topics, or obtain information from everyday sources such as reading the sports pages of a tabloid newspaper. Reading information from unfamiliar sources and about unfamiliar topics can be problematic. Functional literacy is related to the ability to engage in specific activities including work, and includes a range of skills relevant to the culture. With the digital age, information literacy or technology is now a component of functional literacy, as shown in the focus box 'Examples of functional literacy'.

BOX 13.1

EXAMPLES OF FUNCTIONAL LITERACY

- A reading age of approximately 11 years old, which is the age for being able to complete a basic form and read and understand a tabloid newspaper.
- Understanding the instructions on a medicine container.
- Reading stories to children.
- Reading a newspaper story or a map.
- Reading correspondence from a bank or government agency.
- Filling out an application for work.
- Reading the safety instructions for operating machinery.
- Applying effectively for jobs.

Literacy in Australia

The Program for the International Assessment of Adult Competencies (PIAAC) is an international survey coordinated by the Organisation for Economic Co-operation and Development (OECD) that aims to understand current skills and competencies of the adult population in a range of countries (OECD 2013, 2017). Australia participated in data collection in 2011 and 2012 (ABS 2013; AIHW 2018). The program measures three **information processing skills**: literacy, numeracy and problem solving in technology rich environments (PSTRE) and provides competencies for people aged 15–74 years. In this chapter, numeracy and problem solving are considered in the broader context of health literacy.

Information processing skills
A set of skills comprised of literacy, numeracy and problem solving in technology-rich environments.

Skill levels from the *Survey of Adult Readers Skills: Reader's Companion* (OECD 2013) are based around six levels of literacy and numeracy proficiency, ranging from below Level 1 to Level 5. Around 3.7 per cent of Australians aged 15–74 years (620 000 people) had literacy skills below Level 1, and 6.1 per cent of Australians (1.1 million people) had numeracy skills below Level 1. PSTRE groups information technology scores in four skill levels from below Level 1 to Level 3. In Australia, there were 13 per cent (or 2.2 million people) with scores below Level 1 for PSTRE. Individuals with poor literacy, numeracy and PSTRE skills are disadvantaged when it comes to full participation in employment, education and training, and in social and civic life. Low levels of PSTRE skills also have implications for health. Literacy characteristics and skills associated with each level are outlined in Table 13.1.

TABLE 13.1 OECD literacy level by text characteristics and skills

OECD literacy levels	Text characteristics	Skills required
Below Level 1	Brief texts, familiar topics Locating a single piece of information No competing information No use of features specific to digital texts	Locate information in short continuous texts Basic vocabulary knowledge No understanding of the structure of sentences or paragraphs required
Level 1	Short digital or print text Continuous, non-continuous or mixed texts No competing information	Locate a single piece of information Enter personal information onto a document Knowledge and skill in recognising basic vocabulary, eliciting meaning of sentences Reading paragraphs of text
Level 2	Digital or printed texts Continuous, non-continuous or mixed texts Some competing pieces of information	Make matches between text and information Paraphrasing, low-level inferences Integrate two or more pieces of information based on criteria Compare and contrast or reason about information requested Navigate digital texts to access and identify information from various parts of the document
Level 3	Dense and lengthy texts Continuous, non-continuous or mixed texts Multiple pages of text Presence of competing information Minimum level for meeting complex demands of everyday life.	Understanding text and rhetorical structures Navigating complex digital texts Identify, interpret and evaluate one or more pieces of information Varying levels of inference Construct meaning across multiple chunks of text Perform multi-step operations to formulate responses Disregard irrelevant or inappropriate content
Level 4	Complex or lengthy continuous, non-continuous, mixed or multiple type texts Competing information is present and is often as prominent as the correct information	Perform multiple step operations to integrate and synthesise information Complex inferences Application of background knowledge Identifying and understanding one or more specific, non-central ideas Interpret persuasive discourse relationships Dealing with conditional information
Level 5	Dense texts Complex or lengthy continuous, non-continuous, mixed or multiple type texts Competing information is present and is often as prominent as the correct information	Search for and integrate information across multiple dense texts Synthesise similar or contrasting ideas or points of view Evaluate evidence based on arguments Application and evaluation of logical and conceptual ideas Evaluating reliability of evidence Selecting key information Awareness of subtle rhetorical cues Make high-level inferences Use specialised background knowledge

Source: Adapted from OECD Program for the International Assessment of Adult Competencies 2013.

Reflect and apply

Descriptors of each OECD literacy level by text characteristics and reader skills required are shown in Table 13.1. Literacy assessment of the skills of adults with low levels of proficiency is covered by an assessment of reading components, including text vocabulary, sentence comprehension and passage fluency.

An adult at below Level 2 for literacy would be able to:

- recognise and understand basic vocabulary
- locate a single piece of information in a short piece of text
- enter personal information in a document
- read single words and up to a paragraph of simple text.

How would you tailor immunisation information for parents with this level of literacy, compared with an adult with Level 3 literacy?

IT literacy

Information technology literacy (**IT literacy**) is the ability to decide which information is required and then to be able to access that information, usually via online digital resources, and finally to evaluate the usefulness of that information for its required purpose. It involves the ability of an individual to access, manage, integrate and evaluate information to solve a problem, answer a question or source information. The technology characteristics and skills required for the four IT (PSTRE) levels are described in Table 13.2.

IT literacy
Ability to recognise information is needed, and to locate, evaluate and effectively use this information using digital or online methods.

TABLE 13.2 OECD PSTRE levels by characteristics and skills

OECD levels for problem solving in technology-rich environments	Technology characteristics	Skills required
No computer experience		**No prior computer experience**
Below Level 1	Well-defined problems Use of only one function Use of generic interface	One explicit criterion with no categorical or inferential reasoning No transforming of information Few steps
Level 1	Widely available and familiar technology applications—e.g. Facebook, Google, email Few steps Minimal operators Simple matching of content and operators	Little or no navigation Problem may be solved without using specific tools and functions Easily identified task Explicit criteria Simple reasoning such as categorisation

TABLE 13.2 Continued

TABLE 13.2 Continued

Level 2	Use of generic and specific technology applications Novel online forms Navigation across pages and applications	Navigation across pages and applications is required to solve the problem Use of tools Multiple steps and operators Higher monitoring demands Evaluating relevant items Discarding distractors Integration and inferential reasoning
Level 3	Use of generic and specific technology applications Navigation across pages and applications	Use of tools Multiple steps and operators Criteria to be met may be explicit or not be explicit High monitoring demands Unexpected outcomes occur Evaluating the relevance and reliability of information Discarding distractors Integration and inferential reasoning required

Literacy data for the Australian population

Australia participated and collected data as part of the OEDC survey in 2013. Scores for the Australian population for literacy, numeracy and PSTRE from the OECD survey are shown in Table 13.3.

TABLE 13.3 Literacy, numeracy and PSTRE scores by level for the Australian population

Literacy	Numeracy	PSTRE
Below Level 1 3.7% (620 000)	Below Level 1 6.5% (1.1 million)	Below Level 1 13% (2.2 million)
Level 1 10% (1.7 million)	Level 1 15% (2.5 million)	Level 1 31% (5.3 million)
Level 2 30% (5.0 million)	Level 2 32% (5.4 million)	Level 2 25% (4.1 million)
Level 3 38% (6.3 million)	Level 3 31% (5.2 million)	Level 3 3.2% (540 000)
Level 4 14% (2.4 million)	Level 4 11% (1.8 million)	
Level 5 1.2% (200 000)	Level 5 1.4% (230 000)	

For the Australian population, 83 per cent of adults had literacy scores at Level 2 or above, over 75 per cent had numeracy scores at Level 2 or above, and nearly 59 per cent had PSTRE scores at Level 1 or above. This means that a significant proportion of the Australian population is functionally literate. However, it should be noted that the OECD survey was unable to classify the PSTRE score for 25 per cent of respondents, or 4.5 million people.

People with functional literacy, numeracy and IT skills (Level 2 and below) would have the ability to:

- recognise and understand basic vocabulary
- locate a single piece of information in a short piece of text
- enter personal information in a document
- read single words and up to a paragraph of simple text
- do problem solving that did not require specific tools or functions
- do simple reasoning such as categorisation.

People at Level 2 or below would be able to manage little or no computer navigation, and be unable to transform information. Around 50 per cent of Australian males and females scored Level 3 or above for literacy and numeracy. This is an average skill level indicating functional literacy. Less than one-third of the population for both males and females have technological scores above Level 2. These results have implications for access and use of written and online resources, as well as for technology-enabled health monitoring.

Health literacy

The World Health Organization (WHO) defines **health literacy** as the cognitive and social skills that determine the motivation and ability of individuals to gain access to understand and use information in ways which promote and maintain good health (Nutbeam 1998). Health literacy is the degree to which individuals have the capacity to obtain, process and understand basic health information and services (Ferguson & Pawlak 2011). Health literacy has three components:

- functional literacy: the ability to actually read and comprehend information
- conceptual literacy: the ability to seek out, evaluate and use health information
- literacy as empowerment: where individuals understand their rights, their ability to navigate the healthcare system, and their ability to act as informed consumers for health risks, products or treatment options (Kanj & Mitic 2009).

Health literacy
The ability to access, read and understand health-related information and to use this information to promote and maintain good health.

Health information is more likely to be read if it appears easy to read, interesting, brief and important. **Readability** is also important for health literacy, as the more readable a document is, the more easily it is understood. Health literacy also encompasses knowledge related to health matters such as drugs, alcohol, disease prevention and treatment, safety and accident prevention, first aid, emergencies and staying healthy.

Readability
The difficulty related to reading and comprehending text; it is measured by sentence length and vocabulary.

From a functional and conceptual point of view, literacy in healthcare is what enables people to more easily access and understand information that is provided to them in relation to their health. Increasing a person's capacity to understand health information will improve their health literacy and also enhance their capacity to successfully engage with the healthcare system. To do this successfully, health information needs to be presented in such a way as to make it accessible to people with many different literacy abilities (Beauchamp et al. 2015).

E-health literacy The ability to understand and use information and communication technologies for health care.

E-health literacy is increasingly evident in the literature and is an extension of the traditional understanding of literacy as it relates to the capability for seeking, understanding and using online health information (Griebel et al. 2018). For the purposes of discussion here, we do not distinguish literacy and e-health literacy, both of which involve information seeking and information behaviours, but which occur in different settings (i.e. online versus non-online). A related concept is a person's capacity to assess the quality of health information.

Reflect and apply

The University of California San Francisco (2019) has developed a resource for assessing the quality of health information. It can be accessed at: www.ucsfhealth.org/education/evaluating_health_information.

- Use the information on this site to evaluate a health resource that is considered to be credible—for example: www.healthdirect.gov.au or www.healthnavigator.org.nz. What did you find?
- Now conduct a random internet search for a website that contains information about a health concern relevant to your profession. What is the quality of information on these sites compared with those provided by government organisations?

Implications of poor health literacy

Health literacy is a significant problem affecting health outcomes (Cornett 2009; Pirisi 2000; WHO 2014). People with limited health literacy have higher healthcare costs, use healthcare services more frequently, have poor understanding of chronic disease management, underuse preventive health services and tend to be less knowledgeable about health-related topics (Wallace 2006). Low health literacy is associated with poorer health outcomes and less effective use of healthcare services (Berkman et al. 2011). Implications of poor health literacy are experienced by patients, healthcare professionals and the healthcare system itself.

1 Patients

Health literacy includes being able to manage personal health, with similar findings originating from the United States, the United Kingdom and Australia. In the United States, it is estimated that 12 per cent of 228 million adults have adequate skills to manage their own healthcare (Agency for Healthcare Research and Quality 2007), while in the United Kingdom a study of functional health literacy by von Wagner et al. (2007) found 11.4 per cent of participants had marginal or inadequate health literacy for managing their health. Patients with inadequate health literacy have difficulty understanding diagnoses, medication instructions, health forms and instructions before a medical procedure or surgery, in addition to being unfamiliar with medical terminology used by healthcare professionals. The stress of a new diagnosis or treatment and information overload can contribute to limitations in health literacy and lead to poorer health outcomes.

Low health literacy leads to poorer health outcomes (Adams et al. 2009; Williams, Davis, Parker & Weiss 2002). Limited literacy affects health-related behaviours, decision making and health outcomes. The ability to read does not necessarily indicate functional health literacy, as people who can read may be 'illiterate' in terms of understanding health-related or disease-specific information. Poor literacy is associated with less use of preventive health services, increased hospitalisations, reduced knowledge of their chronic disease and poorer health outcomes (Baker et al. 2007; DeWalt et al. 2004; Gazmararian, Williams, Peel & Baker 2003; Sudore et al. 2006). People with low literacy may be reluctant to engage with healthcare services for fear of stigmatisation or may disengage completely if their literacy needs are not supported (Batterham et al. 2016).

The impact of low literacy on health condition management and outcomes has been identified among a number of patient groups including individuals with hypertension, type 2 diabetes, mental health conditions, as well as patients in emergency departments (Boylston Hendon, Chaney & Carden 2011; Cho, Lee, Arozullah & Crittenden 2008; Francis et al. 2002; Kandula et al. 2009; Pandit et al. 2009). Cutilli, Simko, Colbert and Bennett (2018) have documented how poor health outcomes, including decreased physical and cognitive functioning, less preventive care and increased mortality, are associated with low health literacy in older adults. In some communities, however, health-related communication and information, and even decision making, are shared among family and community members. This behaviour can have a positive impact on health literacy, not just at individual level, but also for the broader community (Batterham et al. 2016).

2 Healthcare professionals

Health literacy is impacted upon by healthcare professionals. There can be a lack of awareness by healthcare professionals about the problems faced by patients with low literacy. Healthcare professionals may also be unaware of other barriers to health literacy, such as culture, language, environment (e.g. rural or underserved populations), socioeconomic status and age-related factors. Healthcare professionals may lack confidence in their ability and have limited knowledge of what strategies to use to communicate effectively with people who have low levels of health literacy (Ali, Ferguson, Mitha & Hanlon 2014; Coleman et al. 2017). Literacy level impacts upon high-quality healthcare by affecting safety, effectiveness, timeliness, patient-centredness and equitable treatment (Abrams, Klass & Dreyer 2009). If one considers the low levels of health literacy in the Australian community, it is imperative that healthcare professionals be alert and sensitive to the diverse range of health literacy needs they may encounter in practice (Batterham et al. 2016).

3 System factors

Constraints within healthcare systems impact upon health literacy. Patients often experience short consultation times, care fragmentation, and the need to complete increasing amounts of medical paperwork (Ferguson & Pawlak 2011). There is medication complexity and increased self-care demands with shorter hospital stays, while care plans are often ineffectively communicated. Communication breakdown can occur when a patient with low literacy is responsible for relaying information between different specialists. Consent forms have been developed for legal protection for healthcare service providers and the patient may find them unreadable or incomprehensible. There is no incentive to check literacy or comprehension because of medical reimbursement plans that focus on diagnoses and treatment. The stigma related to low literacy levels negatively impacts upon patients, who may not seek health services or comply with treatment or management protocols (Coleman et al. 2017). This results in health services being underutilised by those patients with real need.

Health implications of low literacy, numeracy and technology skills

From the OECD research, nearly half of the Australian population has reading and mathematical skills at a functional level and limited technology skills. These results have implications for health outcomes and the provision of health services for this population. There is a digital divide in the usage of information technology. People with limited literacy, English as a second language and those on low incomes, for example, use IT less than people with higher literacy levels, university education and high incomes (AIHW 2018).

Patients with low levels of literacy

In Australia, 61 per cent of respondents who reported excellent or very good health had OECD Level 3 literacy; 50 per cent had Level 3 numeracy; and 34 per cent had Level 2 and higher for problem-solving technology (OECD 2013). For each age range, people with poorer health had lower scores in all three OECD areas, suggesting patients with complex and chronic illnesses are more likely to have low literacy, numeracy and PSTRE levels. There were few differences between males and females for people with poor health for literacy, numeracy and PSTRE at all levels. People who are older, or do not have English as their first language and have fair or poor health, have considerable problems with the application of literacy, numeracy and IT. These low levels have implications for healthcare access, compliance and services for these adults. Details are shown in Table 13.4.

When providing resources that require application of literacy, numeracy and IT skills, the healthcare professional should consider the age of the person, whether they were born in Australia and if their first language is English, in order to ensure comprehension, compliance and engagement with the health information.

TABLE 13.4 Health differences in Australia based on demographic characteristics and health literacy levels

Demographics	Health status	Literacy level	Numeracy level	PSTRE level
Male		Level 2 44% Level 3+ 54%	Level 2 49% Level 3+ 49%	Level 1 29% Level 2+ 29%
Female		Level 2 45% Level 3+ 53%	Level 2 59% Level 3+ 38%	Level 1 44% Level 2+ 27%
15–24 years	Good/excellent	Level 3+ 62%	Level 3+ 50%	Level 2 43%
	Fair/poor	Level 3+ 45%	Level 3+ 28%	Level 2 36%
65–74 years	Excellent/good	Level 3+ 38%	Level 3 32%	Level 2 6.7%
	Fair/poor	Level 3+ 18%	Level 3 16%	
Born in Australia (all levels)		Level 3+ 57%	Level 3 46%	30%
Born outside Australia (all levels)		Level 3+ 49%	Level 3+ 40%	24%
First language English		Level 1 12%		
First language not English		Level 1 25%		

Source: Adapted from OECD 2013.

Skills in practice

Demographics and health literacy

Kelly is a student attending placement at an acute care facility. She observes Claire, a social worker, interviewing an elderly Chinese woman, Mrs Chan, who is unsteady on her feet and has been admitted following a fall. Claire has some brochures about resources available to Mrs Chan to assist her to remain living in her own home. As she attempts to hand them to Mrs Chan her son, Eric, who has accompanied her to the hospital, quickly snatches them away and tells Claire that he will 'take care of it'. Claire assumes this is the end of the matter, but watches with interest as Kelly asks Eric about Mrs Chan's ability to read and understand English. She explains to

Eric that promoting Mrs Chan's independence is essential to her wellbeing. Eric begins to relax and assists Claire to engage Mrs Chan in the conversation.

What's happening here?

Claire has maintained both professional and therapeutic approaches to communicating with Eric and Mrs Chan in this exchange. It would have been easy for Claire to shift her communication entirely to Eric in the interest of expedience, or to have expressed frustration at Eric for attempting to take control of the discussion. Instead, she maintained respect for both Mrs Chan and Eric and demonstrated understanding, without judgment, of Mrs Chan's ability to understand the material presented to her. In doing so, she was able to ensure that both Mrs Chan and Eric understood the options available to them to promote positive outcomes for Mrs Chan.

ICT for health

Information and communications technology (ICT) is an increasingly important component of healthcare provision. Healthcare providers and patients are able to access and use information for self-care, connecting with healthcare providers, communicating with others with similar conditions and accessing their personal health records. However, the literacy level, content and format to access most health information technology is often higher than the literacy level of much of the population, as indicated by the OECD survey.

There are advantages in using health ICT for low literacy populations. Individuals are able to access and manage their own healthcare information, source information on a range of topics via the internet, engage with more visual and interactive learning opportunities compared with paper-based information, enter information, obtain personalised feedback and receive monitoring and follow-up by healthcare providers. Websites provide health information on many topics, as well as message boards, chat rooms and web portals for information and social connectedness.

Social media platforms such as Facebook can also be used to provide health information. For example, Australia's National Prescribing Scheme (NPS), MedicineWise, communicates targeted health information through its Facebook page, with resources including videos, challenges, key facts and interactive forums.

Reflect and apply

Access the MedicineWise Facebook page at www.facebook.com/npsmedicinewise and explore the range of resources available on this site. You can see that this site offers a number of opportunities for individuals to obtain and also contribute information. Who may access the information on this site, and how might it be used? How might this site be a valuable resource for your specific area of professional practice?

Below we explore some other examples of how ICT software platforms and electronic devices can support efforts to improve health literacy and communication.

Touchscreen kiosks

Touchscreen kiosks are often available in health centres, shopping centres or other public locations. They contain educational resources about specific health conditions, such as diabetes, with one idea or question per screen, and only essential information for the health condition is presented. As another example, a computer kiosk for a particular condition may use a 'teach back' option, where the client answers multiple-choice questions with immediate feedback about the correct response.

Handheld technologies

Handheld technologies are more accessible, as reliance on text is minimal, design features are geared to adults with limited literacy, and they include large keys, letters on all keys and simple navigation.

Personal wireless devices

Personal wireless devices include smartphones or tablets that are small, portable and private. Users are able to send and receive messages confirming appointments, send and receive emails, host games and use the internet.

Home monitoring equipment

Home monitoring equipment is tied to an information system, and requires action by the client or caregiver, such as the administration of medication. For easily accessible home-use devices, the information display needs to be readable and comprehensible; compact; easy to operate with a limited number of steps, large keys and clear icons; self-calculating; able to store test results, have simple function buttons and automatic calibration. Content from such equipment needs to support literacy by being readable and age- or culture-appropriate; it should also use instructions that reiterate and review the main steps. Other design features include using numbered steps to describe procedures, describing steps in the order they will be performed, illustrating each step, emphasising critical aspects or warnings, and providing a phone number for client support. Principles for designing accessible health ICT are shown in the focus box 'Accessible health ICT'.

ACCESSIBLE HEALTH ICT

BOX 13.1

Principles for ensuring accessible health ICT include:

- using plain and clear language: short, simple, familiar vocabulary using one- or two -syllable words. No jargon, acronyms or abbreviations

- explaining unavoidable medical or technical terms
- using short sentences
- using active voice not passive voice
- consistent word usage
- keeping the reading level at Grade 6 level, or OECD Literacy Level 3.

Design rules for web pages include a simple home page, prioritised information, minimal amount of text per screen, and simplified searching. Navigation needs to be simple and consistent, minimising the need for scrolling and using links and hyperlinks for additional information; printer-friendly options; audio transcription options; and contact information that is easy to find. For ethnically and linguistically diverse groups, content needs to be culturally appropriate and sensitive for users, with community members and their cultural objects being portrayed accurately in photos and graphics. Translation from English needs to be accurate in meaning, context and use of appropriate idioms and expressions.

Specific adaptations that make IT information accessible to individuals with low literacy levels include:

- justifying the left margin only
- formatting that is easy to read and understand
- using bullets, questions and answers to break up the text
- restricting numbers and percentages to one number per point, making sure they require no calculations or inferences and use simple phrasing such as '1 in 10 adults' rather than '10 per cent'
- using colour coding and pictographs to explain a process
- explaining the diagnosis or treatment using more diagrams than words
- using non-verbal reminders and prompts
- featuring content that appeals to diverse racial, ethnic and age groups
- featuring content that has been tested and revised
- ensuring pilot materials have been tested with prospective users.

As well as using specific format and design principles, the use of plain English boosts the readability of written text for people with low literacy levels.

Plain English Language that ensures that information is easily readable and understood by people with low literacy levels.

Plain English

Plain English (or plain language) is simple and unambiguous. It is written so that people can understand information that is important to their lives. Plain English is understood by its audience because it is based on their requirements, characteristics and expectations; see Table 13.5.

TABLE 13.5 Factors contributing to plain English

Audience	Characteristics	Expectations
Age range	Reading abilities	Image of self
Gender	Maths abilities	Attitude towards topic
First language	Familiarity with special/ technical language	Motivation
Family structure	Physical challenges	Mental or emotional challenges
Education	Financial challenges	Specific concerns
Cultural traditions	Specific interests	Biases

Plain English is a process, rather than a certain style. It is not absolute and depends on the reader's understanding of the information they think they need. It is a reader-based rather than text-based analysis of a writing style. To prepare a plain English document, the objectives and outcomes need to be considered as well as the literacy level of the intended audience; see Table 13.6.

TABLE 13.6 Preparing a plain English document

Objectives	Questions to ask
Identify your audience	In what situation or environment will this be used? Who are the readers or users of the document?
Clarify your purpose	What is the reader to do after reading the document?
Determine parameters or constraints	What constraints are there in producing the document?

Reflect and apply

Write 100 words about a chronic disease such as diabetes or cardiovascular disease, using as much medical, technical and jargon vocabulary as you can. Describe how it is caused, and treatment and management options for the patient.

Now rewrite your paragraph, using the principles of plain English, for an adult who can read at OECD Level 1.

Strategies for low literacy health communication

Communication is an important component of health promotion and disease prevention. However, health information is often written for a Year 10 reading level (Safeer & Keenan 2005). It is estimated that more than 50 per cent of the target audience cannot read at this level and will not understand the message that is being delivered. Studies first identified a problem with health literacy in the 1990s, indicating a gap between the readers and the materials (see, for example, Davis et al. 1991; Williams et al. 1995).

Poorly educated adults with low literacy levels also suffer from the highest rates of morbidity and mortality from chronic diseases. When a person is ill or stressed, their attention decreases, as does their reading comprehension, even for those individuals with high health literacy.

For content relevant to a particular audience, such as a health or illness group, accessible health information needs to:

- assume little or no background knowledge
- be relevant for users
- deliver a limited number of messages
- use graphic illustrations to clarify text
- aid comprehension with a format that has a lot of white space—that us, fewer words, less dense text, short line length, 40–50 characters, and similar information grouped under subheadings
- use dark text on a light background
- use large, familiar and easy-to-read fonts such as 12 point Arial, Verdana or Times New Roman with consistent font and style
- use both upper-case and lower-case letters, as all capitals can be difficult to read
- be easy to use and navigate
- have content that is appropriate, acceptable and applicable for its use. Participants will want to choose to use the application.

The need for a framework to improve literacy levels of health information has been identified in areas such as improved health information and a focus on the users of this information (Hill & Sofra 2018). Effective and ineffective interventions to improve health literacy have also been identified (Visscher et al. 2018). To improve the readability of health-related information in written or electronic text the guidelines shown in Table 13.7 are suggested.

TABLE 13.7 Guidelines for written materials to accommodate health literacy requirements

Words	Sentences	Format	Meaning
Avoid long words	Short, focused materials	Single sheet of paper folded in half or thirds	Culturally appropriate
Avoid technical language and jargon	Avoid complex sentences	Graphics—solid print	Clear core message
Use personal pronouns—e.g. I, we, you	Be direct; avoid ambiguity	Keep pages clear and uncluttered	Emphasise desired behaviours
Use verbs instead of nouns for actions	Keep sentences to around 25 words	Organise content with use of headings, subheadings and summaries	Positive, non-judgmental tone
Keep the subject and verb close together at the beginning of the sentence	Use active voice	12 point clear fonts such as Arial, Times New Roman, Verdana	Appropriate cultural and language concepts for the audience
Write acronyms or abbreviations in full	Identify the person and the action	Avoid jumbo print	Use illustrations instead of lengthy descriptions
Define or describe examples of technical words	Use positive words and sentence construction	Illustrations must fit the message being delivered	Prioritise information and place the most important information first
Use everyday language	Explain only one idea in each sentence	Visual, age-appropriate appeal	Positive, non-judgmental tone
Use graphics such as bar charts, line graphs, pie charts, diagrams, line drawings, logos, maps and illustrations instead of all words	Comfortable eye movements for text are line lengths of 10–20 cm (40–70 letters/characters). Shorter lines make it harder to keep your eye on the correct line	Use graphics, charts and pictures to reinforce key facts	Only one idea in each sentence
Lists of 3–7 items	Check readability	The eye is attracted by the largest, most dominant material on the page	Lists help to focus information: include 3–7 items
	Use plain English	Avoid excessive variety in sizes, styles and weight of typeface for heading levels Avoid using all capital letters	Colour psychology affects reading. Reds, oranges and yellows give a feeling of warmth. Greens, blues, violets are perceived as cool colours. Younger audiences respond to warm colours, while older audiences prefer cool colours.
		Ragged right margins make text easier to read. Justified margins stretch the text to the right margin and make it harder to read	Avoid obvious 'dumbing down'
		Align headings and sub-headings on the left margin, not centred	

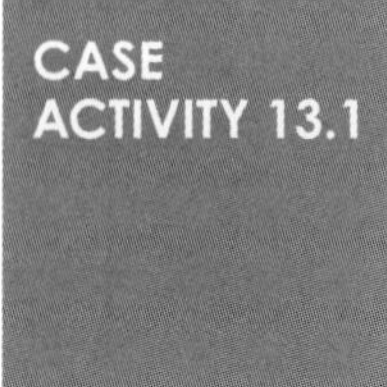

Strategies for low health literacy

DENISE

Denise is a 73-year-old retired woman who has just been diagnosed with type 2 diabetes. Prior to diagnosis, she had symptoms indicating hyperglycaemia and fasting blood glucose levels of 6.7–7.3 mmol/L. Denise is overweight, bordering on obese, with a BMI of 30. Her diet history reveals excessive carbohydrate meals, especially pasta.

JOHN

Upon diagnosis of type 2 diabetes, John would take a proactive approach to his disease. He would read all information given to him by his doctor, and check recommended websites such as Diabetes Australia for relevant information. An appointment with a dietician would be arranged and kept, and he would develop a plan to modify his diet and learn how to read dietary information on items in the supermarket. John would modify his diet accordingly, and look for low GI recipes. He would look on the internet to find local sports near where he lives, and engage in exercises suitable for his age. John is keen to learn how to monitor his blood sugar levels at home.

BILL

After being diagnosed with type 2 diabetes, Bill would not take a proactive approach to his disease. He would not be interested in learning about his condition or measures he could take to improve his health. He is unlikely to read the information given to him by the doctor, and the doctor has possibly not assessed his literacy level. Bill would not search for information through other sources such as the internet, and he possibly does not have computer access or the ICT literacy skills to access information online. He would not understand the importance of diet and blames his poor eyesight for not reading grocery food labels. Bill is unlikely to test his blood sugar at home, instead thinking that knowing the numbers isn't going to do anything for him. He does not seek out exercise options or modify his diet, and says 'I like eating pasta'.

1. Of the three people described, who is likely to have the better health outcome—Denise, John or Bill?
2. Why would this be the case?
3. What strategies could you employ to assist Dennis, John and Bill with their health literacy?

Readability

Readability formulas were first developed in the United States in the 1920s for measuring the reading level of school textbooks, and many were more recently updated for use by the US Navy to determine the readability of their technical manuals. Readability can be calculated using simple formulas that are readily available online. Most readability formulas are designed as mathematical equations that correlate with measurable syntactic and semantic elements of writing. Readability incorporates document design, such as font, spacing, line length and white space, as well as comprehension of language—that is, the meaning of the written text. Readability is defined as the difficulty of text as measured by sentence length and complexity of vocabulary.

Readability can be improved in written text by:

- explaining abbreviations and acronyms the first time they are used
- keeping sentences short
- avoiding symbolic language such as metaphors
- avoiding complicated words
- using vocabulary from the end-user's perspective and experience.

Readability formulas do not help evaluate how well the reader will understand the text, as readability does not equate with understanding. A readability score is not an exact science, as it only gives an indication, and does not consider paragraphs or actual content with words from a specific domain. Information, flyers and websites may follow all the guideline recommendations but still be inaccessible to people with low literacy levels if the content is difficult to comprehend. Readability measurement methods also only work for a specific language: each different language version of the text will have its own readability criteria. Measuring readability is now able to be completed automatically online.

Measuring readability and literacy levels

A number of techniques are available to assess the readability of a text or written materials. It is suggested that informal readability measures are used to ensure that individuals with low literacy levels are able to read and understand information related to their health.

Formal measures may be used to select information for a client or a textbook for health students in a course being taught. A broader range of domestic and international students is entering universities by a variety of alternative pathways. It cannot always be assumed that their literacy levels are at a standard to deal with technical and health-related vocabulary and jargon. To ensure comprehension, it is suggested that subject texts are selected based on readability. After all, it is the content we want students and consumers of health services to understand and master, rather than simply being able to read the text.

Examples of formal readability measures include the following:

- Fry readability formula
- Flesch reading ease formula and Flesch–Kincaid Readability tests

- Gunning Fog Index
- SMOG
- Dale–Chall readability formula
- Spache readability
- cloze technique.

A selection of these readability measures are now discussed.

1 Flesch reading ease formula and Flesch–Kincaid readability tests

The Flesch formula is the easiest formula to use and makes adjustments for the higher end of the scale, so it is useful for measuring the readability of tertiary education texts and complex health information. Scores measure reading from 100 (easy to read) to 0 (difficult to read). A zero score indicates the text has more than 37 words in each sentence and the average word has more than two syllables. The plain English score has been identified as 65. Flesch–Kincaid is the readability statistic used in Microsoft Word, so it can be calculated automatically from a piece of text.

Higher scores indicate material is easier to read; lower scores mean it is more difficult. Scores range from 90–100 *very easy*, to 0–29 *very confusing*. Scores between 90 and 100 are easily understood by an average Year 5 reader. A score between 60 and 70 is acceptable reading ease for the Year 8 or 9 level. Scores between 0 and 30 are considered easily understood by university graduates.

A readability graph was developed in 1963 and has now been converted into a computer program: https://readability-score.com.

2 SMOG

SMOG is a measure of readability that estimates years of education needed to understand a piece of writing. SMOG is an acronym from Simple Measure of Gobbledygook, and is used widely for checking the readability of health messages. It is a more accurate and easily calculated substitute for the Gunning Fog Index. To calculate SMOG:

- count at least 30 sentences
- within these sentences, count the number of polysyllabic words with three or more syllables
- SMOG grade = 3 + square root of polysyllable count.

See Table 13.8 for a SMOG scoreboard. An automatic calculation can be completed using the formula on: www.readabilityformulas.com.

TABLE 13.8 SMOG score and their equivalent grade levels

Total number of polysyllabic words in text sample	Grade level (US)
1–6	Grade 5
7–12	Grade 6
13–20	Grade 7
21–30	Grade 8
31–42	Grade 9
43–56	Grade 10
57–72	Grade 11
73–90	Grade 12
111–132	Undergraduate tertiary level
133–156	Grade 15 (Postgraduate level)

Source: www.readabilityformulas.com.

3 Cloze technique

In a cloze test, every fifth word is deliberately omitted and readers have to select the correct word to go into each space from a given list. The number of correct words added to a text is used to assign a level of difficulty for the text. The advantage of a cloze technique is that it tests both word recognition and comprehension of the read material for a particular audience.

Reliance solely on readability measures from text statistics should be treated with a degree of caution, as measures:

- may fail to capture poor grammar and nonsensical meaning
- may fail to capture poor or unusual punctuation
- may include difficult words with only one syllable, such as medical, technical or scientific words
- overlook the impact of typographical cueing, such as headings, dot points, font, highlighting
- fail to detect contradiction and inconsistency
- are dependent on pronunciation for syllable count, which may vary with polysyllabic words
- may include easy polysyllabic words if they are common words, while a short word may be difficult if it is not used by many people—this includes technical or medical words
- assume that a person's education level or years of schooling is equivalent to their literacy level.

For these reasons, it is important to always assess multiple views of a person's literacy using a variety of formal and informal approaches.

Reflect and apply

Locate a short passage in a published journal article on the topic of diabetes. Select something that is written specifically for a healthcare professional. Perform a readability analysis on this material using one of the methods described in this chapter.

Now rewrite the text in language suitable for use by Denise, John or Bill to address their health literacy needs as described in Case activity 13.1.

Tests of health literacy

Informal check

Checking on a person's literacy level may be explored informally through several techniques. Informal literacy assessment may include the following strategies:

1. Teach back: ask the person to explain what they have been told to check for comprehension.
2. Hand upside-down information fliers to the individual and ask a question related to information in the flier. This should reveal those who cannot read, but avoids embarrassing them.
3. Ask a screening question. For example, 'How confident are you filling out medical forms by yourself?' has been identified in research as being closely aligned with inadequate health literacy when also measured by S-TOFHLA and REALM (Chew et al. 2008). (S-TOFHLA and REALM are discussed in more detail below.)
4. Newest Vital Sign (NVS) (Weiss et al. 2005) is a validated, quick and accurate screening test for limited literacy. It takes three minutes to administer, involves reading a nutrition label and answering six questions about information on the label. Individuals with fewer than four correct answers indicate limited literacy, while those with lower than two correct answers have inadequate literacy. NVS identifies those requiring assistance with literacy-related management of their condition.

Formal assessment

A number of formal assessments have been designed to measure functional health literacy in adults. These include the Test of Functional Health Literacy in Adults (TOFHLA) (Parker, Baker, Williams & Nurss 1995) and a shortened form, S-TOFHLA (Baker et al. 1999). The TOFHLA takes about 20 minutes to administer and contains 50 health-related items assessed using the cloze technique. Every fifth to seventh word in a passage is omitted and the reader is given four similar choices, one of which is correct. This technique assesses comprehension. Numeracy is also tested with 17 items requiring a patient's ability to use hospital forms, labelled prescriptions, glucose monitoring or maintaining clinic appointments, with scores calculated out of 50. The reading and numeracy scores are added to obtain an overall score out of 100, with a score of 75+ indicating adequate health literacy; 60–74 marginal health literacy; and 0–59 reflects inadequate health literacy.

The REALM, or Rapid Estimate of Adult Literacy in Medicine (Davis et al. 1991), is a 66-word item recognition test of health-related vocabulary that has been validated and field tested, and takes less than five minutes to administer. It measures word recognition for common medical words, body parts and illnesses, but does not measure comprehension. Scores range from zero with no words correct to 66 with all words pronounced correctly. Final scores indicate a person has literacy skills below third grade with a score of 0–18, fourth to sixth grade 19–44, seventh to eighth grade 45–60, and greater than ninth grade 61–66.

A shortened form or REALM-SF (Arozullah et al. 2007) has been developed as a seven-word item recognition screening test. Words contain two or three syllables and are relatively common health or medical-related vocabulary. It only takes a couple of minutes to administer.

The Medical Achievement Reading Test (MART) (Hanson-Divers 1997) has been developed to measure medical literacy in a non-threatening way. It has been modelled and validated against the Wide Range Achievement Test, which is a leading reading test to measure general reading ability. The test comprises 42 medical words written in small font and placed on a prescription bottle. Individuals are told the print is small and the glare from the label may make it difficult to read to make the test less intimidating. A score is obtained from the number of words read correctly, but, more importantly, it indicates those with poor literacy who are unable to read many words.

Conclusion

A significant proportion of the adult population have low literacy levels. Health information provided in written or oral form therefore may not be easily and readily understood by people with low literacy. Literacy and IT literacy levels are indirectly related to patient health. If a patient does not have functional literacy, they will have difficulty reading medication instructions and information related to their health condition. This may have consequences for their wellbeing. Measures of readability help to assess the reading (accessibility) level of written materials and health information resources. Written instructions and health information provided in plain English promote readability and comprehension. Information to assess a person's literacy level can be readily obtained when collecting other demographic information. Healthcare professionals should be aware of the consequences of low literacy levels on health outcomes when working with individuals and developing health resources.

SUMMARY POINTS

- Literacy comprises reading, numeracy and IT skills. Skills involved include decoding written words and sentences, comprehension, interpretation and evaluation of written and numerical text.
- Australia's population has a range of literacy levels, which are influenced by age, gender, socioeconomic background and health status.
- In Australia, 83 per cent of the population is functionally literate. Literacy figures for IT are lower, and this has implications for access and use of written and online resources and technology-enabled health monitoring.
- Readability is defined as the difficulty of a text as measured by sentence length and complexity of vocabulary. Readability should be ascertained by both formal and informal measures.
- Healthcare professionals should consider literacy levels, and match these with the readability of educational resources to ensure that individuals are able to understand, access and engage with health information.
- Plain English makes information easily readable by people with low literacy levels. Plain English is language that is understood by its audience; it needs to consider the requirements, characteristics and expectations of the intended audience.

CRITICAL THINKING QUESTIONS

1. Reflect on your own writing. How do factors such as the intended reader and the purpose of the message influence how you write? How might readability be impacted on by these factors? Review some of your writing (e.g. assessment tasks, emails, etc.) and critique them in light of what you have learnt from this chapter.
2. Susan, a woman in her 20s with Down syndrome, has been diagnosed with type 2 diabetes. She is currently hospitalised and you are required to brief her before discharge about management issues and compliance with medication and diet.
   a. How will you determine Susan's literacy level? Describe three methods for assessing her skills.
   b. Write discharge notes in a form that Susan is able to read and understand.
   c. Write a diet plan for Susan using plain English and other strategies to assist readability.

Group activity

Promoting health literacy

In your study groups or via your subject discussion site, develop a role play scenario between a healthcare professional and a person with limited health literacy who is in need of health information. In presenting the role play back to the group, detail how the individual in need of health information was assessed, and the strategies used to ensure that adequate, tailored information was provided. As a group, discuss any additional strategies that could be employed to promote health literacy in each scenario.

WEBLINKS

Health literacy

Agency for Healthcare Research and Quality:
www.ahrq.gov/topics/health-literacy.html

Australian Bureau of Statistics:
www.abs.gov.au/ausstats/abs@.nsf/PrimaryMainFeatures/4228.0?OpenDocument

Health Literacy and Health Behaviour (WHO): who.int/healthpromotion/conferences/7gchp/track2/en

Health Literacy: Implications for Australia:
www.medibankhealth.com.au/files/editor_upload/File/Medibank%20Health%20Literacy%20Implications%20for%20Australia%20Summary%20Report.pdf

Quick Guide to Health Literacy (US Government):
https://health.gov/communication/literacy/quickguide/factsbasic.htm

Readability

Grammarly: How to use readability scores in your writing:
www.grammarly.com/blog/readability-scores

Wylie Communications: 10 free readability calculators:
www.wyliecomm.com/2018/11/10-free-readability-calculators

ICT and Health Literacy

The Role of Health Literacy in Health Information Technology:
www.nap.edu/read/13016/chapter/5

REFERENCES

Abrams, M.A., Klass, P. & Dreyer, B.P. (2009). Health literacy and children: Recommendations for action. *Paediatrics*, 124(3), S327–S331.

Adams, R.J., Appleton, S.L., Hill, C.L., Dodd, M., Findlay, C. & Wilson, D.H. (2009). Risks associated with low functional health literacy in an Australian population. *Medical Journal of Australia*, 191, 530–4.

Agency for Healthcare Research and Quality. (2007). *National Healthcare Disparities Report*. Retrieved from www.ahrq.gov/research/findings/nhqrdr/index.html.

Ali, N.K., Ferguson, R.P., Mitha, S. & Hanlon, A. (2014). Do medical trainees feel confident communicating with low health literacy patients? *Journal of Community Hospital Internal Medicine Perspectives*, 4(2). doi:10.3402/jchimp.v4.22893.

Arozullah, A.M., Yarnold, P.R., Bennett, C.L., Soltysik, R.C., Wolf, M.S., Ferreira, R.M.… Davis, T. (2007). Development and validation of a short-form, rapid estimate of adult literacy in medicine. *Medical Care*, 45(11), 1026–33.

Australian Bureau of Statistics. (2013). *Programme for International Assessment of Adult Competencies, Australia 2011–12, cat. no. 4228.0*. Canberra: ABS.

Australian Institute of Health and Welfare. (2018). *Australia's Health 2018. Series no. 16, AUS 221*. Canberra: AIHW.

Baker, D.W., Williams, M.V., Parker, R.M., Gazmararian, J.A. & Nurss, J. (1999). Development of a brief test measure of functional health literacy. *Patient Education and Counseling*, 38, 33–42.

Baker, D.W., Wolf, M.S., Feinglass, J., Thompson, J.A., Gazmararian, J.A. & Huang, J. (2007). Health literacy and mortality among elderly persons. *Archives of Internal Medicine*, 167(14), 1503–9.

Batterham, R.W., Hawkins, M., Collins, P.A., Buchbinder, R. & Osborne, R.H. (2016). Health literacy: Applying current concepts to improve health services and reduce health inequalities. *Public Health*, 132, 3–12.

Beauchamp, A., Buchbinder, R., Dodson, S., Batterham, R.W., Elsworth, G.R., McPhee, C., … Osborne, R.H. (2015). Distribution of health literacy strengths and weaknesses across socio-demographic groups: A cross-sectional survey using the Health Literacy Questionnaire (HLQ). *BMC Public Health*, 15(1), 678.

Berkman, N.D., Sheridan, S.L., Donahue, K.E., Halpern, D.J. & Crotty, K. (2011). Low health literacy and health outcomes: An updated systematic review. *Annals of Internal Medicine*, 155(2), 97–107.

Boudard, E. & Jones, S. (2003). The IALS approach to defining and measuring literacy skills. *International Journal of Educational Research*, 39(3), 191–204.

Boylston Hendon, J., Chaney, M. & Carden, D. (2011). Health literacy and emergency department outcomes: A systematic review. *Annals of Emergency Medicine*, 57(4), 334–45.

Chew, L.D., Griffin, J.M. Partin, M.R., Noorbaloochi, S., Gill, J.P., Snyder, A., … VanRyn, M. (2008). Validation of screening questions for limited health literacy in a large VA outpatient population. *Journal of General Internal Medicine*, 23(5), 561–6.

Cho, Y.I., Lee, S.-Y.D., Arozullah, A.M. & Crittenden, K.S. (2008). Effects of health literacy on health status and health service utilisation among the elderly. *Social Science and Medicine*, 66, 1809–16.

Coleman, C., Hudson, S. & Pederson, B. (2017). Prioritized health literacy and clear communication practices for health care professionals. *HLRP: Health Literacy Research and Practice*, 1(3), e91–e99.

Cornett, S. (2009). Assessing and addressing health literacy. *OJIN: The Online Journal of Issues in Nursing*, 14(3), Manuscript 2.

Cutilli, C.C, Simko, L.C., Colbert, A.M. & Bennett, I.M. (2018). Health literacy, health disparities and sources of health information in US older adults. *Orthopaedic Nursing*, 37(1), 54–65.

Davis, T.C., Crouch, M.A., Long, S.W., Jackson, R., Bates, P., George, R.B. & Bairnsfather, L.E. (1991). Rapid assessment of literacy levels of adult primary care patients. *Family Medicine*, 23, 433–5.

DeWalt, D.A., Berkman, N.D., Sheridan, S., Lohr, K.N. & Pignone, M.P. (2004). Literacy and health outcomes. *Journal of General Internal Medicine*, 19(12), 1228–39.

Ferguson, L.A. & Pawlak, R. (2011). Health literacy: The road to improved health outcomes. *Journal for Nurse Practitioners*, 7(2), 123–9.

Francis, C., Pirkis, J., Dunt, D., Blood, R.W. & Davis, C. (2002). *Improving Mental Health Literacy*. University of Melbourne: Centre for Health Program Evaluation.

Gazmararian, J.A., Williams, M.V., Peel, J. & Baker, D.W. (2003). Health literacy and knowledge of chronic disease. *Patient Education and Counseling*, 51, 267–75.

Griebel, L., Enwald, H., Gilstad, H., Pohl, A.L., Moreland, J. & Sedlmayr, M. (2018). eHealth literacy research—Quo vadis? *Informatics for Health and Social Care*, 43(4), 427–42.

Hanson-Divers, E.C. (1997). Developing a medical achievement reading test to evaluate patient literacy skills: A preliminary study. *Journal of Health Care for the Poor and Underserved*, 8(1), 56–69.

Hill, S.J. & Sofra, T.A. (2018). How could health information be improved? Recommended actions from the Victorian Consultation on Health Literacy. *Australian Health Review*, 42, 134–9.

Kandula, N.R., Nsiah-Kumi, P.A., Makoul, G., Sager, J., Zei, C.P., Glass, S., Stephens, Q. & Baker, D.W. (2009). The relationship between health literacy and knowledge improvement after a multimedia type 2 diabetes education program. *Patient Education and Counselling*, 75, 321–7.

Kanj, M. & Mitic, W. (2009). *Health Literacy and Health Promotion: Definitions, Concepts and Examples in the Eastern Mediterranean Region. Individual Empowerment—Conference Working Document.* Geneva: WHO.

Nutbeam, D. (1998). Health promotion glossary. *Health Promotion International*, 13(4), 349–64.

Nutbeam, D. (2000). Health literacy as a public health goal: A challenge for contemporary health education and communication strategies into the 21st century. *Health Promotion International*, 15(3), 259–67.

Organisation for Economic Co-operation and Development. (2013). *The Survey of Adult Skills: Reader's Companion*. Paris: OECD Publishing. http://dx.doi.org/10.1787/9789264204027-en.

Organisation for Economic Co-operation and Development. (2017). *Building Skills for All in Australia: Policy Insights from the Survey of Adult Skills. OECD Skills Studies.* Paris: OECD Publishing. https://doi.org/10.1787/9789264281110-en.

Pandit, A.U., Tang, J.W., Bailey, S.C., Davis, T.C., Bocchini, M.V., Persell, S.D., Federman, A.D. & Wolf, M.S. (2009). Education, literacy and health: Mediating effects on hypertension knowledge and control. *Patient Education and Counselling*, 75, 381–5.

Parker, R.M., Baker, D.W., Williams, M.V. & Nurss, J.R. (1995). The test of functional health literacy in adults (TOFHLA): A new instrument for measuring patient's literacy skills. *Journal of General Internal Medicine*, 10, 537–42.

Pirisi, A. (2000). Low health literacy prevents equal access to care. *The Lancet*, 356(9244), 1828.

Safeer, R.S. & Keenan, J. (2005). Health literacy: The gap between physicians and patients. *American Family Physician*, 72(3), 463–8.

Sudore, R.L., Yaffe, K., Satterfield, S., Harris, T.B., Mehta, K.M., Simonsick, E.M. … Schillinger, D. (2006). Limited literacy and mortality in the elderly: The health aging and body composition study. *Journal of General Internal Medicine*, 21(8), 806–12.

UNESCO. *UNESCO Education Sector Position Paper*. Paris: UNESCO. Retrieved from http://unesdoc.unesco.org/images/0013/001362/136246e.pdf.

University of California San Francisco. (2019). Evaluating health information. Retrieved from www.ucsfhealth.org/education/evaluating_health_information.

Visscher, B.B., Steunenberg, B., Heijmans, M., Hofstede, J.M., Deville, W., van der Heide, I. & Rademakers, J. (2018). Evidence on the effectiveness of health literacy interventions in the EU: A systematic review. *BMC Public Health*, 18, 1414.

von Wagner, C., Knight, K., Steptoe, A. & Wardle, J. (2007). Functional health literacy and health promoting behaviour in a national sample of British adults. *Journal of Epidemiology and Community Health*, 61(12), 1086–90.

Wallace, L. (2006). Patients' health literacy skills: The missing demographic variable in primary care research. *Annals of Family Medicine*, 4(1), 85–6.

Weiss, B.D., Mays, M., Martz, W., Castro, K.M., DeWalt, D.A., Pignone, M.P., Mockbee, J. & Hale, F.A. (2005). Quick assessment of literacy in primary care: The newest vital sign. *Annals of Family Medicine*, 3(6), 514–22.

Williams, M.V., Davis, T., Parker, R.M. & Weiss, B.D. (2002). The role of health literacy in patient–physician communication. *Family Medicine*, 34(5), 383–9.

Williams, M.V., Parker, R.M., Baker, D.W., Parikh, N.S., Coates, W.C. & Nurss, J.R. (1995). Inadequate functional health literacy among patients at two public hospitals. *JAMA: Journal of the American Medical Association*, 274(21), 1677–82.

World Health Organization. (2014). *Health Literacy and Health Behaviour*. Geneva: WHO. Retrieved from http://who.int/healthpromotion/conferences/7gchp/track2/en.

CHAPTER 14

ACADEMIC WRITING AND COMMUNICATION SKILLS

JESSICA H. STONE AND MELANIE BIRKS

LEARNING OBJECTIVES

After reading this chapter and completing the activities, you will be able to:

- state the aims and goals of academic writing and communication
- explain the language and components of academic writing and communication
- debate and delineate the differences between academic and other forms of writing and communication
- apply the principles of academic writing to professional development and practice.

KEY TERMS

Academic writing
Argument
Attribution
Contract cheating
Plagiarism
Thesis statement
Three-act structure

Introduction

It is common to hear groans from students when they are faced with the task of writing and presenting an academic paper. It does not seem to matter if the work is an essay on the meaning of life, a report on the popularity of the current government, or the findings of a longitudinal study on the impact of global warming on the mating habits of the common wombat—many writers, students and advanced scholars alike, tremble at the thought of writing an academic paper. Why? Let us examine this concept a little further.

Academic writing Written communication designed for scholarly audiences, with the aim of educating and furthering knowledge.

There is a widely shared misconception that **academic writing** is dry, hard to understand and boring. On the other hand, commercial writing (i.e. for purposes such as business, advertising or entertainment) is often intended to be fun and easy to read. Commercial writing deals with subjects that are either simple or familiar. Students, and even professional academics, sometimes think that because the subject matter of academic writing is often complex and challenging, the writing itself must be complex and highly structured, and therefore must use extremely formal, complicated language. However, this need not be the case.

You will understand from previous chapters that communication is the act of sharing information with others. It sounds simple, but we all know that presenting information, and getting others to understand *what* we are offering, can be anything but simple, especially when the information we want to share is, by its nature, particularly complex and challenging. Fortunately, there are methods and techniques that can strengthen communication across all types of writing. These techniques are available to writers of both academic and non-academic literature.

In this chapter, we discuss the differences between academic and other forms of writing. We examine the important components of academic writing, explore the techniques that lead to strong communication, and discuss how the basic principles of academic writing can be applied to professional development and practice.

Clarity is crucial

Academic writing should be precise, impersonal and objective, and it does require the use of discipline-specific, semi-formal language. However, this writing does not need to be cumbersome or uninteresting. There are significant differences between academic and commercial writing. However, all writing, regardless of its genre (category), shares one common goal: to communicate. If the language used is stiff, overly formal or too complicated, this will hamper communication and, as a result, the writer, the audience and the work will suffer.

Physicians subscribe to the dictum: First, do no harm. These simple words remind medical professionals to honour, respect and put patients first. Writers too, have an oath: First, be clear. The message is the same: honour, respect and put readers first. The most important job—and number one goal—for all writers is to produce clear writing. Clear writing presents material in a way that conveys information correctly. In other words, clear writing *communicates* the message the writer intended. Clear writing is dependent on the following components: purpose, audience, structure, tone, language and voice.

Purpose

A key difference between academic and other forms of writing is the intended purpose of the communication. Often the purpose of commercial communication is to entertain. This may be the case across a number of genres: advertising, plays, films, novels, music, poetry, etc. The primary purpose of academic writing is to contribute to the growth of knowledge, to enhance understanding, and to advance professional growth and development. This applies to all categories of academic communication, including essays, research reports, dissertations and oral presentations. When such writing is being undertaken as part of a program of formal study, a key purpose is to evaluate the student's understanding of a concept or set of concepts. In the process of writing, students develop this understanding through evaluating and presenting both sides of an argument (Listyani 2018). The process of academic writing in such cases is therefore both a means and an end in itself.

There are instances when the purposes of providing entertainment and offering information overlap. For example, an advertisement for laundry soap might be entertaining (funny), informative ('available at supermarkets everywhere') and certainly persuasive ('Buy our soap—it's the bubbliest!'). In the same way, academic communication might offer entertaining, informative and persuasive elements within the same piece of writing. Consider a tutor reading a student's paper; they will be looking to see that the student had met the aims of the assigned writing task, but the process of evaluating that piece of work is made much easier when the writing is clear and engaging. In the same way, a presenter at a professional conference might start a discussion with light humour related to the topic, then present key content in the body of the work, and may end with a persuasive call for additional research efforts. Even with the potential for overlap, the main purpose of academic writing—to inform—helps to shape the work and distinguishes it from commercial communication.

Audience

A significant difference between academic and other forms of writing is the intended audience: the people who will read or attend to a given piece. The audience plays a huge role in guiding the design, structure and production of a piece of writing, whether the writing is commercial or academic. When considering either a reading, viewing or listening audience, writers need to ponder three major questions:

1. Who are the members of the audience?
2. What do the members of the audience expect from the work?
3. What does the writer want the audience to do with the communication?

Who is the audience?

Whether the work is delivered through written, verbal or electronic media, academic communication almost always appeals to a narrow, specific and well-informed audience. Individuals seeking information through academic communication are usually well educated and, much of the time, are either specialists in a given field or students working towards a specialty. These readers often have an advanced understanding of the subject matter, are familiar with the relevant terminology and are aware of at least some of the prevailing literature in the field. Where the work is being submitted for assessment as part of a program of study, the audience will be an academic who fully understands the topic area and its purpose in promoting and evaluating student learning.

Because the audience for academic writing and communication can be narrowly defined, writers may need to focus their work towards the specific informational needs and comprehension levels of that audience. In this way, academic writers are free to use more exacting terminology, refer to complex theories and hone in on important details without fear of 'losing' this particular audience.

Commercial communication appeals to a broad audience (which is why it is sometimes called 'mass communication') whose members vary widely in terms of their comprehension levels. Most such communication today is written for Year 8 to Year 12 comprehension levels. Although writers of commercial literature try to segment audiences into groups by demographics (gender, age, income), the groups will remain large and diverse. Commercial writers are not free to use exacting terminology or to venture into complex themes without the risk of alienating much of this broad and diverse audience. For example, romance novels (boy and girl meet, mess around, break up, get back together) and cosy mysteries (the murder happens behind the scenes) are generally written to appeal to particular audiences (e.g. females, teenagers, adults). Thrillers and war stories, on the other hand, may appeal more to male readers. This is not to say that women do not enjoy a good, fast-paced thriller, or that men do not like to curl up with a cosy novel now and again, but commercial writers, directors and publishers must position their work to appeal to the largest segment of the target mass audience.

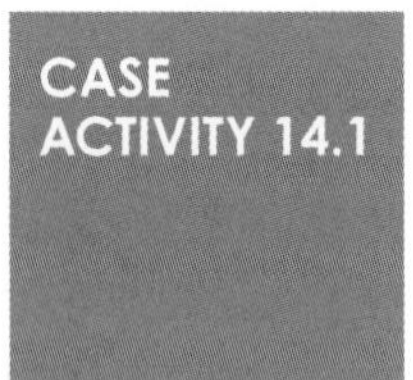

Writing for an audience

Terri is a first year speech pathology student. She has an online blog where she writes short stories with a science fiction theme. Terri has been enrolled in her studies for just a few weeks and is enjoying making new friends and learning new concepts. She is confident that she will do well in her studies because of her skills in writing short stories.

1. What skills in short-story writing will serve Terri well in undertaking academic writing for her studies?
2. What problems might she encounter as she attempts to negotiate writing for a different audience?

What does the audience expect?

Readers of academic writing select pieces of work with the intention of expanding their knowledge of the concepts and theories within a given discipline. They expect a review of the relevant literature and a discussion of the research findings of others within a specific field. In addition, they hope to add to their own body of research and knowledge. The academic audience expects precision, accuracy and an advanced level of sophistication from the writer. This is particularly the case where the audience is reviewing work submitted by a student for assessment. In such cases, the academic has an expectation that the student will achieve a certain standard in respect of specific learning objectives in the context of the broader program of study. Usually, these learning outcomes will inform marking criteria that is used to assess the work produced by the student.

Commercial writing commonly deals with universal humanistic or human nature themes of love, family, crime and death. Audiences of this work do not seek such writing with the express intention of expanding their knowledge. Although films, novels and plays can, and do, educate audiences, the primary expectation of this type of communication is entertainment. Precision, accuracy and sophistication are often not as important as the entertainment value of a piece of commercial work. In these cases, the audience expects a return on the investment of their time and possibly money.

What do you want the audience to do?

Writers, directors and publishers of commercial communication hope that audience members will be entertained and recommend the piece to their friends, colleagues and family—the more, the better. Academic writers anticipate that their readers will use the work to test concepts and theories, to improve performance in a given field, and to advance professional practice and development. Of course, all writers—regardless of genre—hope readers will appreciate their writing, and then share their enthusiasm with others. In the case of work submitted by a student, the hope is that the audience (the person who grades it) will find that the work achieves the goals of the assessment task.

Skills in practice

Expectations of the audience

Suzanne has just received her first assignment back from her tutor. She wasn't happy with her grade. She looked at the feedback provided and disagreed with a number of comments made by her tutor. Suzanne went on to tell her fellow students that the tutor 'didn't know what she was talking about'. She then made comments on the subject online forum about the assessment task, asking whether other students 'had been given the wrong mark' by this tutor.

What's happening here?

Had Suzanne taken the time to reflect on the situation, she may have responded differently. Suzanne should have considered who her audience was, what they expected from her and what she wanted from them. Her audience in this case was her tutor, whose role is to examine the work Suzanne submitted and provide feedback based on established assessment criteria. Suzanne's role is to consider the feedback and use it to improve her writing skills. If she does not agree with the feedback, she has the opportunity to discuss her concerns with the tutor, using communication skills described in earlier chapters. Taking positive steps such as these would help to address the issues. Making disparaging comments about the tutor to her colleagues and online is counterproductive and detracts from the main issue and Suzanne's ability to find a solution to her concerns.

Structure

Structure provides a foundation for writing. Just as a strong foundation stabilises a building, a strong structure grounds written material. Structure helps writers organise the presentation of information. A strong, clear structure gives readers confidence that the material has merit and that the writer is competent. A good structure will be evident to the reader through the logical flow that is apparent in the writing. One of the things that beginning students often struggle with is organising their understanding of how concepts and ideas fit together, and therefore how, and in what order, to best present each point in a way that makes sense to the reader.

Three-act structure Simple format used in academic writing, plays, novels and films. It has an introduction, a body and a conclusion (or summary).

The easiest organisational structure to follow for both writer and reader is the **three-act structure**. This structure has three basic parts: An *introduction* (sometimes known as a set-up); the *body* (where the bulk of the information is offered); and a *conclusion* or *summary* (in works of fiction this section is known as the denouement).

Introduction

The introduction, in all forms of writing, is the writer's opportunity to grab the readers' attention and invite them to stay with the material. In a mystery novel, for instance, the introduction—synonymous with the first act—might present a scenario involving a dead body and ask the big question: Who killed Prince Farthengill? The big question is the essence of a mystery and will by intent, and almost by default, hold readers' interest.

Thesis statement A statement that presents the writer's main idea and primary claim.

In a piece of academic writing, the introduction should funnel the reader into the body of the piece through a broad opening sentence, leading to a narrower and focused description of the topic area, and finish with an overview of what is to follow. The introduction should also contain a statement that presents the writer's main idea and primary claim, such as a single sentence or short paragraph. This is known as a **thesis statement**. The thesis statement provides clear information about the work to follow and, when written with skill, will encourage readers to stay with the piece.

Body

Much as the body—or Act II—of a mystery novel contains the search for clues, potential suspects and motives, the body of an academic paper offers supporting evidence for the writer's primary claim. This supporting evidence is known as the writer's **argument**. Just as a fictional detective collects evidence to make their case, the writers of academic papers collect and organise evidence to convince readers of their claim and their interpretation of the data.

Argument
A collection of evidence that supports the primary idea or claim in a piece of written or oral communication.

In academic writing, the argument is a critical examination and discussion of the evidence about the topic of concern. This critical discussion can be thought of as a debate where all sides of the issue are considered. The job of the writer is to clearly show the reader where they stand on a given topic and convince them that they have considered all other positions. To do this, arguments need to include supporting evidence in the form of primary research undertaken by the writer or from secondary sources that are written by others. These secondary sources can be found in academic journals, policy documents, government reports, books, websites or oral presentations. An important consideration when using these sources is their validity and quality. Sometimes it is easy to identify when evidence is unreliable, but in many cases the onus is on the writer to check the source and evaluate its credibility. Creating a strong argument in favour of the writers' thesis is dependent on the clearly organised presentation of relevant, reputable supporting evidence.

Conclusion

Act III is the conclusion. In the mystery novel, Act III answers the big question posed in the first act (the introduction). In such cases of fiction, it was most likely that the butler did it. In an academic paper, the writer will usually tie all supporting evidence from their argument together in the conclusion. Just as the introduction funnels the reader into the body of the work, the conclusion funnels them out again. Bartley (2016) uses the metaphor of a journey over a mountain when talking about structuring an academic paper She suggests that the reader needs to be given information about where they are going (the introduction), an effective route to a comprehensive understanding of the concepts being discussed (the body) and a way back down the mountain (the conclusion). A standard conclusion usually involves restating what has been done, revisiting the thesis statement and finishing with a broad statement that positions the work in the broader context of the evidence. Bartley (2016), however, suggests that rather than looking backwards, the conclusion is an opportunity to send the reader on their way with a new understanding of the concepts discussed in the work. While the writer should avoid introducing new material at this late stage (imagine how frustrating it would be in a mystery novel to have a viable suspect introduced in the conclusion), it is possible to use the conclusion to directly question a reader about their thoughts on a given issue, or ask them to consider the implications for their own practice.

Again, while there are several organisational structures available to academic writers, the three-act structure is one of the easiest to use and to understand. This ease of use and familiarity makes the three-act structure an excellent choice when preparing almost any kind of scholarly communication.

Reflect and apply

Obtain a piece of academic writing such as a journal article. Can you clearly identify the thesis statement, introduction, body and conclusion? Is the article written logically? Does the writer present a clear and convincing argument?

Tone, language and voice

Tone

The creepy music in a horror movie conveys to the audience a warning that something bad is about to happen. Much like that music, the tone of a piece of written communication gives readers a sense of the subject matter and genre of the work. When the subject matter is meant to appeal to a wide audience, for example, the tone is generally relaxed. Commercial writers use conversational language, colloquial or familiar expressions and stereotypes to set scenes and time frames. These writers are free to abbreviate words and use slang or dialect. Writers of commercial communication are also free to include their own opinions, experiences and biases in their work. All of these elements make up the general tone or feel of the work—for example, whether it is friendly and warm, or serious and cold, questioning, or perhaps attacking and confrontational.

Academic writing should convey a serious tone that says: This work is intended to inform and convince'. Scholarly material is presented in an impersonal and objective manner. The personal opinions and biases of the author should not be apparent and the language is semi-formal and exacting. However, impersonal and objective writing does not have to be dull, stuffy or cold. And semi-formal language does not have to be convoluted or obtuse. Again, clear writing leads to clear communication, and clear communication should be the key goal of all writers.

Language

The language of commercial writing, particularly fiction, can be fanciful and imaginative. Literary devices such as the use of metaphor or simile are intended to enhance the scene that is being created by the writer. For example, it is reasonable for a writer of fiction to describe the moon as a 'glowing tangerine tossed against a velvet cloth'. In contrast, the language used in academic writing must be exact, precise and reliably measurable. In other words, the language selected for academic communication—whether written or spoken—needs to clearly say exactly what it is intended to mean. The tools available for use in commercial writing such onomatopoeia (words that describe sounds), slant (imperfect) rhyme and alliteration (words that start with the same sound) are not appropriate for academic writing.

Academic writers also need to be mindful of precision and accuracy in their work. Precision refers to the use of correct terminology and exacting word choice. These writers need to pay close attention not only to the words used in a paper, but also to how the words are used. It is not enough to say, for example, 'The water cooled'. A more precise sentence might read, 'The water cooled to 4.44°C'. Thus academic writers must pay close attention to the correct presentation of facts, quotes, statistics and other data. Numbers, dates, times and measurements should be triple-checked before the work is finally submitted for review or publication. Commercial writers are free to play around or be loose with their words and even with their statistics. The sentence, 'He was surrounded by thousands of beautiful women', would be fine in a spy novel. In an academic paper, however, readers need to know exactly how many women and exactly what 'beautiful' means.

Voice

Academic writers have traditionally tended to use a formal voice to make their work sound more objective and scholarly. Examples of how this is done include using third person and passive voice (Hyland & Jiang 2017). Third person refers to language that describes situations from the perspective of an observer and so tends to use personal pronouns like 'he', 'she' and 'they', whereas first person uses pronouns such as 'I' and 'we'. Third person is distinct from writing in the first person, as the latter speaks from the perspective of the individual who is writing the story or academic paper.

Passive voice occurs when the thing acted upon (the receiver of an action) forms the subject of a sentence. For example, 'the rock is thrown'. In active voice, the actor who performs the action becomes the subject of the sentence: 'The boy throws the rock.' Notice how much stronger and more forceful the words sound in an active voice.

While using third person and the passive voice may appear to be formal, it also results in writing that sounds weak and lacks authority. Hyland and Jiang (2017) suggest that using less formal writing styles, such as first person and the active voice, enhances engagement and relationships with readers. Ultimately, writing in this way intentionally makes for communication that is more convincing and more credible.

Skills in practice

Tone, language and voice

Let's look at how tone, language and voice can be used to change the impact of a piece of writing.

Example 1

A major problem facing healthcare providers in the current climate is the cost of healthcare. The literature suggests that these costs are escalating at a significant rate. The implications for individual healthcare professionals and clients are potentially significant. Health economists and policymakers are encouraged to consider the hidden costs associated with inadequate resourcing.

Example 2

It's absolutely unacceptable. Whoever is making these funding decisions should be ashamed. Even beginning healthcare professionals like me can see that the cost of poor care goes beyond the financial. And it's just getting worse. How can we be expected to provide quality care under these conditions? The people responsible need to take a good hard look at themselves.

What's happening here?

We can see that the first example is more formally written and suggests that the writer has an understanding of the evidence underlying the issue being discussed. The second example is more emotive and intended to produce an emotional response in the reader. Perhaps the ideal narrative lies somewhere in between these two examples. It is possible to use engaging language while still presenting an argument underpinned by evidence.

Reflect and apply

Which of the two examples described in the 'Skills in practice' feature is better? Consider how the readers might react differently to each example. What is the writer expecting the reader do in each case?

Try to rewrite the message above to capture the best elements of both approaches.

Attribution

Attribution
The practice of giving full credit to the author or source of work cited in a piece of academic writing.

Attribution, the practice of giving full credit to the source of a work cited within a piece of writing, is another key difference between academic and commercial writing. Other than attributing a direct quote to its author, writers of commercial work—especially fiction—are freer to borrow from the ideas of other writers without acknowledging or giving full credit to the source. In academic writing, regardless of its purpose, this is *never* the case. Scholars must be scrupulous about citing the work of other writers and must never submit work that is not original as their own and without indicating the source. In addition, the method or style used to cite work must follow discipline-specific referencing and citation guidelines.

There are several major style guides to choose from when citing sources within an academic paper. Style guides vary between disciplines, so writers will need to learn which guides are acceptable within their field. Popular style guides used in academic writing include the following:

- *The Publication Manual of the American Psychological Association* (American Psychological Association (APA); see https://apastyle.apa.org/manual)
- *The Harvard Citation Style Guide* (numerous versions online; e.g. see https://libguides.jcu.edu.au/harvard)
- *The MLA Handbook for Writers of Research Papers* (Modern Language Association; see https://style.mla.org)
- *Chicago Manual of Style* (University of Chicago Press; see www.chicagomanualofstyle.org/home.html)
- *Scientific Style and Format: The CSE Manual for Authors, Editors, and Publishers* (Council of Science Editors; see www.scientificstyleandformat.org/Home.html).

Reflect and apply

Consider the style guide used in your field of study or practice. How familiar are you with the style? What resources (e.g. online manuals or library guides) or bibliographic tools (e.g. Endnote®) are available to assist you with managing referencing of your work?

Plagiarism and contract cheating

Plagiarism
Using someone else's writing without attribution or permission; stealing intellectual property.

Plagiarism is the act of using another's writing as if it were your own—that is, using another's ideas, words, concepts or data without giving full credit where it is due. Plagiarism is a form of stealing. Writers of commercial communication will most likely be sued if they steal from another writer. Again, ideas and themes are fair game to commercial writers, but using material verbatim is against the law. You may be familiar with cases of copyright infringement in respect of music. Plagiarism is the scholarly equivalent of this type of breach and is considered a very serious transgression in academia.

Academic writers who are still studying stand to be suspended or expelled from university if they plagiarise another's work. Scholarly writers working in the field stand to lose their academic standing and positions for the act of plagiarising, and will severely tarnish their professional reputations. It is quite easy to avoid the penalties associated with plagiarism. Writers simply need to do their own work and give proper credit to the source when using the work of another scholar. In fact, using the work of others to support your ideas and arguments is expected in academic writing. Referencing your own writing shows that you have undertaken research and have considered all the different points of view in respect of a particular topic, and are therefore well informed about all sides of the argument. Only then can you present a well-considered, critical discussion about a topic.

Contract cheating Soliciting the services of another person or organisation to prepare an assessment task that is submitted for grading.

Universities globally are becoming increasingly concerned about the trend towards plagiarism and other forms of cheating involving copying from online sources or purchasing assignments from online essay writing services. This latter activity is known as **contract cheating**. As academics, we often become aware of students engaging others to prepare an assessment task for them to submit as their own. In some parts of the world, this practice is illegal; certainly it is at all times immoral.

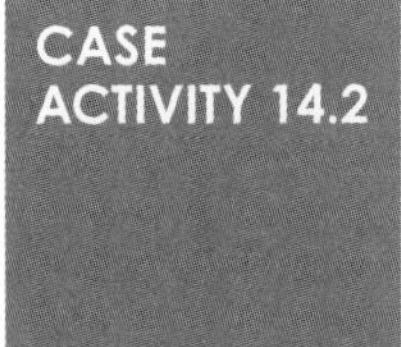

Contract cheating

Terri is struggling to keep on top of her study load. She is working part-time as a carer at a residential aged care facility and needs to find a new apartment to live in as her lease is ending. Terri has received an unsolicited email from an essay writing service. She has a paper to write for a subject that she doesn't think is really important to her future career as a speech pathologist. Terri knows of a few other students that have bought assignments in the past and wonders whether it would be okay to buy her assignment 'just this once'.

1. If you were to speak to Terri about her temptation to buy this assignment, what advice would you give her?
2. Consider how you might use the skills you acquired in Part 1 of this text to encourage Terri to reflect on this situation and to support her to manage her current circumstances.
3. What other action might you take?

It is particularly alarming that students within the healthcare professions would engage in cheating, given the trust that is placed in them by the public. Of particular concern is that cheating in the academic setting has been found to indicate a tendency for a student to also engage in misconduct in the practice setting (Birks et al. 2018).

Grammar, spelling and punctuation

Grammar, spelling and punctuation are fundamental components of language. Spelling and punctuation apply only to the written word, while grammar refers to the correct use of words in both written and spoken language. Even though grammar, spelling and punctuation are separate components of language, they each serve to make its meaning clear. These three components play critical roles in communication.

Grammar

As mentioned, grammar plays a key role in making the meaning of a message clear, which in turn leads to clear communication. But there are other reasons why writers need to pay particular attention to the use of correct grammar. First, good grammar shows a respect for both readers and listeners. Remember the writer's oath? First, be clear. Poor grammar makes text and the spoken word confusing. Double negatives, for example, are puzzling and make readers pause, shake their heads and reread. Two negatives result in a positive, so when faced with a double negative, readers are unnecessarily interrupted and have to work out what the writer is really trying to say.

Consider, for example, this line from a Pink Floyd song: 'We don't need no education.' Lalwani (2011) explains, 'The emphasis is on the fact that no education is necessary. In literal terms the line means that *we do* need some education'. The same holds true for lines such as, 'I can't get no sleep' by Faithless, and 'I can't get no satisfaction' by the Rolling Stones. Rock stars might be able to get away with double negatives, but academic writers should avoid them, as well as avoiding any other grammatical errors that might confuse their readers or audience.

Another argument for the use of good grammar is that where grammar is of poor quality, it brings into question the quality of the work overall. When a writer is trying to make a case through a written piece, poor grammar can suggest deficits in the background research that underpins that work. For students attempting to get a good grade on an assessment task, this may not end well. Criteria that guides the grading of such work almost always assigns marks to fundamental communication issues of style and presentation, including grammar.

Poor grammar signals a lack of sophistication on the part of the writer and demonstrates a lack of respect for the reader. For experienced writers, poor grammar can be a barrier to publication. Although agents, publishers and review boards understand that all writing—commercial and academic—will undergo revision, they are sure to reject writing that is riddled with grammatical errors. Even a great story or a stunning piece of research might be regarded as unacceptable because of grammatical errors in the writing. The most compelling argument for the importance of correct grammar is that, regardless of one's position in life, the use of poor grammar makes the speaker, or writer, sound ignorant (Begala 2000). In academic writing, this is the antithesis of what the writer is trying to achieve.

BOX 14.1

GRAMMAR

Yet another advantage of using good grammar: it helps get dates. What? Yes, good grammar can lead to more dates. Match.com, one of the world's largest online dating sites, encourages its users to use spelling and grammar checkers before posting their profiles because many users filter their choices by the posted language. Use of good grammar, spelling and punctuation in a profile respects the reader and shows an appealing level of education and sophistication. In fact, Match.com even warns its users to, 'Be aware of anyone who makes an inordinate amount of grammar and/or spelling errors' (Match.com 2015).

Spelling

Spelling is the forming of words from letters according to accepted usage. With the advent of spellcheckers, texting and social media, the use of proper spelling has become controversial. Readers understand text messages when words contain only half of their letters. Spellcheckers change words, and words are shortened to stay within the character restrictions of sites like Twitter. Commercial writers increasingly use phonetic spelling when writing dialogue in an attempt to make characters sound authentic. With all these changes, why should academic writers care about spelling words correctly?

The answer has everything to do with the differences between academic and commercial writing. Academic writing must be clear, accurate and precise. Such writing is written for highly educated and well-informed audiences that seek information and advancement in their fields or disciplines. While the use of slang and phonetic spelling may be acceptable as commercial writing meant for a mass audience, academic writing uses a semi-formal tone with the primary intent to inform, not entertain.

Spelling errors signal that a writer is either too lazy or too disinterested to care about the precision of the communication. As is the case with poor grammar, this may indicate the writer's lack of interest in the subject matter and may call into question the accuracy of the research undertaken to support any assertions made. Students who submit academic papers filled with spelling errors and shortened words are likely to be penalised accordingly as, once again, prescribed grading criteria will usually include reference to spelling. Work submitted by experienced writers for publication will not make it past an editorial review board and will certainly not be published if the writer has not bothered to address fundamental errors in spelling. Most importantly, correct spelling leads to clear communication. While commercial communication may be left open to artistic interpretation, writing intended for professional development or advancement requires clarity.

Punctuation

Punctuation is the use of symbols to organise and structure text. Without correct punctuation, communication can, and does, get very confusing. As we have discussed, poor grammar gives the impression that the writer lacks sophistication and education, and poor spelling makes the writer appear lazy or disinterested in their work. But incorrect punctuation can lead to severe misunderstandings that, in research papers and other academic writing, could have serious repercussions. A single misplaced comma or full stop can change the meaning of an entire message. When writing for academic purposes, whether as a student or a professional, consider the consequences of poor punctuation getting in the way of the point being made. For a student, the outcome could be less marks, but for a professional, the entire thesis of the paper could be lost.

Reflect and apply

Read the two 'Dear John' letters below, and note how punctuation changes the entire meaning of the messages (Moore 2015).

Letter 1

Dear John,

I want a man who knows what love is all about. You are generous, kind, thoughtful. People who are not like you admit to being useless and inferior. You have ruined me for other men. I yearn for you. I have no feelings whatsoever when we're apart. I can be forever happy—will you let me be yours?

Jane

Letter 2

Dear John,

I want a man who knows what love is. All about you are generous, kind, thoughtful people, who are not like you. Admit to being useless and inferior. You have ruined me. For other men, I yearn. For you, I have no feeling whatsoever. When we're apart, I can be forever happy. Will you let me be?

Yours,

Jane

Write two letters to the CEO of the local healthcare provider asking for permission to undertake a field excursion in their facility. Use the same words but use different punctuation to obtain completely different effects. Discuss the impact your letters might have on your professional development.

Revision and editing

There are two more important steps to complete before an academic writer can be confident about presenting a scholarly paper or a formal presentation. The first step is revision, and the second is editing. Some academic writers start with editing and move on to revision. Still others edit and revise simultaneously. It does not matter which method is selected; the key is that each piece of written work should be carefully revised and thoroughly edited before presentation or submission.

Revision

While revising a piece of writing, a writer reads along looking for flow, tone and use of language. Most professional writers read their work out loud to listen for the words that bump into each other or the lines that don't make sense. Some writers read from the conclusion to the introduction when revising. Reading in reverse order changes things around enough to prevent the writer from reading so quickly that errors are missed. These are tips that beginning writers can also employ to assist in revision of their work.

Most commercial writers, like novelists and memoirists, employ copyeditors to assist with revision work. These editors look for story, continuity and flow. They look for places where language goes astray. The equivalent of a copyeditor for an academic writer might be a trusted colleague working in the same or similar discipline. A copyeditor working with scholarly material should have a familiarity with the topic, the research methodology (when necessary) and, if possible, the larger body of related work. This editor should be able to assist the writer in discovering gaps in the work, either in the writing or in the research itself. Having said this, often a lay person (friend of family member) can offer a fresh perspective on a piece of work and often picks up issues that might otherwise be overlooked by others who are immersed in the subject matter itself.

Students, on the other hand, need to do their own revision. Not only do they often lack the resources to engage a professional editor, they are required to produce original work when preparing an assessment task. The time invested in this process is not wasted, however, as it provides an opportunity to develop skills in revision and refinement that enhance the quality of writing and promote efficiency in the production of future work.

Editing

Revision and editing differ slightly. Revision looks at the whole picture—the forest, if you will. Editing examines the individual letters in a word, tests every punctuation mark, sounds out each phrase, and searches for grammatical errors. Editing looks at the trees in the forest. Editing is important to address all of the potential issues we have discussed in the preceding sections of this chapter. It can ensure that spelling and grammar are correct, and that punctuation is used effectively in service of the thesis or work being presented.

Often professional writers will engage editorial services, and graduates may employ editors to review large pieces of work such as a dissertation. While this practice is acceptable and often necessary, when a writer has skills in editing it promotes quality and control throughout the process. Developing skills in editing your own work is therefore important, particularly given the significance of written communication in everyday life.

Oral presentations

Scholars from all disciplines—from palaeontology to art history—will, at some point in their careers, need to give an oral presentation of their work. Presentations may be offered at seminars, professional conferences, meetings with colleagues and fundraisers. University students are frequently asked to show their work to teachers and classmates through oral presentations.

Public speaking can be a frightening experience for even the most sophisticated communicators. However, there are a few things to keep in mind, and a few simple tasks that will make the experience more pleasant—or at least tolerable—for you, the speaker, as well as more enjoyable for your audience. These methods include knowing your thesis, understanding your audience and presenting a clear argument. We have already looked at these as they relate to written academic communication; now we will apply them to oral presentations.

The first step towards offering a clear and interesting oral presentation is to know your material—to *really* know your material. This does not mean memorising what you are going to say; it means knowing and understanding your material so well that you could give your speech to friends while relaxing over a coffee. Become so comfortable and familiar with your material that you do not need to refer to notes. The best way to know your material—that is, your thesis, the case you are making—is to practise. Practise your speech while walking to class, while driving, while taking a shower. Give your speech to the family dog 50 times. Dogs are forgiving; they won't mind.

Next, consider your audience. What are the expectations of your audience? What do they hope to gain from listening to your presentation? What do you hope they will take away from your presentation, and what do you hope they will do with the communication you have offered? The answers to these questions will help you decide on the tone and language to use in your presentation.

CASE ACTIVITY 14.3

Oral presentations

Terri has to give a presentation to her fellow students on the topic 'Communicating with children' as part of the assessment for her first year Human Development subject.

1. What does she know about her audience that may help her to prepare for this session?
2. How might this information influence the content, tone and style of her presentation?
3. What are the potential pitfalls in presenting to this audience?

When preparing an oral presentation, start by creating a written outline of the material you wish to present. Break your outline into three parts, in much the same way you organise your written communication. Include an introduction, body and conclusion. An easy way to think about the three-act structure in terms of oral communication is to follow these steps:

1. Say what you are going to say.
2. Say it.
3. Say what you have said.

Your introduction should capture and hold the attention of your audience. Use topic-related humour, startling statistics, interesting anecdotes or thought-provoking questions to engage your audience. Then, clearly tell your audience what you intend to share with them. In other words, present your thesis statement, tell your audience that you will offer supporting evidence, and that you will conclude with what you want them to take away from the presentation. There are many different things audience members might take away from a presentation, including a greater understanding of concepts, new methods of dealing with issues, new directions for study and an interest in supporting further research.

Similar to the organisation of written academic communication, the body of an oral presentation should include compelling evidence to support your argument. However, unlike written communication, oral presentations are offered in short time frames and audience attention must be maintained throughout.

An excellent way to support your argument in an oral presentation—and hold the interest of your audience—is to offer three or so key points of information. You may actually have eight or 12 points of evidence to support your argument and, while these can be shared in a piece of written communication, they will overwhelm and confuse a listening audience. Stick to a few main points.

Finally, offer your conclusion by restating your thesis, recapping and summing up your supporting evidence by asking for something from your audience, and by thanking your audience for their attention. Requests can be as simple as asking the audience to continue to think about the material you have presented, or as complex as inviting the audience to expand the concepts and discoveries through continuing research. Making a request of audience members plants a seed about your thesis that will grow long after the microphone is turned off.

In terms of the practicalities of presenting, there are a few things you can do to ensure the process goes well:

- Where possible, familiarise yourself with the layout of the room where the session will be held.
- Ensure the audio-visual equipment you need is available, and that you know how to use it.
- If using presentation software, don't overload your slides; apply the 6x6 rule—no more than six lines and no more than six words per line on a slide

- use graphics to add emphasis, variety and, where appropriate, humour
- if confident, involve the audience through questioning or inviting comments; an active audience will be much more engaged in your presentation.

Reflect and apply

Reflect on a scholarly presentation you have seen recently, or review an example on an online videosharing platform. Review the suggestions for oral presentations discussed in this section. Which of these guidelines did the presenter adhere to? What were the major strengths of the presentation? Did you pick up any more tips for giving effective oral presentations?

Conclusion

In this chapter we have discussed the aims and goals of academic writing, explained the language and components of scholarly communication, delineated the differences between academic and commercial communication, and shown how the principles of academic writing relate to professional development and practice. You can continue your exploration of these important components of academic writing and communication by reading the work of other scholars, and by considering how successful each writer is in terms of communicating clearly. It is now up to you, as an academic writer, to apply these components to your own work. Most of all, it is up to you to continue to explore, to keep writing and to embrace the writer's oath: First, be clear.

SUMMARY POINTS

- Communication is the act of sharing information with others.
- The number one job for all writers is to produce clear writing.
- In order for writers to write clearly, they must first know the purpose of the writing—their reason for writing the piece.
- Academic and commercial writing differ in purpose. The primary purpose of commercial writing is to entertain. The primary purpose of academic writing is to inform.
- Structure provides a platform for clear writing. The three-act structure is the easiest structure to follow for both writer and reader. The three-act structure offers an introduction, which sets up the piece, a body where the bulk of the information is presented, and a summary where conclusions are drawn and clearly stated.
- Academic writers must offer a thesis statement and an argument. The thesis statement presents the writer's primary claim and main idea. The argument offers evidence that supports that claim and idea.

- The use of correct grammar, spelling and punctuation ensures that a writer's message is received and prevents the impression that the writer is lazy or unsophisticated.
- Writers are often required to give an oral presentation of their work. As with written presentations, oral presentations require the presenter to know their work and their audience, and develop an effective strategy to get their message across.
- Revision and editing is a critical process in ensuring the quality of all writing.

CRITICAL THINKING QUESTIONS

1. Students of practice-based professions often question why they need to develop skills in academic writing. Consider the many occasions where a healthcare professional would benefit from being able to present a sophisticated, clear and logical argument. In particular, think about how such skills would benefit the recipients of their services, both directly and indirectly.
2. As you travel to and from university, make a mental note of the various billboards, public posters and names of shops on view. How many of them contain spelling or punctuation errors?

Group activity

Academic writing and communication skills

In your study groups or via your subject discussion site, discuss the significance of academic writing and communication skills to your specific discipline. What aspects of that professional role would be most dependent on these skills? What are the consequences of poor academic writing and communication?

WEBLINKS

Academic writing

Harvard College Writing Center:
http://writingcenter.fas.harvard.edu/pages/resources

The Purdue Writing Lab:
https://owl.english.purdue.edu

University of Sydney: Writing:
https://sydney.edu.au/students/writing.html

Plagiarism and contract cheating

Contract cheating and assessment design:
https://cheatingandassessment.edu.au

Turn It In: Education with Integrity:
www.turnitin.com

Oral presentations

6 tips for giving a fabulous academic presentation (Wiley Network): www.wiley.com/network/researchers/promoting-your-article/6-tips-for-giving-a-fabulous-academic-presentation

Structuring a presentation (University of Leicester): www2.le.ac.uk/offices/ld/resources/presentations/structuring-presentation

REFERENCES

Bartley, A. (2016). Academic writing as a journey. *Teaching English in the Two Year College*, 44(2), 199–200.

Begala, P. (2000). *Is Our Children Learning—The Case against George W. Bush*. New York: Simon & Schuster.

Birks, M., Smithson, J., Antney, J., Zhao, L. & Burkot, C. (2018). Exploring the paradox: A cross-sectional study of academic dishonesty among Australian nursing students. *Nurse Education Today*, 65, 96–101.

Hyland, K. & Jiang, F. (2017). Is academic writing becoming more informal? *English for Specific Purposes*, 45, 40–51. doi:10.1016/j.esp.2016.09.001.

Lalwani, P. (2011). Double negatives buzzle. Retrieved from http://buzzle.com/articles/double-negative-examples.html.

Listyani (2018). Promoting academic writing students' skills through 'process writing strategy'. *Advances in Language and Literary Studies*, 9(4), 173–9.

Match.com. (2015). *Good Advice: Safety Tips to Follow*. Retrieved from www.match.com/help/safetytips.aspx.

Moore, S. (2015). A humorous look at the importance of punctuation. Retrieved from www.vappingo.com/word-blog/the-importance-of-punctuation.

CHAPTER 15
DIGITAL COMMUNICATION

NICHOLAS RALPH AND MELANIE BIRKS

LEARNING OBJECTIVES

After reading this chapter and completing the activities, you will be able to:

- discuss the role and impact of electronic forms of communication in the healthcare environment
- explore strategies for managing electronic communication in the healthcare environment
- outline the emerging role of social media in healthcare
- identify and explore contemporary issues with electronic communication in healthcare
- engage professionally when using electronic forms of communication.

KEY TERMS

Alarm fatigue
E-health
Electronic communication
Telehealth

Introduction

The 'digital age' (or 'electronic age') is an expression used to describe the increasing presence of digital technologies in society. The term *digital* refers to the way in which data are expressed on devices to enable a meaningful interface between a machine and its user. For instance, a series of digits such as 0s and 1s may translate to letters, numbers or algorithms that tell a digital device (such as a computer) to do something. Although these digits are nonsensical to the untrained eye, their conversion from digital sequences into everyday language in emails, text messages, pagers, web pages and software programs and the like enable us to work with digital or electronic forms of communication.

Electronic forms of communication have infiltrated nearly every facet of modern society. Devices such as the personal computer (PC) and the smartphone have revolutionised how machines can connect us to the world, resulting in constantly evolving ways in which we communicate. For instance, while **electronic communication** in the social context revolved around early forms of web-based social media such as Facebook, younger technologies are more mobile-orientated with applications (apps) such as Twitter (messaging service) and Instagram (image-sharing application) becoming increasingly prevalent. While these technologies have rapidly engaged users across the world, more formal settings such as healthcare have been slower to employ newer forms of communication (and in some contexts, any form of electronic communication). Although this might lead to the conclusion that healthcare is averse to the adoption of new technology, such a concept could not be further from the truth. Few fields outside healthcare have taken advantage of the technology of new life-saving or life-changing devices such as the cardiac pacemaker, the Cochlear implant and diagnostic medical imaging. Where many technologies fall down in healthcare is at the point of communicating electronically. Healthcare, by nature, is a human-oriented system; it depends on strong interpersonal communication, whether clinicians or patients are involved. For many in the healthcare professions, electronic communication is seen as an impediment to the delivery of patient care, rather than a means of enhancing it.

Electronic communication Communication transmitted via an electronic processor—for example, telephone, fax machine, computer, smartphone, notebook, palmtop; includes data, text, images and video.

In this chapter, we explore ways of working with electronic forms of communication in healthcare settings. We address commonly used forms of electronic communication and how they can be used professionally and meaningfully in delivering quality patient care.

What is electronic communication?

It is appropriate that electronic communication should be defined first. Such is the influence of electronic communication that it now touches almost every part of daily life. When data, text, images or speech are transmitted by wire, cable or wireless connection, it is defined as a form of electronic communication (Australian Law Reform Commission 2006). This definition means that electronic forms of communication encompass a huge array of devices—landlines, computers, smartphones, pagers, fax machines—as well as a plethora of ways to communicate—

for example, data, text, images, speech and video. Relatively recent technologies such as MMS (Multimedia Messaging Service), Twitter, Facebook and YouTube have added further layers of complexity to electronic communication, as a single message can be sent via multiple forms of media.

The general trend of electronic communication is to elicit greater user engagement and interaction with transmitted content, whether as part of a conversation or with created online content. Although the idea of interacting with other people is an inherent aspect of communication, the way that electronic communication has heralded new forms of large-scale, instantaneous, internationalised communications in coordinated ways is unprecedented. For these reasons, communicating electronically is a tremendous benefit to society, as it has connected people with information or content that they previously had difficulty accessing, or could not access at all.

Who uses electronic communication?

Home internet connection rates are high in both Australia (86%) and New Zealand (80%) (Australian Bureau of Statistics 2018; InternetNZ 2017). Electronic communication is similarly used in other developed countries across the globe. Despite broad and increasing uptake of electronic communication, healthcare has been slow to employ it, being one of the last areas to be disrupted by the digital revolution impacting industries across the globe (Hambleton & Aloizos 2019).

However, in most healthcare contexts, clinicians regularly engage with a number of electronic or digital interfaces that are commonly used to communicate with other healthcare professionals, patients and the community. Email, web browsing and software programs are the most frequently used forms of electronic communication, yet increasingly there is an emphasis on employing new forms of communication to facilitate the delivery of quality healthcare. Progressively, initiatives such as electronic health records, wireless patient monitoring and **telehealth** are being adopted in the healthcare sector as technology advances and the need to improve time and cost efficiencies increases. Until recently, the high cost and difficulty of implementing broad-scale communicative technologies has hindered the uptake of electronic communication in healthcare.

Telehealth
Health-related services or information delivered electronically from or between healthcare professionals.

Why use electronic communication?

Communicating electronically has become such a dominant way of sending and receiving information that it has drastically changed the way humans interact with each other. The ease with which transmissions are made across a range of simple-to-use devices has driven the proliferation of electronic communication, along with the connecting networks needed to drive it. In 2017 on one telecommunications network alone, 308 text messages were sent per second in Australia (McIntosh 2019). This statistic (which does not include messaging apps) illustrates how deeply electronic communication has penetrated the fabric of society and shaped the connections people make with each other using technology.

Human beings have always endeavoured to communicate efficiently, whether through Aboriginal rock art, Native American smoke signals, town criers, the invention of the printing press, or the discovery of the first broad-based electronic communication: telegraphy (Table 15.1). However, it was not until the establishment of the internet in the public domain that efficient, instantaneous and international electronic communication became a possibility.

TABLE 15.1 Key developments in communication

Pre-3500 BCE	Indigenous paintings communicated cultural information
3500 BCE	Development of cuneiform and hieroglyphic writing in the Middle East
1600 BCE	Phoenicians develop an alphabet
105 CE	Paper is invented in China
1450	Johannes Gutenberg builds a printing press in Germany
1831	The electric telegraph is invented
1876	Use of the first electric telephone, in Boston, United States
1925	First television signal is broadcast in the United Kingdom
1957	First communications satellite launched into space: *Sputnik 1*
1969	ARPANET, the ancestor of the internet, is established
1972	Electronic mail or 'email' is developed
1973	The first handheld mobile phone is demonstrated by Motorola
1989	A prototype of the World Wide Web is built
1992	The first SMS (text message) is sent
2004	Facebook is launched
2006	Twitter is founded
2007	Dropbox is established
2012	Pinterest becomes the third-largest social network
2013	LinkedIn reports over 300 million users across the globe
2016	Smartphone ownership equals 63% of the global population
2019	Facebook reports 2.41 billion users worldwide

People embrace technology because it is efficient, immediate, broad-reaching, easy to use and cost-effective. It enables people to select a device and target an information transmission in order to enhance the quality of electronic communication. As personal use of technology increases throughout the world, there appears to be an increasing tendency to harness it for professional reasons. Although the reasons why electronic communication is gradually permeating the professional environment are complex, its instantaneousness and traceability bring efficiency and accountability to the professional environment. It also connects professionals who may be separated geographically. For instance, some surgeons may operate on a patient under the guidance or advice of a colleague watching the procedure thousands of kilometres away on video teleconferencing. Communicating via electronic media will become increasingly common, and it shows how connecting with others electronically can facilitate immediacy, efficacy and safety in professional contexts.

Reflect and apply

List all of the ways in which you communicate electronically. Identify each device you use, and complete this table to show how you predominantly use it.

Type of device	Who do you contact with it? (e.g. friends/family/lecturer)	Communication type (e.g. professional/social)

What are the risks of using a single device across several contexts to communicate with people? Which form of electronic communication do you use the most? How do you use it, and with whom do you communicate?

Brainstorm ideas for how electronic communication could be used in the healthcare setting. Identify at least three uses where the technology you have selected could facilitate the delivery of care.

Electronic forms of communication have been gradually implemented globally across most developed healthcare systems. As the technological literacy of the healthcare workforce improves, the possibilities of developing healthcare initiatives, designed to improve the delivery of care through electronic communications, is becoming an increasingly researched subject area. Many of these technologies are classified under the banner of **e-health**, which involves technologies that use electronic means—hence the 'e' in 'e-health'—to facilitate the delivery of healthcare. The term 'e-health' can be used to encompass every conceivable technology that is supported by electronic means. Alternatively, a more targeted definition can be applied to denote approaches to healthcare over the internet. However, defining e-health is of less importance than evaluating the benefits and potential pitfalls that electronic communication can bring to healthcare. Examples of several key studies across different forms of electronic communication are discussed below.

E-health
Technologies that use electronic means to facilitate the delivery of healthcare.

E-health initiatives

The healthcare environment is increasingly characterised by the influx of electronic communications technology as healthcare professionals work towards becoming more efficient and improving safety. The various types of technology used are extensive. However, some forms of electronic communication, such as electronic health records (EHRs), are becoming more commonplace in healthcare. Allen-Graham et al. (2018) used adverse drug events as a measure of completeness and consistency through an audit of 200 patient records. These authors found that electronic records were used to varying degrees in the five studied institutions, resulting in similar variations in the quality and quantity of data captured. This research suggests that, used correctly, EHRs can be a valuable asset in the provision of safe, quality healthcare.

While the outcomes of technology such as EHRs will depend on how well it is used, the impact of other forms of electronic communication such as telehealth is better understood. Telehealth has particular application in regional and remote areas where access to specialist healthcare professionals may be limited. Cottrell and colleagues (2019) used a retrospective audit to compare telehealth models of advanced physiotherapy care with fly-in, fly-out services. These authors found that the telehealth model resulted in cost savings while not impacting the quality of service delivery.

Aside from benefiting the delivery of patient care, electronic communications technology has also been found to benefit collaborative practice among healthcare professionals. Rankin, Truskey and Chisolm (2019) undertook a systematic review of the use of social media in interprofessional education (IPE). These authors found that existing literature suggested that blogs, wikis and virtual reality platforms had a positive impact on students and recommended expanding the use of social media to promote collaborative learning. While the usefulness of social media to healthcare professionals is well established, its value in educating patients is also gaining traction. Attai and colleagues (2015), in a pilot study, demonstrated that Twitter was a useful medium for increasing knowledge and reducing anxiety among breast cancer patients.

CASE ACTIVITY 15.1

Social media in patient education

Jacob is a registered healthcare practitioner at a large general practice clinic in a rural town with a population of 2500. The clinic is about to launch a drive to improve influenza immunisation rates to 60 per cent within the community, and is unsure whether the use of electronic communication will be effective. Jacob is undertaking further education to broaden his scope of practice and decides to commence a project with a researcher at a nearby regional university to realise the clinic's goal of improving influenza immunisation rates. A recent local census recorded the email addresses of 45 per cent of its citizens and the town has a Facebook page that 2200 people 'like'. Jacob knows that the local high school has experienced some recent success on social media in relation to reducing harmful drinking behaviours among students, by using Twitter messages. However, Jacob is not sure about what approach to use. Conduct a review of the literature to assist in responding to the following questions.

1. What are the advantages and disadvantages of using Facebook and Twitter to achieve the desired immunisation rates?
2. What challenges might Jacob face in using social media for this purpose?
3. What strategies could Jacob employ to address these challenges?

Despite early receptiveness to social media among healthcare professionals and consumers, surprisingly little research has been conducted on the use of email in the healthcare sector. Seth et al. (2016) found the majority of patients surveyed in their study were comfortable receiving communication from their healthcare provider via email. While concerns about confidentiality remain, the increasing prevalence of electronic forms of communication, as noted by these authors, has increased acceptability of this mode of information exchange.

The proliferation and advancement of mobile-based communications, such as smartphones, have contributed to the frequent usage of email in society. The healthcare environment was an early user of mobile technology in the form of pagers and this trend has intensified in recent times. While many clinical environments restrict the use of mobile devices in clinical areas, there is evidence that these can be a valuable tool in student learning while on clinical placement. Maudsley et al. (2019) undertook a systematic review of the use of mobile devices by a wide variety of healthcare profession students and found a number of benefits for their educational experience. These included opportunities to log clinical information, record achievement of competencies, self-regulated learning and just-in-time access to evidence to support practice. It is clear that mobile devices will offer benefits to healthcare professional and patient education at an increasing rate.

Once area of health management that is gaining increasing traction is the use of smartphone apps to promote, track, manage and even communicate health activities. Many people own smartwatches and fitness trackers that monitor movement and activity to detect trends and assess health status. While the most common of these trackers monitor physical activity, there are an emerging number of apps that aim to promote mental health. The intention of all such fitness apps is to promote wellbeing, although there is a need to ensure the quality of these products. Torous et al. (2019) propose a number of standards in respect of issues such as effectiveness, experience and security of the more than 10 000 commercially available apps purporting to support mental health. In the absence of regulation of such apps, caution in their use is recommended (Wisniewski et al. 2019).

How to use electronic communication

Despite the advances in electronic communication, knowing how to use it is important, as the context of communicating in a connected environment can be unique. Online environments offer the user the chance to communicate speedily and globally, sometimes with a relative degree of anonymity.

Freedom of communication and expression on the internet is a good example of how electronic communication has changed the face of modern society. With over half the global population now connected to the internet, the sheer number of users drives the massive array of different, easily accessible content available to individuals browsing online from any point on the planet. Although the benefits of using electronic mediums of communication in this context may be obvious, the unparalleled freedom to communicate in the online environment brings certain responsibilities to users. As UNESCO (2019, n.p.) states, the internet:

> provides an unprecedented volume of resources for information and knowledge that opens up new opportunities and challenges for expression and participation. The principle of freedom of expression and human rights must apply not only to traditional media but also to the Internet and all types of emerging media platforms, which will contribute to development, democracy and dialogue.

As a matter of course, members of the public have a legal responsibility to avoid engaging in illegal conduct online. However, the boundaries are much blurrier when people's private and professional lives intersect. As was discussed in Chapter 10, numerous regulatory and industry bodies have developed guidelines and policies designed to clarify personal and professional boundaries in respect of the use of social media and to ensure that healthcare professionals are aware of their responsibilities. The very nature of the work of healthcare professionals requires a high standard of personal and professional behaviour and these guidelines and policies reflect this expectation.

Reflect and apply

Conduct an internet search to locate social media policies produced by your relevant professional, regulatory and industry bodies. Review the content of each. What elements of these documents surprise you? Are they sufficient to address the rate at which advancements in technology are occurring?

Skills in practice

Social media and professional behaviour

Thomas is a final year psychology student on placement at a regional health service. He posts on his Facebook page that he is 'bored out of his mind' and that 'nothing ever happens in this place'. Thomas subsequently applies for a graduate placement at the health service. As part of their routine processes, the recruitment manager conducts a search of social media activity of applicants for all graduate positions. Thomas receives a letter advising that his application for a position was not successful.

What's happening here?

The health service is justified in obtaining publicly available information to assess the suitability of applicants for a position in their health service. Where competition is particularly high, as can happen in regional areas with limited graduate opportunities, a seemingly innocent comment on a publicly available site can be the difference between success and failure. Even when social media settings are 'private', the potential for sharing of postings makes the potential for broader dissemination high.

The unique characteristics and contexts of communicating electronically give rise to a number of complex issues that must be considered. For instance, users of electronic communication should recognise that electronic communication might not provide important verbal or physical cues that give context to what has been said. Therefore, the 'tone' of electronic communication can be misconstrued. Because of the absence of hand gestures, facial expressions and physical positioning, users can take messages to be threatening where the intent was jovial, or abrupt where the intent was clarity. Because of these perceived issues, 'emoticons' (short for 'emotion icon') were introduced to offer users greater clarity. Emoticons include smiling and frowning faces, as well as depictions of many other expressions. However, these emoticons are rarely used in professional communications; they are mainly used in social interactions.

Another important point when using electronic communication is to understand that it can be an isolating and impersonal experience, often prompting users to say things they otherwise would not, in order to be heard. Social media can be particularly vulnerable to this phenomenon as 'likes' (Facebook) and 'retweets' (Twitter) and various other voting systems reflect the popularity or controversy of the communication. This context has a particular impact in open forums of communication, as dissenting or alternative viewpoints are often suppressed or negatively received. Because of the relative anonymity of the online environment, the lack of an identifiable person sending an electronic communication can either embolden someone to make a statement or refute a statement that can result in the tone of the conversation significantly deteriorating.

The technological literacy skills of the user can significantly contribute to the deterioration of some communications. Sometimes these skills can affect the clarity of communications and result in conflict because of misinterpretation or misunderstanding. Poor written literacy is not uncommon in electronic communication, and spelling and grammar mistakes can distort and confuse the intent of the message. For instance, omitting a salutation in emails can be perceived as rude, while poor capitalisation or grammar can roll sentences and paragraphs into one incomprehensible collection of words. Technological illiteracy can also result in a decrease in the quality of communications as users struggle to send or reply to messages, resulting in unclear transmissions.

In view of these points, it is worth noting that electronic communications are unlike most other conversations because they are asynchronous—that is, there can be large gaps of 'silence' between messages, leaving the users to interpret the length of silence in falsely negative or even positive ways. In normal communication, silences often reflect meaning, as they may be for consideration, contemplation and even contempt. However, when individuals fail to appropriately engage in a timely and regular fashion with those who are trying to interact with them, it can leave participants open to attaching the wrong meaning to gaps in communication.

The following recommendations are made to guide approaches to communicating electronically as a professional, whatever medium is used:

1. *Be clear:* To facilitate a meaningful exchange of ideas and/or information, both parties should be clear about the outcome of communication. For instance, you may be designing a web page for health consumers or carrying out an e-health assessment. To ensure clarity, plan the communication according to what needs to be *achieved*.
2. *Be brief:* For consumers of health and healthcare, information overload can result in decisional uncertainty and regret. Communication from healthcare professionals should be only as long as needed to give an explanation and confirm it has been understood. This principle applies to any form of website, telehealth, EHR or messaging service. Access should also not require complicated authentication processes or content-heavy online information.
3. *Be simple:* Lay people want to be spoken with in a way that is simple and familiar. Avoid vague and technical words. Talk with the patient, not at them

or above them. Similarly, when planning to use e-communication, ask this simple question to validate whether to proceed: 'Will it make the delivery of healthcare a better experience for patients/consumers?' If the answer is 'no', do not use the latest, greatest health app that only adds a further layer of complexity to healthcare.

4. *Be timely:* Healthcare is often time-dependent. Electronic communication should therefore facilitate timely communication and not hinder it. Ask yourself, 'When does this patient need communication? What are the consequences of not communicating this information now? Will it affect their mental state if they are made to wait? What support can be provided to them until results are available?'
5. *Be inclusive:* Electronic communication should not be available only to those who can afford or proficiently use a smartphone, a tablet or a laptop. Social determinants of health such as low socioeconomic status can predict access to and use of technology. Be sure to understand your target population before designing or delivering health-centred communication. If they are not users of smartphones or computers, electronic communication may not be appropriate.
6. *Be discreet:* Health information is sensitive, even when you think it might not be. Communication should *always* be targeted and reflective of social and cultural responses to health and illness. For instance, a group email including certain cultural groups regarding health information such as contraception may have negative implications for them, particularly if that communication was intercepted.
7. *Be accurate:* Proofread your information to ensure accuracy and structure. Information should be devoid of under- or over-exaggeration.
8. *Be appropriately formal/informal:* Health consumers derive support from each other. Create or allow space for them to ask questions, compare their experiences and demonstrate the human side of health and illness. Effective communication results when health consumers are able to engage with each other online in an informal way, free from the interference of healthcare professionals. Similarly, where appropriate, ensure formality for electronic communication. Health consumers can implicitly demand formality to elicit feelings of confidence that the care or advice they are receiving can be trusted.
9. *Be giving:* Communication is incomplete without giving people an opportunity for response. Ask for feedback from users of electronic information to ensure they are given an opportunity to comment on the quality of the communication. Additionally, be the kind of healthcare professional who supports question prompt lists, particularly where the nature of communication is shaped by technology and alters the way communication can naturally occur face-to-face. Coming prepared to a consultation may facilitate patient care. A recent review in the world's top-ranked cancer journal found that 'question prompt lists can increase

the number of questions asked by patients without increasing consultation length and may encourage them to reflect and plan questions before the consultation' (Licqurish et al. 2019).

10. *Be listening:* Listening is a vital feature of effective communication. Allow space in online verbal communication for people to say what they need to say. Listen to understand and not just to respond. Follow-up with them to inform them their feedback has been addressed (adapted from Business Communication Articles 2019).

Although these tips for working with electronic forms of communication are by no means exhaustive, they address some of the key issues experienced in using such contemporary ways to interact and inform others. Knowing how to safely and professionally use electronic communication is as equally important as knowing when to do so.

Reflect and apply

Conduct an audit of your last five electronic communications across each of the different types of message or information transfers you have made: SMS, phone, email, social media, blog or websites. Note how you communicate, and reflect on how the way you use technology to speak with others would change as a healthcare professional.

Explore the online environment and determine how private your online identity is. Could a patient locate your whereabouts? Could a potential employer form a negative judgment about you from your social media presence?

Contemporary issues with using electronic communication in healthcare

While healthcare has been slow to embrace some forms of electronic communication, other arguably less noticeable forms of electronic communication are intractably embedded in modern healthcare. Patient monitoring is a key example of a situation where a machine is communicating health-related messages to clinicians. Increasingly, there are concerns around the interface between people and machines, with commentary centred on topics such as alarm fatigue and the reliance on digital messages at the expense of comprehensive patient assessment.

An important safety issue in contemporary healthcare is **alarm fatigue** (The Joint Commission 2016). Medical device alarms contribute to a cacophony of sounds in the clinical environment. These alarms are usually designed to communicate to the clinician that the patient has strayed from acceptable physiological parameters.

Alarm fatigue
A phenomenon that results from healthcare workers being exposed to alarms on medical equipment with such frequency that they become desensitised and less likely to respond.

However, when these machines perpetually sound because of a physiologically unstable patient or incorrectly set parameters, clinicians can become immune to the alarms, or may silence them. This response is largely because the sounding alarm is perceived to be more a source of annoyance than a meaningful message.

Several strategies to overcome alarm fatigue have been proposed: establishing clearer alarm parameters; standardising the characteristics of alarm sounds; and improving the interface between clinicians, medical devices and patients. For instance, Turmell et al. (2017) trialled a multiphase approach to alarm management that included daily electrode change, customisation of alarm parameters and timely removal of telemetry. As a result of these interventions, alarms were reduced by up to 30 per cent.

However, the human factor in alarm fatigue remains an issue, as getting the interface between the patient, the machine and the clinician to work is key to overcoming some of the difficulties with this form of electronic communication. Desensitisation and apathy are the main contributors to alarm fatigue (Turmell et al. 2017). Strategies to address the problem need to therefore be innovative if they are to be successful. Short and Chung (2019) investigated the use of a smartphone app to filter and bundle clinically significant alarms. Through the use of this technology, nurses were able to recognise and reconcile alarms in real time, reducing redundancy and enhancing efficiency.

Apart from issues around alarm fatigue, some concerns exist around the perceived overreliance on machines at the expense of a thorough and comprehensive assessment (Phillips & Barnsteiner 2005). While little literature exists on this issue, even today, the fundamental lessons of dealing with electronic communication still apply. As in the case of written online communication versus face-to-face discussion, physical and vocal cues are not present in the former. Similarly, the interface between the patient, the machine and the clinician can potentially obscure some of the vital cues that impact on the quality and timeliness of care delivery.

Issues inherent to the uptake of telehealth and other mobile technologies question whether the access that some technology provides is being gained at the expense of a comprehensive assessment. For example: Can a thorough consultation be made over a telephone? Can a pressure ulcer or wound infection be assessed via videoconferencing? Can remote patient monitoring replace seeing and assessing the patient in person? All of these questions target the nexus between the tools healthcare professionals have (look, listen, touch, smell, feel, push, prod, poke) and the technologies they can access. The human factor is at the centre of discussions around the use of technology at the clinical interface; for this reason, it will be humans who need to not only communicate using electronic communication but also communicate *about* electronic communication. Advocating for the effective, sensible application of technology where appropriate will ultimately come down to healthcare professionals determining whether the technology is an enabler or a barrier to the care they can provide.

For these reasons, recognising the place of electronic communication in the healthcare environment is of paramount importance, whether it is sending an email or responding to a machine alarm. There will continue to be a need to utilise electronic communication in efficient and effective ways by respecting the contexts where electronic communication contributes to the quality of care, rather than detracts from it.

Conclusion

This chapter has provided an overview of some of the key points about working with electronic communication. The complexity and array of technologies used to facilitate the transfer of electronic communication limits the potential to address the topic exhaustively; however, it can be seen that some general rules apply. Before electronic communication was conceived, effective and efficient means of communication were those that conveyed a message in a clear, concise and powerful way. Such forms of communication—whether smoke signals or ancient hieroglyphs—used new technologies to articulate a message so that humans were listened to, rather than focusing on the technology itself. Technology will continue to evolve; however, in working with electronic forms of communication, the need to be clear, concise and respectful of the human factors at play in the healthcare environment will continue to be a priority.

SUMMARY POINTS

- Electronic communication plays a significant role in daily life; however, its use in improving the quality of communication in healthcare will continue to evolve.
- The context of electronic communications is complex; however, approaching it strategically can significantly enhance the safety, quality, efficiency and effectiveness of communication.
- Electronic forms of communication should be an adjunct to strong interpersonal face-to-face communication skills in the healthcare environment, not a replacement.
- The use of electronic communication in healthcare is an under-researched field. As evidence builds, the implementation and integration of electronic communication in the healthcare environment will become better targeted and more helpful to healthcare professionals.
- The emergence of social media will pose significant opportunities and challenges in the healthcare environment and create new ways of connecting stakeholders.
- While electronic communication offers many potential advantages to users in healthcare, there are drawbacks that healthcare professionals should be aware of, such as alarm fatigue and the potential for decreased emphasis on patient contact.

CRITICAL THINKING QUESTIONS

Table 15.1 outlines key developments in communication in history. Think about how communication patterns have altered since that time.

1. Compile a list of other intentional and unintentional consequences that have arisen as a result of changes in communication.
2. Put on your futuristic hat and imagine what might happen to communication patterns over the next 20 years. Construct a similar table to Table 15.1.
3. How might these futuristic happenings impact upon healthcare efficiencies and effectiveness?

Group activity

Social media usage

In your study groups or via your subject discussion site, discuss your use of social media. List five uses of social media that may benefit care delivery and list a further five that may hinder it. Compare and compile lists between groups and discuss the implications of your ideas in the context of the standards for practice applicable to your profession.

WEBLINKS

Electronic communication and health

Statement on use of the internet and electronic communication (Medical Council of New Zealand):
www.mcnz.org.nz/assets/standards/9fcbd84fb3/Statement-on-use-of-the-internet-and-electronic-communication-v2.pdf

Telecommunications and media

Communications Report 2017–18 (Australian Communications and Media Authority):
www.acma.gov.au/theACMA/communications-report

Telehealth

NZ Telehealth Resource Centre:
www.telehealth.org.nz

Telemedicine in Australia (Australian Institute of Health and Welfare):
www.aihw.gov.au/reports/hospitals/telemedicine-in-australia/contents/summary

Telemedicine in Australia (Venture Insights):
www.ventureinsights.com.au/product/telemedicine-in-australia

Social media

Australian Health Practitioner Regulation Agency (AHPRA) Social Media Policy:
www.ahpra.gov.au/Search.aspx?query=%27theand%20social%20media%20policy%27

Social media use may have employment repercussions:
www.odt.co.nz/business/social-media-use-may-have-employment-repercussions

REFERENCES

Allen-Graham, J., Mitchell, L., Heriot, N., Armani, R., Langton, D., Levinson, M., Young… & Wilson, J.W. (2018). Electronic health records and online medical records: An asset or a liability under current conditions? *Australian Health Review*, 42(1), 59–65.

Attai, D.J., Cowher, M.S., Al-Hamadani, M., Schoger, J.M., Staley, A.C. & Landercasper, J. (2015). Twitter social media is an effective tool for breast cancer patient education and support: Patient-reported outcomes by survey. *Journal of Medical Internet Research*, 17(7), e188.

Australian Bureau of Statistics. (2018). *Household Internet Access*. Retrieved from www.abs.gov.au/ausstats/abs@.nsf/0/ACC2D18CC958BC7BCA2568A9001393AE?Opendocument.

Australian Law Reform Commission. (2006). *Documentary Evidence: Electronic Communications*. Retrieved from www.alrc.gov.au/publications/6.%20Documentary%20Evidence/electronic-communications.

Business Communication Articles. (2019). *10 Most Important Principles of Effective Communication*. Retrieved from www.businesscommunicationarticles.com/principles-of-effective-communication.

Cottrell, M., Judd, P., Comans, T., Easton, P. & Chang, A.T. (2019). Comparing fly-in fly-out and telehealth models for delivering advanced-practice physiotherapy services in regional Queensland: An audit of outcomes and costs. *Journal of Telemedicine and Telecare*. doi:1357633X19858036.

Hambleton, S.J. & Aloizos, J. (2019). Australia's digital health journey. *Medical Journal of Australia*, 210(6), S5–S6. doi:10.5694/mja2.50039.

InternetNZ. (2017). *State of the Internet 2017: The State of the Internet in New Zealand*. Retrieved from https://internetnz.nz/sites/default/files/SOTI%20FINAL.pdf.

Licqurish, S.M., Cook, O.Y., Pattuwage, L.P., Saunders, C., Jefford, M., Koczwara, B., Johnson, C.E. & Emery, J.D. (2019). Tools to facilitate communication during physician–patient consultations in cancer care: An overview of systematic reviews. *CA: A Cancer Journal for Clinicians*. doi:10.3322/caac.21573.

Maudsley, G., Taylor, D., Allam, O., Garner, J., Calinici, T. & Linkman, K. (2019). A Best Evidence Medical Education (BEME) systematic review of: What works best for health professions students using mobile (hand-held) devices for educational support on clinical placements? BEME Guide No. 52. *Medical Teacher*, 41(2), 125–40.

McIntosh, B. (2019). The evolution of the text message—25 years on. Retrieved from www.vodafone.com.au/red-wire/text-message-25-years.

Phillips, J. & Barnsteiner, J.H. (2005). Clinical alarms: Improving efficiency and effectiveness. *Critical Care Nursing Quarterly*, 28(4), 317–23.

Rankin, A., Truskey, M. & Chisolm, M. S. (2019). The use of social media in interprofessional education: Systematic review. *JMIR Medical Education*, 5(1), e11328.

Seth, P., Abu-Abed, M.I., Kapoor, V., Nicholson, K. & Agarwal, G. (2016). Email between patient and provider: Assessing the attitudes and perspectives of 624 primary health care patients. *JMIR Medical Informatics*, 4(4), e42.

Short, K. & Chung, Y. (2019). Solving alarm fatigue with smartphone technology. *Nursing2019*, 49(1), 52–7.

The Joint Commission. (2016). *National Patient Safety Goals.* Retrieved from www.jointcommission.org/assets/1/6/2016_NPSG_HAP.pdf.

Torous, J., Andersson, G., Bertagnoli, A., Christensen, H., Cuijpers, P., Firth, J., … Mohr, D.C. (2019). Towards a consensus around standards for smartphone apps and digital mental health. *World Psychiatry*, 18(1), 97.

Turmell, J.W., Coke, L., Catinella, R., Hosford, T. & Majeski, A. (2017). Alarm fatigue: Use of an evidence-based alarm management strategy. *Journal of Nursing Care Quality*, 32(1), 47–54.

UNESCO. (2019). *Freedom of Expression on the Internet.* Retrieved from https://en.unesco.org/themes/freedom-expression-internet.

Wisniewski, H., Liu, G., Henson, P., Vaidyam, A., Hajratalli, N.K., Onnela, J.P. & Torous, J. (2019). Understanding the quality, effectiveness and attributes of top-rated smartphone health apps. *Evidence-based Mental Health*, 22(1), 4–9.

GLOSSARY

Academic writing
Written communication designed for scholarly audiences, with the aim of educating and furthering knowledge.

Active listening
An intentional attending skill designed to understand the other.

Advocacy
The 'combination of individual and social actions designed to gain political commitment, policy support, social acceptance and systems support for a particular health goal or program' (WHO 1998).

AIDET
A mnemonic outlining the framework that improves communication between clinicians and recipients of care: A = Acknowledge; I = Introduce; D = Duration; E = Explanation; T = Thank.

Alarm fatigue
A phenomenon that results from healthcare workers being exposed to alarms on medical equipment with such frequency that they become desensitised and less likely to respond.

Argument
A collection of evidence that supports the primary idea or claim in a piece of written or oral communication.

Attribution
The practice of giving full credit to the author or source of work cited in a piece of academic writing.

Burden of disease
A measurement of the impact of disease and disability on quality and quantity of life.

Bureaucracy
The forms and processes that characterise an organisation and its administration.

CALD
Culturally and linguistically diverse.

Client
A person engaging with a health service, usually for the purpose of maintaining or promoting health.

Clinical handover
The transfer of professional responsibility and accountability for some or all aspects of care for a patient, or group of patients, to another person or professional group on a temporary or permanent basis (ACSQHCS 2012).

Code of conduct
Set of principles that govern how an individual, group or organisation should behave and practise.

Code of ethics
Set of guidelines prepared by an organisation or professional body to inform its members how they should conduct themselves to meet certain ethical and integrity standards.

Communication literacy
The ability to understand and apply principles of communication in order to effectively convey meaning.

Communication skills
The ability to convey and share information with another effectively and efficiently using verbal, non-verbal and written skills.

Communication triggers
Words, facial expressions and voice intonation or behaviour that stimulates a response in another (usually a negative response).

Community
A group of individuals who are linked geographically through location, or conceptually through values, beliefs or interests.

Compassionate intention
Genuine care, consideration and attention to others; these are the goals of communication.

Confidentiality
Implicit protection of personal information provided by individuals in the course of a professional healthcare interaction or relationship.

Conflict
An inevitable aspect of human interaction when two or more individuals or groups pursue mutually incompatible goals; if managed well, conflict can be beneficial.

Conflict management
Minimising the negative aspects of conflict while increasing the positive aspects.

Consumer
A person engaging with healthcare, usually with a high level of involvement and decision making in their own care.

Context
The physical and psychosocial environment that provides the setting in which communication exchanges occur.

Contract cheating
Soliciting the services of another person or organisation to prepare an assessment task that is submitted for grading.

Cooperation
The process of working together to achieve an outcome satisfactory to all parties.

Cross-cultural communication
An exchange of information in a context comprising two or more cultures.

Cultural competence
An awareness of cultural diversity and the ability to communicate effectively and respectfully during interactions with people of different cultural backgrounds.

Cultural knowledge
Familiarity with culture-related evidence and issues.

Cultural self-awareness
Being conscious of our personal reactions to people who are different from ourselves. We need to recognise our own values and biases as well as the values and biases of colleagues and patients, and be consciously aware of our own reactions and the reactions of others who are from diverse cultures.

Cultural sensitivity
Acknowledging the legitimacy of cultural difference and embracing those differences during interactions with people from diverse cultures.

Cultural value dimensions
These include individualism and collectivism; power; distance; uncertainty; avoidance; masculinity; and femininity.

Culturally diverse
The presence of multiple diverse cultures in a population.

Culture
A cluster of societal elements held in common by a particular group of people.

Design thinking
A non-traditional, non-linear approach to problem solving that is creative, solutions-focused and human-centred.

Discrimination
Behaviour that prevents members of one group having access to the opportunities available to others.

E-health
Technologies that use electronic means to facilitate the delivery of healthcare.

E-health literacy
The ability to understand and use information and communication technologies for health care.

E-health record
An electronic version of a person's healthcare record.

Electronic communication
Communication transmitted via an electronic processor—for example, telephone, fax machine, computer, smart phone, notebook, palmtop; includes data, text, images and video.

Emotional intelligence
The awareness of one's own emotions and those of others. Includes having the aptitude to manage these emotions to enhance interactions with others.

Empathy
A conscious awareness of another person's perspective, feelings and behaviours.

Ethnocentrism
Using one's own culture to evaluate another culture; one's own culture is generally considered to be superior.

Facilitational advocacy
Advocacy that empowers disadvantaged groups to lobby for change by providing individuals and communities with the skills to tackle health issues.

Feedback
Constructive information in response to a specific work activity or overall performance.

Feminine culture
Gender-based cultural/societal preference or focus on nurture, care, sharing, quality of life, people and relationships.

Fidelity
To behave in a way that means the healthcare professional keeping the promises made as part of the professional role,

whether that is to provide safe and competent patient care, to act ethically, or simply as part of the relationship with patients or clients.

Fourth Industrial Revolution
A period of societal disruption brought about by the advent and increasing use of digital technologies.

Functional literacy
The ability to understand short and familiar texts, and to obtain information from everyday sources.

Health literacy
The ability to access, read and understand health-related information and to use this information to promote and maintain good health.

Health policy
'Includes actions or intended actions by public, private and voluntary organizations that have an impact on health… policy may refer either to a set of actions and decisions, or to statements of intent' (Palmer & Short 2010).

Identity
A conscious awareness of how a person's individual characteristics and culture combine to form a realisation of how they see themselves.

Individual advocacy
Partnering with individuals to advocate on their behalf or to foster self-advocacy so that people can speak for themselves, asserting their own needs when they face specific difficulties.

Information processing skills
A set of skills comprised of literacy, numeracy and problem solving in technology-rich environments.

Interprofessional communication
When students or practitioners from different professions are self-aware and communicate effectively with each other in a collaborative, responsive and responsible manner.

Interprofessional relationships
The interactions between people from different professional groups that incorporate the principles of respectful communication.

IT literacy
Ability to recognise information is needed, and act effectively to locate, evaluate and effectively use this information using digital or online methods.

Legislation
A collective body of laws or a single law (known as a statute).

Liminal space
A space of transition or uncertainty where knowledge is tacit and transformational.

Literacy
Ability to read and write and to use language proficiently.

Masculine culture
Gender-based cultural/societal preference for assertiveness, ambition, control, competition, achievement and technical expertise.

Mediation
A method of negotiation where a mutually acceptable third party helps people find a solution to a conflict that they cannot find by themselves.

Mindfulness
A state of having complete awareness of oneself in the present moment.

Models of communication
A collection of agreed terms and ideas that form a framework on which communication practice can be based.

Negotiation
The process of communication and bargaining between people seeking to arrive at a mutually acceptable outcome on issues of shared concern.

Non-verbal communication
Communication without spoken words.

Numeracy
Ability to work with numbers and apply basic principles of mathematics.

Open communication
Communication that is transparent and accessible; includes the concept of freedom of expression.

Organisational communication
The flow of information between individuals and groups at various levels of hierarchy and across different locations within an organisation.

Othering
The identification of people as being different from oneself and responding accordingly.

Patient
A person receiving healthcare, usually in a clinical environment.

Patient-centred care
Healthcare that respects and responds to individual people's preferences, needs and values, and ensures that the patients' values and involvement guide all decision making.

Personal autonomy
An ethical principle that people should be allowed to be self-governing and make decisions for themselves.

Person-centred communication
Communication that empowers others to participate positively.

Plagiarism
Using someone else's writing without attribution or permission; stealing intellectual property.

Plain English
Language that ensures that information is easily readable and understood by people with low literacy levels.

Policy advocacy
Efforts on a broader population scale (community, national or international) to influence policy and enhance health outcomes.

Prejudice
Preconceived opinions or attitudes held by one group about another; often without basis in fact and often resistant to change despite the availability of new information.

Privacy
The right of an individual to keep information about themselves from being disclosed to others.

Professional communication
The exchange of information in the context of inter- and intra-professional relationships with the aim of achieving positive outcomes for the recipients of healthcare services.

Professional identity
The personal and social identity that develops in a professional as a result of their work activities.

Professional presence
A combination of communication, professional etiquette, behaviour, attitude and appearance to produce the optimal version of oneself in a professional context.

Quality
The systematic application of continuous improvement processes and procedures that mitigate a recognised or perceived risk to enable a high standard of care.

Racism
Prejudice based on the physical characteristics of an ethnic group.

Readability
The difficulty related to reading and comprehending text; it is measured by sentence length and vocabulary.

Reciprocity
A situation in which each party in a relationship or exchange mutually benefits from the process.

Reflection
A series of practices that allow a person to look back on events and analyse what happened and what they might do differently next time.

Reflective practice
A process of analysing one's experiences to improve the way a person works. It is a continuous professional development activity and assists people to become proactive professionals.

Representational advocacy
A type of advocacy that speaks for or represents the needs of vulnerable groups.

Resilience
Refers to the ability to adapt or bounce back in difficult situations.

Respectful communication
Incorporates full disclosure and transparency in all interactions with others, including patients/clients, families and other members of the healthcare team.

Safety
Awareness, planning and performance of conscious acts to eliminate or minimise the potential for harm to individuals.

SBAR
A mnemonic employed in healthcare communication between healthcare professionals: S = Situation; B = Background; A = Assessment; R = Recommendation.

Self-awareness
A state of being mindful of one's thoughts and motivations, including how one engages with others, and the effect this has on them.

Self-care
A conscious practice of undertaking purposeful actions to sustain and maintain one's own holistic well-being.

Self-efficacy
Belief in oneself to meet challenges or complete a task.

SOAP
A mnemonic used to help clinicians structure progress notes in a problem-specific clinical decision-making order:
S = Subjective; O = Objective; A = Assessment; P = Plan.

Social contract
The bargain struck between a profession and society to provide specialised skills and a guaranteed commitment to

professional attributes (integrity, altruism, etc.), in return for autonomy in practice and the privilege of self-regulation. The 'profession' is then trusted to provide specific services to society.

Social media
A collective term given to online websites and applications (such as Facebook, Twitter, Instagram, etc.) that enable people to communicate, create and share information and ideas.

Stakeholder network
A set of individuals and organisational groups that are linked together by a common interest.

Stereotype
Fixed and inflexible ideas about a social group.

Supervision
A process that allows a person an opportunity to discuss and resolve workplace issues and dilemmas.

Telehealth
Health-related services or information delivered electronically from or between healthcare professionals.

Therapeutic communication
The exchange of information between healthcare providers and patients, clients or consumers of healthcare services, with the aim of developing a relationship that benefits the well-being of the individual.

Therapeutic relationships
Collaborative relationship between the healthcare professional and client that empowers and fulfils the client's needs.

Thesis statement
A statement that presents the writer's main idea and primary claim.

Three-act structure
Simple format used in academic writing, plays, novels and films. It has an introduction, a body and a conclusion (or summary).

Transitions of care
The process of transferring all or part of a patient's care delivery transferred between healthcare providers or care locations.

Verbal communication
All communication that is spoken (including words and other sounds).

INDEX